AN INTRODUCTION TO NEUROGENIC COMMUNICATION DISORDERS

Fourth Edition

An Introduction to Neurogenic Communication Disorders

Fourth Edition

ROBERT H. BROOKSHIRE, Ph.D., CCC/SP

Director, Speech Pathology Section
Neurology Service
Department of Veterans Affairs Medical Center
Professor, Department of Communication Disorders
University of Minnesota
Minneapolis, Minnesota

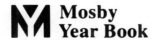

Mosby
Year Book

St. Louis   Baltimore   Boston   Chicago   London   Philadelphia   Sydney   Toronto

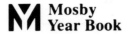
Mosby
Year Book

Dedicated to Publishing Excellence

Sponsoring Editor: David K. Marshall
Assistant Editor: Julie Tryboski
Associate Director, Manuscript Services: Frances Perveiler
Production Project Coordinator: Carol Reynolds
Proofroom Manager: Barbara Kelly

Mosby−Year Book, Inc.
11830 Westline Industrial Drive
St. Louis, MO 63146

3 4 5 6 7 8 9 0 CL MAL 96 95 94 93

Library of Congress Cataloging-in-Publication Data
Brookshire, Robert H.
    An introduction to neurogenic communication disorders / Robert H.
Brookshire. — 4th ed.
        p.   cm.
    Rev. ed. of: An introduction to aphasia. 3rd ed. c1986.
    Includes bibliographical references and index.
    ISBN 0-8151-1295-5
    1. Communicative disorders.   2. Speech disorders.   3. Aphasia.
I. Brookshire, Robert H.   Introduction to aphasia.   II. Title.
    [DNLM: 1. Aphasia.   2. Communicative Disorders.   3. Nervous System
    Disorders.   WL 340 B873i]
RC423.B74   1991
616.85'52—dc20
DNLM/DLC
for Library of Congress

91-28054
CIP

For Lisa
The autumn wind touches the mountain ————————————————
The spring leaf falls to earth

PREFACE

I have written this book to provide its readers with a basic understanding of neurogenic communication disorders—their causes, symptoms, and treatment. I have tried to be practical about what I have included in this book. I have included material that I consider both important and useful to those who are beginning their study of neurogenic communication disorders. My selection of what to include and what to leave out no doubt reflects my personal biases about who, how, and why we treat. However, it also reflects my experiences in approximately 20 years of teaching university students about neurogenic communication disorders, and my sense of what has seemed important to them.

This book is neither a training manual nor a source of techniques. Reading it will not make the reader competent to evaluate, diagnose, or treat patients with neurogenic communication disorders. No book or collection of books can do that. Clinical competence comes from knowledge of the scientific and clinical literature, supplemented and elaborated by clinical experience, both supervised and independent. This book will help the student get started on the road to clinical competence by providing a basic understanding of what neurogenic communication disorders are, and how they are measured and treated.

A reviewer of the manuscript for this book commented, "I was somewhat nonplussed by the opinions that Brookshire puts forth as facts. There are many controversies surrounding many of the issues covered in the text, and few of them are specifically targeted as controversial issues." My purpose herein is to provide an overview of neurogenic communication disorders together with basic concepts about their causes, diagnosis, assessment, and treatment. It may be that I have not identified areas of controversy, and it is certain that I have often presented my opinions as "facts." One "fact" is, I think, inescapable—that there are few "facts" in the domain treated by this book. Even such seeming "facts" as the pyramidal system and apraxia of speech are in one sense matters of opinion or convenient fictions. The situation is somewhat like the story of the commencement speaker at a medical school graduation ceremony, who closed his speech by saying,

> "And last of all I want to tell you some good news, followed by some bad news. Half of everything you've been taught in medical school is wrong. And that's the *good* news. The *bad* news is—We don't know *which* half is wrong!"

It may be that half (or more) of everything in this book is "wrong," in some sense, and it may be that there are few, if any, true and enduring "facts" in it. The content of this book represents my best guess about what is likely to prove true over time, and I hope that I will have guessed right more often than not. Perhaps this book may be best treated as a sort of springboard from which its readers may launch themselves into more extensive and in-depth reading of the scientific and clinical literature. That literature may help the reader to decide what can be called "fact" and what should be called "opinion." Finally, we must all remember that treatment of neurogenic communication disorders is still as much *art* as *science,* and that empirically-verified "facts" may prove trivial or irrelevant in helping the neurologically-compromised patient become a better communicator.

Finally, an editorial note—I continue to believe that the word "aphasic" is an adjective, and not a noun. I also continue to believe that use of "aphasic" as a noun, in addition to being stylistically deplorable, depersonalizes those for whom we provide services. Therefore the reader will not (I hope) find that I refer to "aphasics" in this book.

Robert H. Brookshire

ACKNOWLEDGMENTS _____

Few of the ideas in this book are truly my own. The influence of colleagues, students, and the patients I have known and worked with permeates the contents. Without them this book would not exist.

My special thanks to Linda Nicholas, M.A., for reading and commenting on portions of the manuscript; to Audrey Holland, Ph.D., for commentary and advice; to Paul Barkhaus, M.D., and John Davenport, M.D., for advice and assistance regarding medical and neurologic matters; to Sandra Lundgren, Ph.D., for commentary and assistance in dealing with neuropsychologic assessment; and to Meredith Gerdin, Don MacLennan, Shirley Porrazzo, Jim Schumacher, and Mary Sullivan, the clinical staff of the Speech Pathology Section, Minneapolis Veterans Affairs Medical Center, for my continuing education in treatment of patients with neurogenic communication disorders.

Robert H. Brookshire

CONTENTS

Chapter 1

Neuroanatomy

Persons attempting to learn neuroanatomy eventually learn three somewhat disconcerting facts. (1) There are lots of different parts in the nervous system. (2) Almost every part has several different names. (3) Most of the different parts aren't really different parts, but convenient fictions invented by humans to make it easier to describe, analyze, and draw the nervous system.

The proliferation of names for parts of the nervous system probably started in the 19th century, during which many people were studying the nervous system. Communication among investigators was not what it is today, and there was a tendency for explorers of the nervous system, like explorers of the planet, to name things they discovered after themselves. Eventually, those investigating the nervous system began to call for more descriptive names, because (1) the old names were difficult to remember, and (2) most of the parts had already been named, so the new people couldn't name things after themselves. Unfortunately, there still remained some gratification attendant upon attaching a name to something, even if that something already had a name, so the proliferation of names hasn't completely stopped, although it has slowed to a crawl. In this chapter, I will give the most common multiple names when I begin to discuss a part of the nervous system. Then I will use what I consider the most descriptive (and easiest to remember) one.

We can't do much about facts 1 and 3. The nervous system is exceedingly complex, and in order to understand how it works, one has to subdivide it, even though the subdivisions may be arbitrary and imaginary. I will occasionally remind readers of this arbitrariness, but not always. To do so would be to use more space for the reminders than for the "facts."

THE GENERAL STRUCTURE OF THE NERVOUS SYSTEM

Descriptions of the nervous system almost always (arbitrarily) divide it into two major parts—the *central nervous system* (CNS) and the *peripheral nervous system* (PNS) (Fig 1–1). The central nervous system is made up of the *brain, brain stem,*

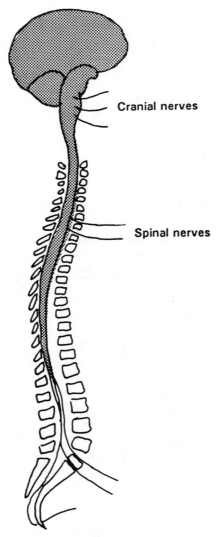

Cranial nerves

Spinal nerves

FIG 1–1.
The central and peripheral nervous systems. The central nervous system consists essentially of everything enclosed by the meninges (the brain, cerebellum, brain stem, spinal cord) and the peripheral nervous system consists of nerve fiber tracts, sensory receptors, and motor end plates outside the brain, cerebellum, brain stem, and spinal cord.

cerebellum, and *spinal cord.* The *peripheral nervous system* is made up of the *cranial nerves, spinal nerves,* and some parts of the *autonomic nervous system.* The autonomic nervous system is responsible for control and regulation of the heart muscles, smooth muscles in internal organs, and glands. Although it is responsible for many vital life functions, it is not directly concerned with communication. Consequently, it will not get much attention in this chapter.

THE CENTRAL NERVOUS SYSTEM

The Meninges.—The central nervous system is enclosed in three membranes, much as a peel encloses a piece of fruit. The membranes are called *meninges*. They are, going from inside to outside, the *pia mater,* the *arachnoid,* and the *dura mater* (Fig 1–2). They cushion and protect the CNS from injury, making the mnemonic *PAD* (for *p*ia, *a*rachnoid, and *d*ura) practical.

The *pia mater* has two layers. The inner layer is nonvascular (contains no blood vessels) and adheres tightly to the surface of the brain. There are veins and arteries on the outer surface of the pia mater, in the space between the pia and the arachnoid. The *arachnoid* is nonvascular and does not conform to the contours of the brain, creating a space between the arachnoid and the pia. This space is called the *subarachnoid space.* The subarachnoid space is greatest over the fissures and least over the convolutions. It is filled with *cerebrospinal fluid,* a clear, colorless fluid that cushions and protects the brain against trauma, and provides a pathway for various metabolic and nutritional compounds to reach the brain.

The *dura mater* is a tough, slightly elastic membrane that serves both as a covering for the brain and spinal cord and a lining for the inner surface of the skull. It has two layers: a tough dense inner layer that is relatively nonvascular, and an outer layer, rich in blood vessels and nerves. Between the two dural sheets are the large *venous sinuses* of the brain. The venous sinuses are a collection system for receiving the venous blood flowing down from the brain and discharging it to the internal jugular vein for return to the heart and lungs.

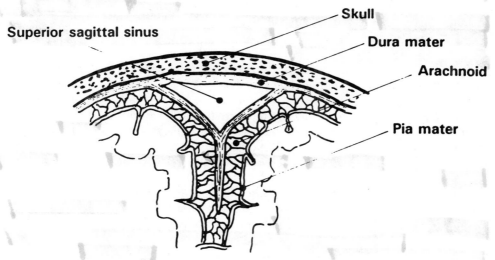

Superior sagittal sinus

Skull

Dura mater

Arachnoid

Pia mater

FIG 1–2.
The meninges. This drawing represents part of a vertical section through the brain somewhere near the middle. The falx cerebri is a tough sheet of dura that projects down into the cleft that divides the two brain hemispheres. The superior saggital sinus is a hollow tube within the dura mater that collects venous blood from the brain.

The Brain.—The brain is the largest component of the central nervous system. It is a gelatinous mass of nerve cells and supportive tissue sitting atop the brain stem within the cranial vault. An average human brain weighs about 3 pounds and is mostly (78%) water. The brain's tissues are made up of *neurons* (nerve cells), *glial cells,* which support and separate the nerve cells, blood vessels, and connective tissue cells. Glial cells are five to ten times more numerous than neurons, and account for about half of the brain's mass. Even so, the brain contains over 10 billion neurons. The brain is a big spender. It contains only about 2% of total body mass, but it receives 20% of cardiac output and consumes about 25% of the oxygen used by the body. The brain is not thrifty. It has no metabolic or oxygen reserves, and is completely dependent on the heart and lungs for oxygen and nutrients, via the blood. The brain is metabolically fragile. People lose consciousness within 10 seconds after the brain's blood supply is interrupted, and the brain will be permanently damaged if its blood supply is interrupted for more than 2 or 3 minutes.

The brain can (arbitrarily) be divided (from upper to lower, and from phylogenetically younger to phylogenetically older structures) into the *cerebrum* (including the cerebral hemispheres and the basal ganglia), the *brain stem* (including the midbrain, pons, and medulla), and the *cerebellum.*

The *cerebrum* is divided into two halves, or *hemispheres,* by a deep fissure that runs from front to back down the center. Visually, the hemispheres appear to be identical mirror images. (As we shall see, they are not identical functionally.) The surface of the hemispheres is covered by a network of convolutions, making it look something like the surface of a pecan. The convolutions (ridges) are called *gyri* (singular = gyrus), and the depressions (valleys) are called *sulci* (singular = sulcus).

The convoluted surface of the brain is called the *cortex.* It is gray in color and rich in nerve cells. It varies somewhat in thickness, from 1.5 mm in the occipital area to 4 mm in the precentral area. It is made up of six layers, each containing different combinations and types of cells. The human cerebral cortex is responsible for planning and carrying out most volitional motor activity, conscious processing of sensory information, and all "higher" mental processes—speech, language, reasoning, and so forth.

Each hemisphere has historically (and arbitrarily) been divided into four *lobes,* named after the parts of the skull that overlie them (Fig 1–3). The lobes are topographic conventions, and do not reflect differences in the structure of the brain. The four lobes are the *frontal lobe,* the *parietal lobe,* the *occipital lobe,* and the *temporal lobe.*

The boundaries of the lobes are based, at least in part, on certain "landmarks" on the brain surface. The two hemispheres are separated by the *longitudinal cerebral fissure* (or *intrahemispheric fissure*), which runs from front to back down the middle of the brain. A rigid sheet of dura protrudes down into the longitudinal cerebral fissure for most of its length. This sheet of dura is called the *falx cerebri.* A prominent sulcus (valley) begins in the vicinity of the longitudinal fissure at approximately the vertex (highest point) of the brain, and progresses laterally (to the side) about halfway down the lateral surface of the hemisphere. (see Fig 1–3). This sulcus is called the *central sulcus* (or *fissure of Rolando*). Another prominent sulcus forms a deep

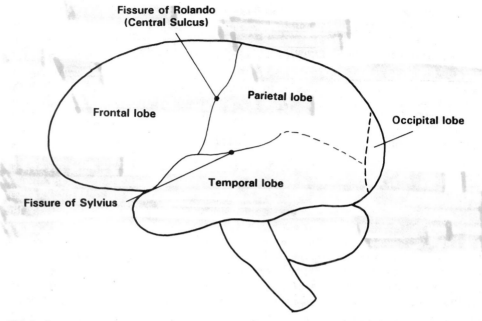

FIG 1–3.
The lobes of the brain. The lobes are arbitrary divisions, and do not represent either architectural or functional differences.

cleft that begins in the inferior frontal region and progresses upward and back, terminating about two thirds of the way back on the lateral surface (see Fig 1–3). This sulcus is called the *lateral cerebral fissure* (or *fissure of Sylvius*). It is also sometimes called the *frontotemporoparietal sulcus,* because it forms the border between these three lobes. The *calcarine fissure* is a less prominent sulcus on the mesial surface at the back of the brain, near the longitudinal sulcus.

The frontal lobes make up about one third of the surface area of the brain, and form approximately the anterior one third of each hemisphere. Their lower boundary is the lateral cerebral fissure (fissure of Sylvius), and their posterior boundary is the central fissure (fissure of Rolando). The *parietal lobes* are behind the central fissure and above the lateral fissure. Their posterior boundaries are imaginary lines, established arbitrarily. The *occipital lobes* are the most posterior and they extend from the imaginary line demarcating the posterior parietal boundary to the longitudinal fasciculus. The *temporal lobes* make up the lowest one third of the brain. The temporal lobes start at the lateral fissure, and extend downward to the mesial surface of the hemisphere. They extend back to the imaginary line marking the anterior border of the occipital lobe.

In addition to the landmarks that allow us to locate the lobes of the brain, there are a number of other landmarks that are important because they allow us to locate important *functions* in the brain. The *precentral gyrus* is a prominent bulge just in front of the central fissure (fissure of Rolando), and the *postcentral gyrus* lies just behind it (Fig 1–4). The *supramarginal gyrus* curves around the posterior end of the lateral (Sylvian) fissure. The *angular gyrus* lies just behind the supramarginal gyrus. There are three major horizontal convolutions in the temporal lobe, called the *superior, middle,* and *inferior* temporal gyri (from top to bottom). The *insula* is an expanse of cortex that is folded beneath the lateral fissure. It can be seen only if the lateral fissure is spread apart. The insula is also called the *island of Reil.*

The Motor, Sensory, and Association Cortex

The first of these functional regions to be identified was the *primary motor cortex.* It lies just in front of the central fissure, and corresponds roughly to the area of the precentral gyrus. The nerve cells in the primary motor cortex are responsible for voluntary movement of skeletal muscles on the *contralateral* (opposite) side of the body. That is, the left hemisphere primary motor cortex controls muscles on the right side, and vice versa. The *primary sensory cortex* lies just behind the central fissure, corresponding roughly to the area of the postcentral gyrus. The primary sensory cortex is responsible for *somesthetic* (skin, muscle, joint, tendon) sensation from the contralateral side of the body. (Gross perception of pain, temperature, and light touch are not the exclusive responsibility of this strip of cortex. Lower structures in the brain can generate these perceptions. More about this later.) The *primary auditory cortex* is located on the upper surface of the temporal lobe, at the border of the lateral fissure, in the transverse temporal gyrus, better known as the *gyrus of Heschl.*

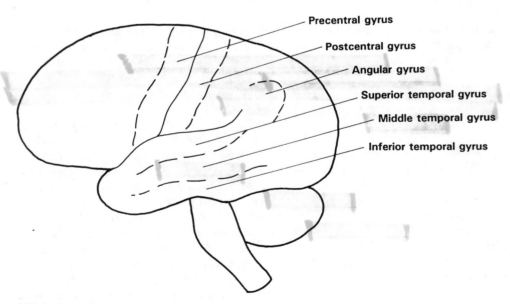

Precentral gyrus
Postcentral gyrus
Angular gyrus
Superior temporal gyrus
Middle temporal gyrus
Inferior temporal gyrus

FIG 1–4.
Often-cited "landmarks" on the brain cortex. There is considerable variability across brains in the location and prominence of the landmarks, sometimes making them difficult to identify.

The *primary visual cortex* is located in the occipital lobe, around the calcarine fissure. Figure 1–4 shows the location of these functional areas.

Neural connections to cortical sensory and motor areas are systematically arranged, and "maps" of sensory and motor functions have been drawn for both human and animal brains. Investigators created these maps after observing the effects of electrical stimulation of the cortex, after observing deficits resulting from surgical *ablation* (removal) of parts of the cortex, and after observing deficits resulting from naturally occurring lesions (in the case of humans), or from experimentally produced lesions (in the case of animals).

As mentioned earlier, the primary motor cortex, located just in front of the central fissure, is responsible for volitional skeletal muscle movements on the contralateral side of the body. The connections between the primary motor cortex and skeletal muscle groups are arranged so that it is possible to create a functional map of the motor cortex, showing which areas are responsible for given muscle groups. Such a map, sometimes called a *homunculus* ("little man"), is shown in Figure 1–5. It can be seen from Figure 1–5 that the voluntary musculature is represented in up-

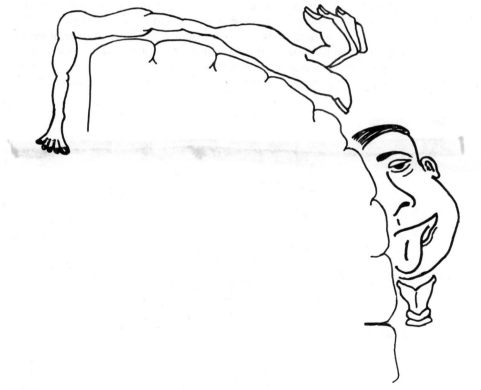

FIG 1–5.
A "homunculus" representing the location of motor function in the primary motor cortex. The size of the body part portrayed represents the amount of motor cortex devoted to that body part.

side-down fashion on the motor cortex, with cortex responsible for the toes and foot located on the superior mesial surface of the precentral gyrus, and representation for the knee, hip, shoulder, elbow, wrist, hand, and face located laterally and downward. The homunculus looks strange because the area of cortical representation for a body part is not commensurate with its size. The cortical areas for the face and hand are larger than those for other parts of the body. These differences in cortical representation appear related to the degree and precision of motor control required for given body parts. The hand, mouth, tongue, and lips, which can perform movements with great dexterity and coordination, receive comparatively large cortical representation relative to other body parts. The primary sensory cortex, immediately posterior to the fissure of Rolando, is arranged as a mirror image of the motor cortex.

In the human cerebral cortex, the primary sensory and motor areas account for only a small proportion of total cortex. Most is *association cortex.* The major association areas include the *frontal association area,* the *parietal or somesthetic association area,* the *temporal or auditory association area,* and the *frontal association area* (Fig 1–6). Association cortex is believed to be responsible for higher mental activity in man. The frontal association area is thought to play a role in the initiation and integration of purposeful behavior. The parietal association area is thought to be important for discrimination and integration of tactile information. The temporal association area is considered important for discrimination and integration of auditory information, and for many language processes. The frontal association area is considered important for planning and carrying out sequences of volitional movments.

Deep Brain Structures

The Ventricles.—Deep within the white matter of the brain lie the four *cerebral ventricles*—two *lateral ventricles,* a *third ventricle,* and a *fourth ventricle* (Fig 1–7).

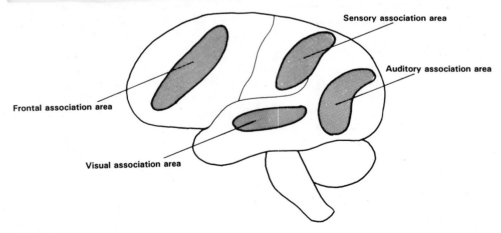

FIG 1–6.
The association areas of the brain. Like the lobes of the brain, these represent somewhat arbitrary functional divisions. No differences in brain architecture mark these divisions, and their size and location vary somewhat, depending on who draws the picture.

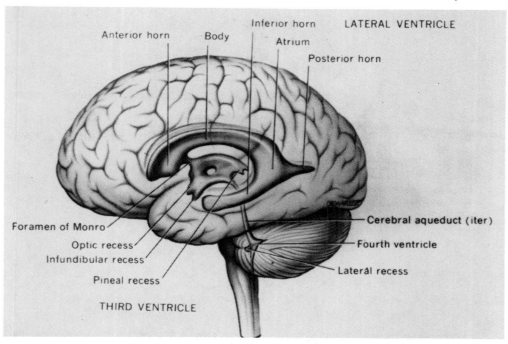

FIG 1–7.

The ventricles of the brain. The ventricles form a fluid-filled space in the center of the brain and brain stem. The cerebral acqueduct is another name for the acqueduct of Sylvius.

They are interconnected and filled with cerebrospinal fluid. The two lateral ventricles (one in each hemisphere) are largest. The corpus callosum forms the roof of the lateral ventricles. The third ventricle is a broad, irregularly shaped disk-like cavity located on the midline below the lateral ventricles, at the top of the brain stem. The fourth ventricle is a narrow tubular cavity extending down into the brain stem. The pons and medulla are in front of the fourth ventricle and the cerebellum is behind it.

The ventricles contain the *choroid plexus,* the body's primary source of cerebrospinal fluid. The cerebrospinal fluid circulates throughout the central nervous system. It flows from the lateral ventricles to the third ventricle via the *foramen of Munro* (or *intraventricular foramen*), and from the third ventricle to the fourth ventricle by way of the *aqueduct of Sylvius* (see Fig 1–7). Cerebrospinal fluid leaves the brain through three openings in the fourth ventricle—one *foramen of Magendie* and two *foramina of Luschka.* We will see later how blockages in these passageways sometimes cause problems within the cranial vault.

The Basal Ganglia and Brain Stem

Several structures involved in movement and sensation are located deep within the brain. The *thalamus* is a pair of large nuclei, one on each side of the third ventricle (Fig 1–8). (Nuclei are collections of nerve cells that are differentiated from surrounding tissue either by cell type or cell density.) The thalamus apparently plays a

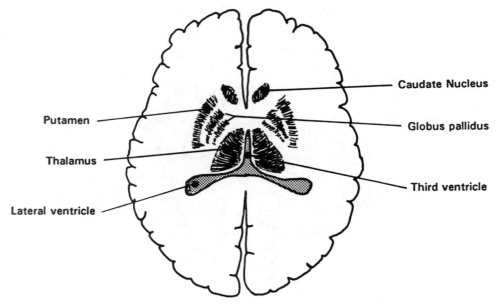

FIG 1–8.
The basal ganglia. The basal ganglia are a collection of structurally distinct bodies deep within the brain. They are important in integration and organization of sensory information and motor output.

role in consciousness, alertness, and attention. It does this by regulating and integrating neural messages traveling between the cortex and lower centers. The *basal ganglia* consist of several nuclei (see Fig 1–8). The *lenticular nucleus* (sometimes divided for descriptive purposes into the *globus pallidus* and the *putamen*) is separated from the thalamus by the posterior limb of the *internal capsule,* which is the major pathway for motor and sensory projection fibers between the brain and lower structures. The *caudate nucleus* is adjacent to the inferior border of the anterior horn of the lateral ventricle. It is separated from the lenticular nucleus by the anterior limb of the internal capsule.

Just below the basal ganglia is a region of the deep brain called the *midbrain* (Fig 1–9). The midbrain is the uppermost (and smallest) part of the *brain stem.* The midbrain contains centers for eye movements and postural reflexes. The next lower division of the brain stem is called the *pons* (see Fig 1–9), easily identified by its forward bulge. The pons contains a number of nuclei concerned with hearing and balance, and several cranial nerves originate here. The lowest division of the brain stem is called the *medulla.* The medulla is structurally homogeneous with the cervical spinal cord, and consists of dense, tightly packed fiber tracts representing all the fibers travelling from the brain and cerebellum to the spinal cord.

The Cerebellum

The *cerebellum* is just behind the pons and medulla (see Fig 1–9). The cerebellum is divided into two hemispheres with an outer layer of gray matter, the *cerebellar*

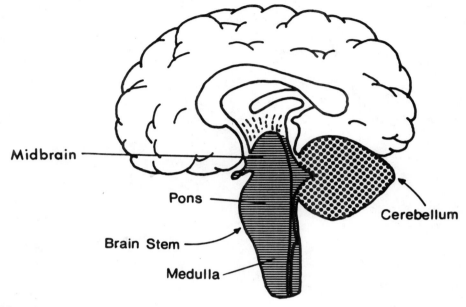

FIG 1–9.
The midbrain, brain stem, and cerebellum. The midbrain and brain stem are composed primarily of motor and sensory nerve fibers. The cerebellum has cortex and fiber tracts, and is important in regulating movement.

cortex. The cerebellum has a central core of white matter and deep nerve cell clusters (the cerebellar nuclei). The cerebellum does not initiate movements, but coordinates and modulates movements initiated elsewhere (primarily by the motor cortex). The cerebellum integrates the output from cerebral motor control centers with feedback from muscles and the vestibular system to coordinate volitional movements and regulate automatic postural adjustments that accompany movement.

NERVE CELLS AND NEURAL PATHWAYS

The Nerve Cell

The activity of the nervous system is produced by nerve cells, or *neurons* (Fig 1–10). Each neuron has a cell body and numerous projections. Most of the projections are short and hair-like. They are the receptors for the neuron, and are called *dendrites.* One of the projections is longer, thicker (usually), and less hair-like. It is the route over which electrical signals from the cell body are transmitted to other neurons, and is called the *axon.* Axons range in length from very short (less than a millimeter) to several feet long. Axons also differ in diameter, and as a consequence they differ in the speed with which they conduct nerve impulses. Those with larger diameters conduct impulses faster than those with smaller diameters. Bundles of axons are called *nerves.*

The point at which the axon of one neuron encounters a dendrite of another is

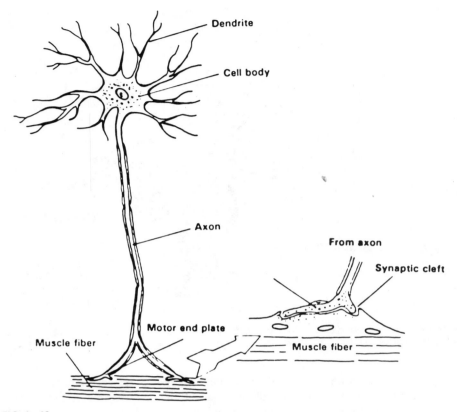

FIG 1–10.
A motor neuron, showing the cell body, axon, and myoneural (muscle-nerve) junction. A motor end plate (the junction between a neuron and a muscle fiber) is shown at the *lower right.*

called the *synapse* (see Fig 1–10). The tiny space between an axon and a dendrite is called the *synaptic cleft.* Transmission of nerve impulses across the synaptic cleft is a chemical process. A transmitter substance (acetlylcholine, epinephrine, dopamine, etc.) is released by the axon and drifts across the synaptic cleft, where it excites the dendrite, generating a change in its electrical charge. This electrical signal will (if it is especially strong, or if it is combined with input from other dendrites) cause the second neuron to fire, sending a signal down its axon. The transmitter substance that started the process is quickly absorbed or neutralized by other chemicals in the second neuron.

Nerve Fiber Tracts

The white matter, which forms much of the central core of the brain, is composed of the axons of nerve cells. The axons are clustered into bundles. These bundles of axons, in turn, make up nerve fiber tracts that make neural intercommunication possible. There are three major categories of nerve fibers within the central nervous system. They are *projection fibers, commissural fibers,* and *association fibers.*

Projection fibers traditionally are divided into two categories, depending on what they do. *Efferent fibers* carry command and control signals from the brain to muscles and glands. They begin at neurons in the motor and premotor cortex and progress downward through the brain, converging as they approach the brain stem, through which they pass to enter the spinal cord, from whence connecting nerve fibers are distributed to various muscle groups. As they progress downward, they form a compact, dense fiber band. At the level of the basal ganglia, this band of fibers is called the *internal capsule.*

Afferent fibers carry sensory information from receptors in the periphery to the brain. They begin in sensory receptor cells scattered throughout the peripheral nervous system. They converge and enter the spinal cord and brain stem throughout the length of those two structures. As they progress upward they form a compact dense band of fibers. They pass through the internal capsule, above which they fan out to their destinations in the brain, primarily in the postcentral gyrus.

Fiber tracts that cross the midline between the hemispheres are called *commissural fibers.* There are commissural fibers at all levels of the nervous system, but those that connect the cerebral hemispheres are the most important for speech and language. The three most important are the *corpus callosum,* the *anterior commissure,* and the *posterior commissure* (Fig 1–11).

The *corpus callosum* is by far the largest commissure. Besides providing the pathway for most interhemispheric communication, it serves as the major structural connection between the hemispheres. If the corpus callosum disappeared, the two hemispheres would tend to fall apart (but if the brain were in its customary place, the hemispheres would be held in place by the meninges and the skull). The corpus callosum is crescent-shaped, with the open side of the crescent facing down. The anterior third is called the *genu,* the central third is called the *rostrum or body,* and the posterior third is called the *splenium.* Fibers crossing through the genu connect cortical areas in the anterior and inferior frontal lobes; fibers crossing through the rostrum connect cortical areas in the posterior frontal and parietal lobes; and fibers crossing through the splenium connect cortical areas in the posterior parietal and occipital lobes.

The *anterior commissure* crosses the midline deep within the brain near the thalamus. The *posterior commissure* crosses at the posterior base of the brain, just below the end of the splenium of the corpus callosum. The anterior and posterior commissures are much smaller than the corpus callosum, and they may not be important for interhemispheric communication, although the extent of their participation is disputed.

Association fibers connect cortical areas within a hemisphere. The cortical areas may be close together or far apart. Short association fibers usually are called simply *association fibers,* but long association fibers get a shorter but harder-to-remember name: *fasciculus* (plural = fasciculi). Fasciculi are long and massive (as fiber tracts go) bundles of nerves connecting widely separated regions within a hemisphere. However, they never cross the midline. (If they did, they would be called commis-

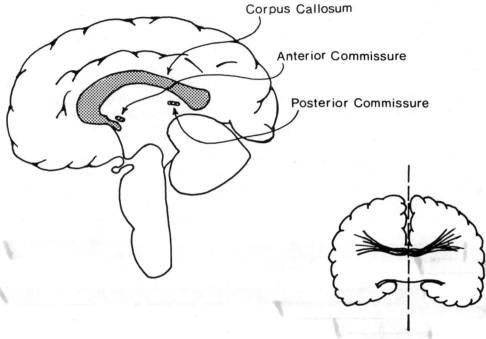

Corpus Callosum

Anterior Commissure

Posterior Commissure

FIG 1–11.
The major interhemispheric fiber tracts. The corpus callosum provides most of the communication between hemispheres, with the other commissures playing lesser parts.

sures.) There are three major fasciculi in the human brain—the *uncinate fasciculus,* the *arcuate fasciculus,* and the *cingulum.* The uncinate fasciculus connects the inferior frontal lobe with the anterior temporal lobe. The cingulum runs along the top of the corpus callosum and connects deep regions of the frontal and parietal lobes with deep regions of the temporal lobe and midbrain. Fortunately, the uncinate fasciculus and the cingulum play no major roles in speech and language, so we can safely forget them. This is not the case for the arcuate fasciculus, sometimes called the *superior longitudinal fasciculus.* It is a crescent-shaped fiber tract that connects posterior and central regions of the temporal lobe with posterior and inferior regions of the frontal lobe. From the temporal lobe it sweeps up and back around the posterior end of the fissure of Sylvius. Then it curves forward and downward to the frontal lobe. Most of the arcuate fasciculus lies about an inch beneath the cortex, within the white matter of the brain. As we shall see, the arcuate fasciculus plays a central role in some models of how the brain deals with language.

The Upper Motor Neuron and the Lower Motor Neuron

The motor system traditionally (and, need we say, arbitrarily) is divided into two levels between the cortex and the muscles—the *upper motor neuron* and the *lower motor neuron.* From a functional standpoint, the upper motor neuron is part of the central nervous system and the lower motor neuron is part of the peripheral nervous system. The cell body of the upper motor neuron is in or just beneath the cerebral cortex, with its axon passing through the midbrain, brain stem, and spinal cord to synapse with the lower motor neuron. The cell body of the lower motor neuron is in the brain stem or spinal cord and its axon passes peripherally in a spinal nerve. The upper motor neuron synapses at a specialized junction called a *muscle fiber motor end plate.* Lower motor neurons are often divided into *cranial nerves* and *spinal nerves.* The cell bodies of the lower motor neurons in cranial nerves are located in the brain stem, in the cranial nerve motor nuclei. The cell bodies of spinal nerve neurons are located in the anterior part of the spinal cord, which is why they sometimes are called *anterior horn cells.*

The Pyramidal, Vestibular-Reticular, and Extrapyramidal Systems

To describe how the central nervous system creates movement, it is customary (and arbitrary) to divide it into three parts—the *pyramidal system,* the *vestibular-reticular system,* and the *extrapyramidal system.*

The *pyramidal system* is the great initiator of volitional movement. It contains the motor neurons in the primary motor cortex and their axons, which project to synapses with lower motor neurons in the brain stem and spinal cord. The pyramidal system initiates and organizes skilled volitional movements. It is a *direct system.* "Direct" means that there are no synapses between the neurons in the primary motor cortex and the motor neurons in the brain stem and spinal cord. (This means that some of the axons in the pyramidal system are from 2 to 3 feet long. The longest are those that synapse with the lowermost spinal nerves.) Injuries involving the (upper) motor neurons in the pyramidal system cause paralysis of muscle groups, disruption of skilled movements, exaggeration of normal reflexes, appearance of pathologic primitive reflexes, and exaggerated muscle tone. Injuries involving lower (peripheral) motor neurons served by the pyramidal system cause paralysis, diminution or abolition of reflexes, and loss of muscle tone.

The *vestibular-reticular system* contains neurons spread throughout the brain stem, cerebellum, and the reticular formation (a system of fibers and nerve cells within the central core of the brain stem). These neurons also synapse with lower motor neurons. The vestibular-reticular system has responsibility for balance and orientation of the body in space, and for maintaining general states of attention and alertness.

The *extrapyramidal system* arises from many locations in the central nervous system (the cerebral cortex, the basal ganglia, the cerebellum, and the brain stem). Neurons in the extrapyramidal system project primarily to cranial and spinal nerves. The primary function of the extrapyramidal system appears to be regulation of automatic, integrative aspects of motor activity. Injuries in the extrapyramidal system cause involuntary movements to appear. These movements are superimposed upon (or replace) voluntary movements.

The vestibular-reticular system and the extrapyramidal system are *indirect sys-*

tems. "Indirect" means that they are multisynaptic, with one or more synapses intervening between the neuron of origin and the lower motor neuron. Because the paths of the pyramidal, vestibular-reticular, and extrapyramidal systems are common throughout much of their course, an injury that affects one system usually affects all three. Therefore, we commonly see combinations of pyramidal, extrapyramidal, and sometimes vestibular signs when the pyramidal system is damaged.

Some people consider the vestibular-reticular system and cerebellar pathways to be a part of the extrapyramidal system. Although they have structural similarities, they appear to have different functions, so they are considered separately here. Because of its diffuseness, the extrapyramidal system is said by some to be a convenient fiction without neuroarchitectural validity. (The same could be said about many other conventional physiologic divisions.) Many neurophysiologists argue that the concept of the extrapyramidal system should be abandoned.

THE PERIPHERAL NERVOUS SYSTEM

The peripheral nervous system contains the cranial nerves, the spinal nerves, and some parts of the autonomic nervous system. We will concentrate on the cranial nerves and the spinal nerves because, as we mentioned earlier, the autonomic nervous system is not directly concerned with speech and language.

Cranial Nerves and Spinal Nerves

The *cranial nerves* (at least most of them) synapse with the central nervous system at the level of the pons and the medulla. There are 12 pairs of cranial nerves (one nerve of each pair on each side). Cranial nerves I (olfactory) and II (optic) are actually fiber tracts of the brain. They don't exit via the brain stem, but they were called cranial nerves in the 19th century and the custom persists. Some cranial nerves serve motor functions. Some serve sensory functions. Some serve both motor and sensory functions. The cranial nerves are labelled, from top to bottom, with the Roman numerals I through XII (another 19th century custom), and each has a name. Some of the names are descriptive and English (e.g., optic [I], olfactory [II], facial [VII]), but most are cryptic and unusual (e.g., trigeminal [V], vagus [X]). The cranial nerves, their names, their motor or sensory functions, and their innervation sites are summarized in Table 1–1. Several mnemomic devices (some obscene) have been devised by students who must memorize the cranial nerves and their names. Although the obscene ones are the most entertaining, they probably are not appropriate in a serious work such as this. Therefore, the following somewhat tortuous mnemonic is passed along.

> On old Olympus's towering tops
> A Finn and German vend at hops.

Calling the accessory nerve the *spinal accessory* nerve makes the mnemomic less tortuous but no more literary:

On old Olympus's towering tops
A Finn and German view some hops.

The *spinal nerves* are bundles of nerve fibers that leave the sp
the brain stem. There are 31 pairs, divided into 5 sets. From top to
cervical nerves (8), *thoracic nerves* (12), *lumbar nerves* (5), *sacral*
coccygeal nerve (1). They often are abbreviated. *C3* stands for th
nerve, *T4* for the fourth thoracic nerve, and so on. Nerves C1 throu
above their correspondingly numbered vertebrae, but nerves C8 through the coccygeal nerve exit from beneath their correspondingly numbered vertebrae. Each spinal nerve has a posterior *dorsal* (sensory) *root* and an anterior *ventral* (motor) *root*.
The spinal nerves conduct motor and sensory impulses to and from the viscera,
blood vessels, glands and muscles.

The Spinal Cord

The spinal cord, when viewed in cross section (Fig 1–12) has an outer layer of
white matter and a central core of *gray matter*. The latter looks somewhat like a but-
terfly. The white matter contains ascending and descending nerve fibers (the axons
of anterior and posterior horn cells—see above). The gray matter contains numerous motor and sensory neurons. The motor neurons are located primarily in the *anterior horns* of the central gray matter, and the sensory neurons in the *posterior
horns* (see Fig 1–12).

TABLE 1–1.

The Cranial Nerves

Nerve	Name	Type*	Function
I	Olfactory	S	Smell, taste
II	Optic	S	Vision
III	Oculomotor	M	Eye and eyelid movement
IV	Trochlear	M	Eye movement
V	Trigeminal	S,M	Sensation from face; motor to masseters, palate, pharynx
VI	Abducens	M	Eye movement
VII	Facial	S,M	Sensation from anterior tongue; motor to facial muscles
VIII	Vestibular	S	Balance, hearing
IX	Glossopharyngeal	S,M	Sensation from posterior tongue, soft palate, pharynx; motor to pharynx
X	Vagus	S,M	Motor to larynx, pharynx, viscera; sensation from viscera
XI	Accessory	M	Motor to larynx, chest, shoulder
XIII	Hypoglossal	M	Motor to tongue

*S-sensory; M-motor.

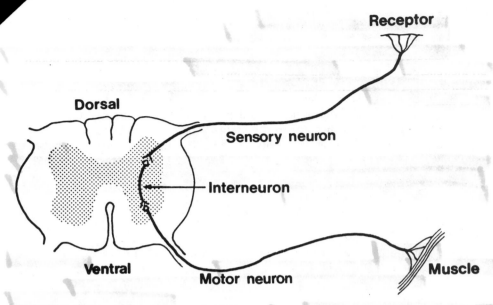

FIG 1–12.
Cross section of the spinal cord, showing the anterior (ventral) and posterior (dorsal) columns. The anterior columns are primarily responsible for motor functions and the posterior columns for sensory function. The three neurons shown make up a reflex arc.

There are two major motor pathways from the head to the peripheral muscles. The *corticospinal* pathway is the pathway of the *pyramidal system* (so named because it begins at *pyramidal* nerve cells in the cerebral cortex, which are called pyramidal cells because they are shaped like pyramids). It begins in the primary motor cortex and ends at synapses with the cranial nerves or spinal nerves. The *spinocerebellar* pathway connects the cerebellum and brain stem with the peripheral nervous system. As we noted earlier, the corticospinal pathway is a *crossed* pathway—lesions in one brain hemisphere cause impairments on the contralateral side of the body. In contrast, the spinocerebellar pathway is *uncrossed*—lesions in one cerebellar hemisphere cause impairments on the same side of the body.

The *sensory pathways* in the posterior spinal cord are complex. The pathway for *pain and temperature* ascends in the lateral spinal cord to the thalamus and parietal lobe. It is a crossed pathway, and the crossing occurs almost immediately where the peripheral nerve joins the central nervous system. The pathway for *proprioception* (position sense) and *stereognosis* (the ability to identify objects by touch) ascends through the dorsal (posterior) spinal cord to the cerebellum and the postcentral gyrus in the parietal lobe. This pathway is also a crossed pathway, but it ascends on the ipsilateral side of the spinal cord and crosses over in the brain stem. The pathway for *light touch* ascends in the ventral (anterior) spinal cord to the brain stem and parietal lobe. This pathway contains both uncrossed fibers and fibers that cross at the brain stem. That is why light touch sensation often is preserved when one side of the spinal cord is damaged.

The Reflex Arc

Some reflexive motor responses can be accomplished at the level of the lower motor neuron, without participation of higher levels. Such reflexive activity depends on the *reflex arc,* which permits rapid movements without the participation of higher neural systems. The reflex arc has five parts—a sensory receptor, an afferent (sensory) neuron, an interneuron, a motor neuron, and an effector, usually a muscle (see Fig 1–12). Stimulation of the sensory receptor causes it to generate an electrical signal, which is transmitted by the afferent neuron to the posterior column of the spinal cord, where the receptor synapses with the interneuron. The interneuron transmits

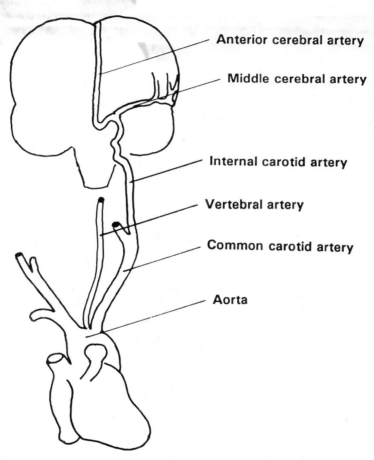

FIG 1–13.

How the blood gets from the heart to the brain. The aorta is the major artery from the heart. The common carotid and vertebral arteries branch off the aorta. The common carotid eventually divides into the external and internal carotid arteries. The external carotid arteries supply blood to the face and the internal carotid arteries supply the middle parts of the brain. The vertebral arteries supply posterior parts of the brain.

the impulse to the motor neuron in the anterior column of the spinal cord. The motor neuron activates a muscle or gland. Injuries in the reflex arc result in diminution or abolition of reflexes served by the arc. The reflex arc usually is under the inhibitory control of higher levels of the central nervous system. Lesions in fiber tracts above the arc may disconnect the reflex arc from this inhibitory control, resulting in exaggerated and hyperactive reflexes.

BLOOD SUPPLY TO THE BRAIN

The brain's blood supply comes from the heart. The heart pumps blood into the *aorta,* the major artery coming from the heart. Above the heart the aorta sends off four arteries toward the brain—two *common carotid arteries* (one on each side) and two *subclavian arteries* (again, one on each side). The common carotids ascend into the neck where they each divide into an *internal carotid* and an *external carotid* artery. (This is going to be complicated. Figure 1–13 may help.) The external carotid

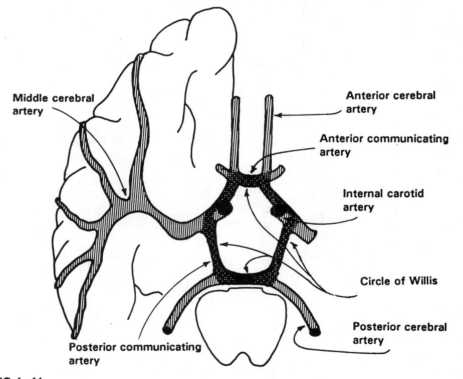

FIG 1–14.
How blood is distributed to the brain by the circle of Willis. Occlusions below the circle of Willis may not cause as much brain damage as occlusions above the circle, because the circle of Willis provides a pathway for blood from unoccluded arteries to reach all the arteries above it.

heads off for the face, and we can ignore it from now on. The internal carotids proceed upward toward the brain on each side of the neck, near the surface, just behind the angle of the jaw. They eventually connect to opposite sides of the *circle of Willis* (more on the circle of Willis later). Now we return to the subclavian arteries (one on each side) and follow them to where they branch into the *vertebral arteries* (again, one on each side). The vertebrals follow the anterior surface of the medulla upward until they *anastomose* (join together) at the base of the pons to form the *basilar artery*. The basilar artery continues upward along the midline of the pons and eventually connects into the posterior part of the circle of Willis.

The circle of Willis is a circular (or heptagonal) set of arteries at the base of the brain approximately at the midline (Fig 1–14). The circle of Willis interconnects the four arteries (two carotids and two vertebrals) that lead from the heart to the brain. Because of this, it may provide an alternative source of blood if one of the four is blocked, because the other three unblocked arteries may provide enough blood flow to maintain cerebral functions. This can occur only when the blockage is *below* the circle of Willis. Prolonged occlusion of a cerebral artery above the circle of Willis al-

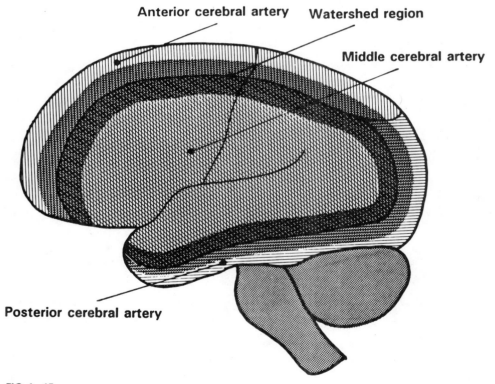

FIG 1–15.
The distributions of the cerebral arteries. The "watershed" areas represent areas in which the distributions of two arteries overlap. Occlusions in these areas may have diminished effects on cerebral functions because of collateral circulation from the distribution of a neighboring artery.

ways causes brain damage, because the cerebral arteries share no common source above the circle of Willis.

Three pairs of cerebral arteries branch upward from the circle of Willis—two *anterior cerebral arteries,* two *middle cerebral arteries,* and two *posterior cerebral arteries.* The anterior cerebral artery supplies the superior and anterior frontal lobes and the front of the corpus callosum. The middle cerebral artery has a fan-shaped distribution, and supplies most of the lateral surfaces of the brain hemispheres. The posterior cerebral artery supplies blood to the occipital lobe and the lower parts of the temporal lobe (Fig 1–15). The areas served by the cerebral arteries slightly overlap at the boundaries of their distributions. Consequently, blockages occurring at the periphery of an artery's distribution may have diminished effects, because of collateral blood supply from the adjacent artery. These areas of overlapping blood supply are sometimes called *watershed* areas.

Chapter 2

The Neurologic Examination

Most patients with neurogenic communication disorders are seen by a neurologist before they are seen by a speech-language pathologist. The neurologist who sees a patient with suspected nervous system pathology usually is concerned with (1) determining the location and extent of the pathology; (2) determining the nature or cause of the pathology; and (3) the course of the pathology—whether it is static, resolving, or growing worse. The primary tools in this endeavor are (1) the patient's medical history; (2) examination of the patient; and (3) interpretation of laboratory findings.

THE MEDICAL HISTORY

The medical history is elicited either from the patient (if he or she is capable of giving it) or from a family member or someone else close to the patient. The history is obtained during an interview. The interview usually covers the patient's *current complaint(s), the onset of the problem(s), the progression of the problem(s),* and the *family history.*

The *family history* is important because some neurologic diseases are hereditary or familial. (*Hereditary* implies a definite genetic inheritance pattern; *familial* implies greater than expected occurrence in families. Huntington's disease, myotonic dystrophy, and Friedreich's ataxia are hereditary. Some cases of Alzheimer's disease and some forms of epilepsy may be familial.) When the diagnosis is uncertain, evidence of a hereditary pattern may help to confirm a diagnosis that could not be made on the basis of the patient's current symptoms alone.

The patient's *current complaint(s)* are probably the most important part of the medical history. The patient's report of *pain, sensory problems, motor problems, incoordination, seizures, dizziness,* or *changes in consciousness or mentation* are important contributors to the diagnosis.

If the patient reports *pain,* its location and distribution may point to the location of the pathology. Localized pain may implicate specific organs, muscles, or nerves. Generalized pain may suggest generalized neuropathy or involvement of major nerve roots or their distributions. Knowing what relieves or exacerbates the pain may also help to determine its source. If the pain is worse with movement or effort, or if it changes with changes in posture, its source often is mechanical (compression of nerves, inflammation of joints). If the pain is unaffected by movement, effort, or posture, its source may be inflammation of peripheral nerves or lesions in the central nervous system that affect sensory pathways (e.g., thalamic pain syndrome).

If the patient reports *sensory or motor problems,* the reported location, severity, and nature of the problems provide information that can be embellished by the physical examination. The neurologist asks the patient to describe the problems, paying particular attention to when they were first noticed, what they were like at onset, and how they may have changed from onset to the present, and whether they now are constant or intermittent.

If the patient reports *seizures,* the neurologist questions the patient about when they began, what they were like, and whether their beginning was concurrent with other medical or physical events (e.g., a fall, headache, changes in mental status). The neurologist also asks questions about the seizures' course (How many have occurred? Are they increasing or decreasing in frequency?) and nature (Are they preceded by an aura? Are they focal or generalized? Do they respond to medication?).

If the patient reports *changes in consciousness or thinking abilities,* the neurologist determines the extent to which consciousness or mentation is compromised, the course of the changes (Are the changes increasing in magnitude? Decreasing? Constant?), and whether they are related to other symptoms or to events in the patient's life. The neurologist determines if the changes affect consciousness and mentation generally, or if they are specific to certain functions, such as speech, memory, or orientation.

The patient's description of the first symptoms receive careful attention, and the patient may be questioned to find out if they actually were the first symptoms. It is not unusual for patients and their families to ignore or discount the importance of early symptoms because they may be innocuous, and may not be perceived as related to the patient's current complaints.

The patient's description of the *progression of the problem* often provides important information for the diagnosis. The neurologist will question the patient to find out if the course of symptom development was steady and regular, or if there were periods of remission or stabilization. Gradual and uninterrupted development of symptoms may suggest dementia, degenerative disease, or a slowly growing tumor. Rapid uninterrupted development of symptoms may suggest a malignant tumor, encephalitis, or amyotrophic lateral sclerosis. Rapid development of symptoms with plateaus in which symptom development stabilizes may suggest thromboembolic disease, especially of the larger arteries. Gradual development of symptoms, with periods of remission, may suggest multiple sclerosis or vascular disease involving small arteries.

THE PHYSICAL EXAMINATION

In the physical examination the *cranial nerves, the motor system, the sensory system, reflexes, coordination, balance, gait, and station, visual fields,* and *higher cortical functions* are all evaluated.

Examination of Cranial Nerves.—The cranial nerves are evaluated by testing the sensory and motor functions of the body parts that are served by each cranial nerve. Cranial nerve testing usually progresses from the top down. The eyes and eye muscles are evaluated by testing visual acuity, visual fields, eye movements, lid movements, and the pupillary reflex (constriction of the pupil when light shines into the eye). The sensory and motor functions of the cranial nerves for the face are assessed by testing facial muscle movements in facial expression (both voluntary and involuntary), whistling, winking, etc., and by testing perception of light touch and pinprick in the face. The cranial nerves serving the tongue and structures involved in swallowing are evaluated by testing tongue and palatal movement, tongue sensation, and the gag reflex. Taste is difficult to evaluate and is, unfortunately, not routinely tested. The muscles of the neck and shoulders are tested by assessing head and neck movements. Hearing acuity and equilibrium are tested to assess the integrity of cranial nerve VIII.

Examination of the Motor System.—The motor system is examined by means of *inspection, palpation, passive movements,* and *active movements.* The patient's posture and general appearance, and the shape, size, and condition of muscle groups are visually assessed. Deformity, atrophy (degeneration of muscles, "wasting away"), and involuntary movements are noted.

Muscle tone, the tension remaining in a muscle or muscle group when it is voluntarily relaxed, is evaluated by palpation and shaking. *Passive movement* is evaluated by moving each limb while the patient maintains the limb muscles in a state of relaxation. *Range of passive movement* is assessed by moving each limb through its full range and noting resistance to movement or pain during movement. There are two kinds of resistance to passive movement. In *spasticity* the muscles of the limb resist stretching. Spastic muscles respond more vigorously to fast stretch than to slow stretch. As the velocity of muscle stretch increases, there usually is a sudden increase in resistance—the "spastic catch." In *rigidity* (more properly, "plastic rigidity") the limb resists passive movement in any direction, although there may be asymmetry between flexor and extensor resistance. (In Parkinson's disease, for example, flexor muscles are more affected than extensors.)

Next the *speed, strength, range, accuracy,* and *coordination* of volitional movements are assessed. *Slowness of movements* (often the only sign of mild paresis), *weakness* (tested by having the patient move the limb against resistance), and *incoordination* (assessed by asking the patient to execute sequences of movements involving a number of muscle groups) are noted. Signs of *myotonia* (persisting, involuntary contraction of a muscle following voluntary movement) and *synkinesia,* the tendency for voluntary movements to generate involuntary movements on the contralateral side (e.g., closing the right hand causes involuntary closing of the left hand), also are noted.

Examination of the Sensory System.—The sensory system is examined to determine whether *anesthesia* (loss of sensation), *hypoesthesia* (decreased sensitivity), or *hyperesthesia* (increased sensitivity to normal stimuli) are present. Both *deep sensation* and *superficial sensation* are assessed. Deep sensation includes joint sense (the ability to tell the position of the limbs without seeing them) deep pain sensation, tested by pinching muscles and pressing on structures that are sensitive to pressure, and sensitivity to vibration. Diminished sensitivity to these forms of stimulation implicates the posterior sensory tracts in the spinal cord. Superficial sensation is assessed by testing the patient's ability to perceive light touch, stroking, or pinprick on the skin, and by measuring the patient's ability to report differences in the temperature of objects placed against the skin. Diminished sensitivity to light touch, pinprick, and temperature implicate the anterior sensory tracts in the spinal cord. *Double simultaneous stimulation* may be used to detect slight impairments in sensory function. In double simultaneous stimulation two symmetrical points on the body are simultaneously stimulated (e.g., the same location on the left forearm and right forearm is lightly touched). If the patient's sensory function is diminished on one side, the stimulation on the less impaired side is reported by the patient while that on the impaired side is not. Inability to detect the stimulus on the impaired side during double simultaneous stimulation is called *extinction,* and is associated with cortical lesions.

Evaluation of Reflexes.—Both *superficial* and *deep* reflexes are evaluated. Superficial reflexes are elicited by stroking, touching, or brushing the surface of body parts. Some are normal, and some signify neuropathology. Normal superficial reflexes include the gag reflex, the corneal reflex (blinking when something touches the cornea), and the plantar reflex (bending downward of the toes when the sole of the foot is stroked). Pathologic reflexes include the *Babinski reflex* and the *grasp reflex.* The Babinski reflex is elicited by stroking the sole of the foot, at which time the toes bend upward and fan out, in contrast with the normal plantar reflex, in which the toes bend downward, and do not fan. The presence of a Babinski reflex suggests a lesion in the upper motor neuron. The grasp reflex is a pathologic superficial reflex, characterized by involuntary grasping of objects placed in the hand or used to stroke the hand. If the grasp reflex is strong, the patient may be unable voluntarily to release objects held in the affected hand (such as the examiner's necktie!).

Deep reflexes are elicited by tapping or suddenly stretching muscles or tendons. Perhaps the best known deep reflex is the *patellar reflex* or knee-jerk reflex, elicited by tapping the patellar tendon, just below the kneecap. Deep reflexes may be *exaggerated* or *diminished.* Exaggeration of deep reflexes suggests damage in the upper motor neuron, which releases the lower levels of the nervous system from the control of the cortex and midbrain structures. Diminution of deep reflexes suggests damage in the peripheral nerves; either the lower motor neuron or in the sensory feedback fibers serving the affected muscle groups.

Throughout the evaluation of cranial nerves, the motor system, the sensory system, and reflex testing, one side of the body is compared with the other. The presence of a pathologic symptom on one side of the body implicates the contralateral brain hemisphere, and helps to determine if the lesion is in the brain, the ipsilateral motor neuron, or if the lesion is in the lower motor neuron. Comparison of motor, sensory, and reflex findings on the two sides of the body helps the examiner determine the location of the damage responsible for the patient's deficits, both in terms of which side of the central nervous system is affected and how high or low the damage is.

Assessment of Coordination, Balance, Gait, and Station.—The patient's limb coordination is assessed by asking the patient to carry out various targeting movements such as repeatedly touching first the examiner's finger and then the patient's nose while the examiner slowly moves his finger back and forth before the patient. Balance is evaluated by asking the patient to stand on one leg with eyes open and with eyes closed. Gait is evaluated by asking the patient to walk away from and then toward the examiner. Station (the patient's standing and sitting posture) is assessed by visually evaluating the patient's posture while he stands or sits passively. Incoordination in limb movements and walking implicates the cerebellum or the extrapyramidal system, the latter being more likely if involuntary movements are also present. Impaired balance may suggest cerebellar or extrapyramidal system involvement, involvement of the vestibular system in the inner ear, or impaired sensory feedback from muscle groups. Abnormal posture may be caused by muscle weakness, spasticity, or the patient's response to pain associated with certain positions.

Assessment of Visual Fields.—Because blindness in parts of the visual fields can be very useful in locating cerebral lesions, the patient's visual fields are often assessed during the neurologic examination. The assessment may be relatively informal, or it may be carried out under controlled conditions, using specialized machines (perimetry). The kinds of visual field deficits observed may suggest (or confirm) the location of the lesion (or lesions) responsible for the patient's deficits. How visual field blindnesses are related to cerebral pathology is discussed later in this book (*see* pages 55–58).

Assessment of Cortical Function.—The neurologic examination usually includes basic screening tests of cortical function (sometimes referred to as "higher cortical function"). Orientation, memory, language, and cognitive abilities are tested. Orientation is assessed by asking questions such as "Where are you now?" "What day of the week is it?" What is the weather like today?" "Why are you here?" Short-term (immediate) memory is assessed by asking the patient to repeat series of digits, words, or sentences. Long-term memory is assessed by asking the patient for biographical information. Cognitive abilities are assessed by asking the patient to draw, copy, spell words, do arithmetic calculations, or define proverbs. These tests give only gross estimates of cognitive abilities. When deficits are identified, they are usually tested more extensively in a follow-up assessment.

INTERPRETATION OF LABORATORY TESTS

The neurologist almost always orders laboratory tests to obtain information about the patient that cannot be obtained from the interview and physical examination. In addition to standard laboratory tests such as analysis of blood and urine, other special tests that are useful in the diagnosis of neurologic disorders usually are ordered.

The *spinal tap* permits assessment of the composition of the patient's cerebrospinal fluid. A hypodermic needle is inserted between the vertebrae in the lower spine, below the level of the spinal cord, and a sample of cerebrospinal fluid is taken for analysis. When the needle is inserted, the pressure with which the fluid flows into the syringe is measured. Increased pressure may suggest blockage in the circulation of cerebrospinal fluid, the presence of space-occupying pathology such as a tumor or abscess, or swelling of brain tissue. The fluid is sent to the laboratory, where it is analyzed for the presence of cells, bacteria, parasites, or viruses, and its chemical composition is determined, including the amounts of glucose and protein in the fluid. The presence of red blood cells or a yellowish color (*xanthochromia*) are signs of bleeding into the ventricles, meningeal spaces, or spinal cord. The presence of bacteria, parasites, or viruses proves infection with those agents. Increased protein content may suggest meningeal inflammation, tumor, or obstructions within the spinal canal. Cerebrospinal fluid glucose levels often are lowered by infections.

The *electroencephalogram* (EEG) is a graphic record of the electrical activity of the cerebral cortex. It is obtained by placing electrodes on the scalp. The electrodes detect the tiny electrical signals that are generated by the brain cortex. The signals are amplified until they are capable of operating pens that record the signals on a moving strip of paper. The activity from a number of electrodes is recorded, so that tracings of the electrical activity at several cortical locations (usually 16) are obtained. The amplitude and pattern of the waveforms in the tracings, and the location of anomalous patterns of activity, permit the neurologist to make inferences about what is happening physiologically in the patient's brain. Localized brain lesions often cause *focal disturbances* in the EEG record in the vicinity of the lesion. The disturbance usually takes the form of abberations in rhythm and amplitude (Fig 2–1). General disturbances of brain function usually cause general abnormalities in the EEG record across all recording sites. Electroencephalography is useful for detecting and localizing seizure activity. In some cases, the EEG may help to distinguish between cortical and subcortical lesions in patients with overt neurologic signs of stroke. If the EEG record from a stroke patient is normal, the stroke is likely to be subcortical; if the EEG is abnormal the stroke is likely to be cortical. When a patient is in deep coma, EEG recordings may be used to estimate the severity of brain injury and predict whether the patient is likely to return to consciousness.

An adaptation of EEG recording is *measurement of evoked cortical potentials,* also called *evoked response testing.* When evoked cortical potentials are measured the patient is placed in a quiet, dark room with scalp electrodes on his head. When the patient's EEG has stabilized, tactile, auditory, or visual stimuli are presented and the electrical activity of the cortex is measured from the scalp electrodes. Most of

R = right	F = frontal	P = parietal	AT = anterior temporal	T = temporal
L = left	O = occipital	Pc = precentral	Pf = posterior frontal	E = ear

Calibration: 50 microvolts (vertical) and 1 second (horizontal).

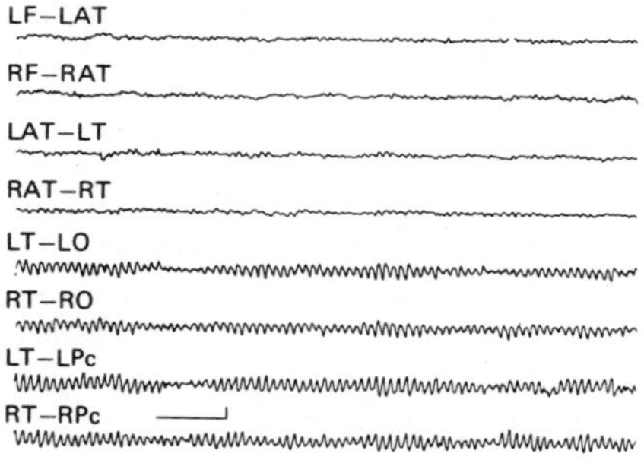

Normal Adult

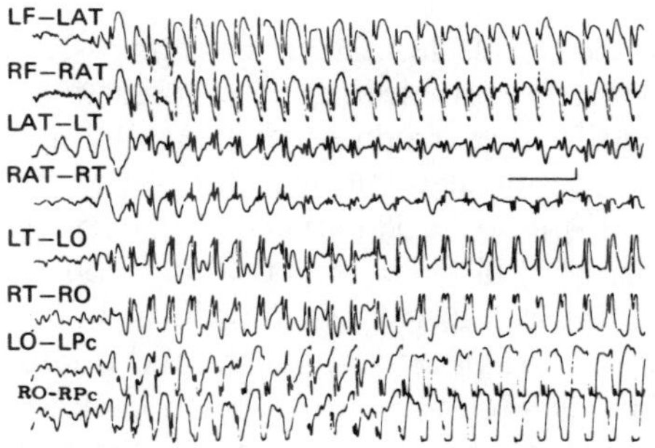

Petit Mal Epilepsy. This 6-year-old boy had one of his "blank spells," in which he was transiently unaware of surroundings and blinked his eyelids, during the recording.

FIG 2–1.

Examples of normal and abnormal EEGs. On the left is a recording from a patient with no EEG anomalies. On the right is a recording from a patient with petit mal epilepsy, showing general disruption of cortical activity. (From DeGroot J, Chusid JG: *Correlative Neuroanatomy.* Norwalk, CT, Appleton & Lange, 1988. Used by permission.)

these signals are quite small, and multiple responses to stimulation must be "averaged" by a computer. The computer calculates the cortical activity occurring at each of many time intervals following each stimulus. Changes in activity that regularly follow each stimulus are added together, and irregular (random) changes are ignored. A graphic printout of the averaged waveform attributable to stimulation is then generated. Alterations of computed waveforms for the *visual evoked response* (generated by visual stimulation), *brain stem evoked response* (generated by auditory stimulation), and *somatosensory evoked response* (generated by weak electrical stimulation of peripheral sensory nerves) suggest damage to the central nervous system conduction pathways serving those sensory modalities—damage that may not be detectable by clinical neurologic examination.

Several radiographic tests (tests that depend on the use of x-rays) may provide information about what is happening within the central nervous system. *Cerebral angiography* (or *cerebral arteriography*) is accomplished by injecting radiopaque fluid into one of the arteries that supply blood to the brain (usually a carotid artery but occasionally a vertebral artery). A sequence of radiographs of the head is then taken. The radiopaque fluid fills the injected artery and its branches and eventually makes its way into the cerebral veins, so that when the radiographs are developed one can visualize the circulation through the larger cerebral vessels. (Angiograms do not show the smallest vessels.)

Angiograms are useful in detecting occlusions of arteries or their branches, because occluded vessels do not fill with the fluid and therefore are not visible on angiography (Fig 2–2). Blood vessels that are narrowed but not occluded fill slowly. Slow filling of vessels is detected by evaluating the progress of the fluid through the vessels across the series of radiographs. Angiography may also show the presence of space-occupying lesions such as tumors or abcesses if the lesion displaces cerebral blood vessels from their customary locations. A recently developed procedure for computer enhancement of angiographic images, *digital subtraction* angiography, provides improved image quality while lessening the amount of radiopaque fluid that must be injected into the vascular system.

B-mode carotid imaging is a noninvasive technique for visualizing superficial (extracranial) blood vessels with ultrasound. It is frequently used to visualize the carotid arteries in the neck. A transducer that emits high-frequency sound waves is placed against the neck over the carotid artery. The sound waves are transmitted into the neck, where some are reflected back, depending on the acoustic absorption characteristics of the tissues beneath the transmitter. A detector picks up the reflected sound waves and a computer analyzes the variations in the waves and generates an image of the tissues scanned. Echo arteriograms are most useful for detecting stenosis or ulceration in the carotid arteries, although it cannot reliably differentiate between severe stenosis and complete occlusion. It cannot be used to image vessels within the cranial vault because of artifacts generated by the skull.

Carotid phonoangiography is another technique for assessing the condition of the carotid arteries. In carotid phonoangiography a sensitive detector is placed over the carotid artery. The detector picks up the sounds of the blood moving through the artery and converts them to electrical signals. These signals are then amplified and converted to a graphic display. Stenosis or roughness in the arterial walls creates tur-

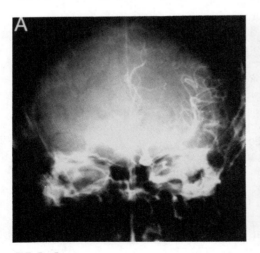 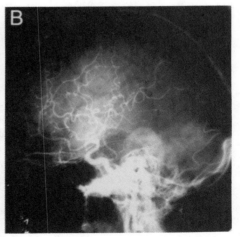

FIG 2–2.
A normal cerebral angiogram. **A,** view taken from the front, showing the anterior cerebral artery proceeding upward on the midline, and the middle cerebral artery proceeding laterally and upward. **B,** lateral view, shows the middle cerebral artery and the posterior branches of the posterior cerebral artery. The carotid artery is visible in the neck in both views.

bulence in the blood flowing through the artery. The turbulence generates sounds (bruits) that, when amplified and converted to a graphic display, allow the neurologist to estimate the amount of stenosis or roughness inside the artery.

Transcranial Doppler ultrasound is an experimental noninvasive technique for measuring blood pressure and flow in the cerebral arteries. High-frequency sound waves are transmitted into the head by a probe attached to a computer. The computer manipulates the characteristics of the sound waves in order to target a particular blood vessel. A detector picks up the reflected sound waves and passes them to the computer. The computer analyzes changes in frequency of the reflected waves (the Doppler effect) and generates a graphic image representing blood pressure and flow within the artery.

Computed tomography (CT scanning or CAT scanning [*computerized axial tomography*]), like evoked response testing, makes use of a computer to process and analyze information. In CT scanning the patient is placed in the center of a circular arrangement of x-ray generators and detectors, which rotate axially around the patient. The x-rays pass through the parts of the patient's body being scanned and are picked up by detectors on the other side of the circle. The signals from the detectors are passed on to a computer that analyzes them and generates photograph-like images that represent cross sections of the body (Fig 2–3). The scanner moves up or down the body in regular steps so that a series of images representing consecutive layers or "slices" of the body are obtained.

By using a narrow beam of x-rays, sensitive detectors, and computer enhancement of signals, soft tissues not visible on standard radiographs become visible on CT scans. In many instances CT scanning has replaced other tests. It provides better visualization of internal structures with less risk to the patient. Computed tomography scanning can almost always distinguish between hemorrhagic and occlusive strokes, but it does not directly show what causes occlusive strokes. The CT scan may be normal if the stroke is recent. Computed tomography scanning also provides good visualization of tumors, abscesses, and hematomas.

Magnetic resonance imaging (MRI; sometimes called *nuclear magnetic resonance imaging* [NMRI]) is a recently developed technique that generates photograph-like images that look somewhat like the images generated by CT scans. Magnetic resonance imaging requires no radioactive tracers and it usually provides images with greater detail than those from CT scanning. Magnetic resonance imaging depends on the fact that the nuclei of some atoms behave somewhat like small bar magnets, so that if they are placed in a strong magnetic field, they will all orient themselves in the same direction, in line with the magnetic field. In MRI the body part to be imaged is placed within such a magnetic field. Then, when the hydrogen nuclei in the body tissues have all aligned themselves with the magnetic field, a short pulse of electromagnetic energy is introduced into the field, causing the hydrogen nuclei to be momentarily deflected from alignment. As the nuclei swing back into alignment with the magnetic field, they emit tiny electromagnetic signals. A set of detectors measures these signals and sends them to a computer that constructs a photograph-like image from the signals (Fig 2–4). Magnetic resonance imaging is sensitive to differences in the chemical composition of tissues, while CT scanning is sen-

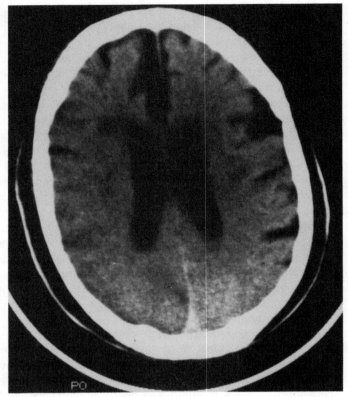

FIG 2–3.
A CT scan of a patient with a long history of neurologic problems. The lateral ventricles are enlarged and the sulci are widened, suggesting shrinkage of brain tissues. *Dark areas* suggest areas of damage in the anterior left hemisphere near the midline and in the lateral aspect of the frontal lobe in the right hemisphere.

sitive to differences in the density of tissues. For this reason, MRI can show differences between tissues that have similar density but different chemical composition, such as gray matter and white matter in the brain—differences that cannot be seen on CT scans. Magnetic resonance imaging is superior to CT in imaging the thalamus, brain stem, cerebellum, and spinal cord. Magnetic resonance imaging is better than CT scanning for detecting arteriovenous malformations and aneurysms, but it usually is less useful than CT scanning for distinguishing among hemorrhages, vessel occlusions, and tumors. Magnetic resonance imaging requires no radiation, and so far there is no evidence that the magnetic fields used are a risk to patients.

Single-photon emission computed tomography (SPECT), sometimes called *regional cerebral blood flow* (rCBF) *measurement* is a procedure for estimating blood flow in various brain regions. Because cerebral blood flow and cerebral metabolism usually are related, measurement of rCBF provides indirect estimates of regional cerebral metabolism, rather than static images of structures. The patient inhales air

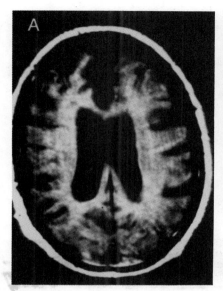 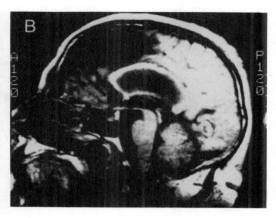

FIG 2–4.
MRI scans of the patient shown in Figure 2–3. The sulci are better visualized, and the areas of damage seen in the CT scan are also seen in this MRI, especially in the lateral view **(B).**

containing small amounts of a slightly radioactive gas (usually xenon 133). The radioactive gas eventually enters the bloodstream. When it reaches the brain a scanner detects the radioactivity emitted by the gas, converts it into electrical signals, and sends it to a computer that analyzes the signals and generates an image representing the blood flow in various brain regions. Studies of rCBF are useful in detecting vasospasm following hemorrhages, and can provide information about collateral blood flow in patients with documented cerebrovascular lesions (Walker-Batson et al., 1987).

Positron emission tomography (PET) measures the metabolic activity of regions of the brain. The patient is given a solution of metabolically active material (usually glucose) tagged with a positron-emitting isotope (oxygen, flourine, carbon, or nitrogen). The glucose eventually makes its way to the brain, where it is metabolized. The glucose and the isotope concentrate at areas of high metabolism (which are the areas of greatest neural activity and greatest blood flow). The positrons emitted by the isotope are picked up by a set of detectors, the signals are amplified, and then sent to a computer that processes them to generate an image representing the regional metabolic activity of the brain. Scanning with PET is at this time primarily a research tool. The PET scans are expensive (the scanning facility needs a cyclotron and associated physicists and chemists to prepare the isotope), and PET scanners are currently found only in large institutions—usually those with large medical research operations. Both PET and SPECT provide estimates of rCBF. However, PET scans also permit visualization of hypofunction in brain regions in which blood flow is not compromised, and in which no structural damage is visible on standard CT scans (Metter et al., 1984; Metter et al., 1983).

Chapter 3

Neuropathology of Aphasia

Aphasia is caused by malfunction of the language-competent regions of the brain. The most common cause of dysfunction in these regions (and of aphasia) is interruption of the brain's blood supply. Aphasia sometimes occurs following traumatic brain injuries, brain tumors, infections, chemical toxicities, or nutritional disturbances, but when it does, other cognitive and communicative impairments usually accompany the aphasic language disturbances. In the following section, the neurologic developments that may compromise the brain's ability to carry on language processes are summarized. It is convenient to divide etiologies into *acute events** and *insidious processes. Acute events* progress rapidly and symptoms are fully developed within a few minutes to a day or two. *Insidious processes* progress slowly and symptoms develop in piecemeal fashion, often taking months or years to be fully expressed.

ACUTE EVENTS

During the first few days after acute injuries to the brain, usually there is generalized disruption of cerebral processes, in which parts of the brain that are not actually damaged may cease to function, or may function poorly. Consequently, one typically sees a pattern of generalized disruption of brain functions immediately after the injury, which gradually resolves to more limited disruption of specific processes, with the pattern of disruption depending on what regions of the brain have actually been damaged or destroyed.

Vascular Incidents (Strokes)

The common technical term for vascular incidents in the brain or brain stem is *cerebrovascular accident.* In more common parlance, the term is *stroke,* which aptly

---

*The term "acute" is sometimes used to denote the initial stages of a pathologic condition. In this sense, "acute" is used in contrast with "chronic," a term denoting the long-term persistent state of a condition.

portrays the sudden and dramatic nature of most cerebrovascular accidents. Stroke is the third leading cause of death in the United States. In 1985, there were an estimated 500,000 strokes, and 152,700 deaths attributable to strokes. There are about 2 million survivors of strokes in the United States (Caplan, 1988). Most cases of aphasia are caused by strokes.

Strokes can be *ischemic* or *hemorrhagic*, although the occurrence of ischemic stroke is far higher (80% ischemic vs. 20% hemorrhagic). In ischemic stroke (sometimes called *occlusive* stroke), an artery is blocked, with consequent loss of blood supply to central nervous system tissues served by the artery. If the occlusion lasts more than a few (3 to 5) minutes, death (*necrosis*) of central nervous system tissue is likely. The medical term for death of tissue caused by interruption of its blood supply is *infarct*.

Ischemic incidents can be either *thrombotic* or *embolic*. In *thrombotic incidents* (cerebral thrombosis), an artery is gradually occluded by a plug of material accumulating at a given site until it closes off the affected artery. In *embolic incidents*, an artery is suddenly occluded by a "plug" of material that moves within the bloodstream.

Cerebral Thrombosis (Ischemic Stroke).—Most cerebral thromboses occur in the large arteries that supply blood to the brain (the internal carotids, the vertebrals, and the basilar artery). Thromboses are much less likely in smaller arteries. (Arteries become progressively smaller in diameter as they progress away from the heart until they reach the capillary level, after which the venous system begins and the veins become progressively larger.) A thrombosis typically begins in areas of slowed blood flow and increased turbulence—at branchings and divisions in the arterial system. Atherosclerotic plaque, composed of lipids (fatty deposits) and fibrous material, begins to accumulate, and gradually thickens over the course of years. The growing layer of plaque gradually fills the *lumen* (open space within the artery). As the size of the lumen diminishes, blood flow decreases. Because slowly flowing blood tends to clot, the risk of clot formation in the narrowed artery increases. Sometimes the plaque in the arterial wall cracks or ulcerates. Blood platelets and fibrin (a protein found in blood) adhere to the ulceration, accelerating clot development. The clot may eventually occlude the artery, or parts of the clot may break off and become emboli traveling through the vascular system, eventually occluding a smaller vessel downstream from the original clot.

In *embolic incidents* (cerebral embolus), an artery is occluded by a fragment of material that travels through the circulatory system until it reaches a blood vessel smaller than its own diameter, where it stops, occluding the artery. The material in the embolus may be a blood clot that has broken loose from its site of formation, a fragment of lining from an artery, atherosclerotic plaque, tissue from a tumor, a clump of bacteria, or other solids that circulate in the bloodstream.

Determining whether the cause of a particular event is thrombotic or embolic often is difficult, so the diagnostician may hedge his or her bets by referring to ischemic incidents as *thromboembolic* events. However, thrombotic and embolic events often differ in their progression. Embolic strokes usually are maximally expressed within a few minutes, but thrombotic strokes usually develop more slowly, and in a stepwise manner. Transient ischemic attacks—transient disruptions of cerebral circulation, which cause abrupt but temporary episodes of sensory disruption, limb weakness, slurred speech, visual complaints, or mild aphasia—may precede actual strokes. Sometimes an embolus may occlude an artery long enough to cause an infarct, then break up or dissolve. When blood flow is restored, the weakened arterial walls in the previously infarcted area may leak, creating a hemorrhagic stroke (see below).

Compromised blood supply to the brain and brain stem may also be caused by *hypoperfusion,* in which blood flow to the brain is lessened, not by occlusion of arteries, but by insufficient blood volume or insufficient cardiac pumping volume. The pattern of cerebral damage is different for hypoperfusion and occlusion. Occlusion causes maximal damage to brain tissue in the center of the circulatory field served by the occluded artery or arterial branch. Hypoperfusion causes maximal damage in the watershed areas (border zones) of the circulatory fields of the major cerebral arteries. The blood tends not to penetrate into these border zones, where vessel diameters are small and flow resistance high.

Rubens (1977) has described some of the physiologic changes that take place after ischemic strokes. During the first few days after the stroke, brain tissue in the region of the stroke swells. If the damaged area is large, the swelling may raise intracranial pressure and cause displacement of brain tissue, with extremely large lesions causing *herniation* (see pages 40, 208–209). By the end of the first week the swelling begins to diminish, and the patient's physical, cognitive, and behavioral states begin to improve. Two other processes also play parts in the disruption of cognition and behavior after ischemic strokes. Blood flow to both hemispheres decreases, and may remain depressed for several months after the stroke. Neurotransmitters are released into the brain substance, not only in the area of the stroke, but throughout the brain and into the cerebrospinal fluid. The presence of these neurotransmitters in the brain substance diminishes neuronal metabolism and may contribute to reductions in cerebral blood flow. Finally, according to Rubens, the phenomenon of *diaschisis* also plays a role in the impairments seen after strokes. Diaschisis refers to decreased responsiveness in brain tissues that are away from the damaged tissue, but are connected to it by neuronal pathways. For many years, diaschisis was an unproven phenomenon, but studies with positron emission tomography have confirmed that destruction of brain tissue in one area is followed by reductions in cerebral metabolism in other areas, primarily those that have substantial neuronal connections to the damaged area (Metter et al., 1983; Metter et al., 1984).

The foregoing events are superimposed upon the actual destruction of brain tissue caused by the stroke, resulting in the characteristic pattern of spontaneous recovery following stroke, as these initial, but transitory, consequences of the stroke diminish with time. During the first 2 to 4 weeks after the stroke, cerebral swelling diminishes, cerebral blood flow to undamaged tissue is restored, and neurotransmitters released as a consequence of the injury are resorbed. As these physiologic repairs are accomplished, the patient gradually improves, with generalized impairments of cognition and behavior resolving to a more specific collection of symptoms that reflect the permanent damage caused by the stroke. It is often difficult to predict a patient's residual level of impairment during the first few days after a stroke, because the effects of the tissue destruction are masked and exacerbated by the transitory effects described above. Consequently, clinicians often hold off making predictions about a patient's eventual level of functioning until these immediate postinjury effects have diminished. In most cases, 2 weeks to 1 month are sufficient for this purpose.

Cerebral Hemorrhage.—*Hemorrhages* are caused by rupture of a cerebral blood vessel. Such ruptures may be caused by weakness of a vessel wall, by traumatic injury to a vessel, or by extreme fluctuations in blood pressure. Cerebral hemorrhages can be divided into two categories—those in which the hemorrhage occurs within the brain or brain stem and those in which a blood vessel in the meninges or at the surface of the brain bleeds into the spaces between the brain and skull. The former are called *intracerebral hemorrhages* and the latter are called *extracerebral hemorrhages.*

Extracerebral Hemorrhages.—Extracerebral hemorrhages can be classified as *subarachnoid, subdural,* or *extradural* hemorrhages, depending on where the blood accumulates. *Subdural* and *extradural hemorrhages* usually are caused by traumatic head injuries in which dural blood vessels are torn or lacerated. *Subarachnoid hemorrhages* are the most common extracerebral hemorrhage. They typically are caused by leaking or ruptured blood vessels on the surface of the brain, brain stem, or cerebellum. Subarachnoid hemorrhages frequently are caused by ruptured aneurysms. *Aneurysms* are balloon-like malformations of weakened areas of arterial walls. They are very susceptible to rupture. The most common sites for aneurysms are at arterial bifurcations at the base of the brain. Most aneurysms occur in the internal carotid (30%), the anterior cerebral (30%), or the middle cerebral arteries (25%). The basilar artery is the next most frequently involved (10%) (Caplan, 1988). If an aneurysm is diagnosed before it ruptures it may be surgically repaired. Sometimes this can be done even after the aneurysm begins to leak. However, many patients with subarachnoid hemorrhage die or suffer irreversible brain damage before this can be done.

Intracerebral Hemorrhages.—The most common sites for spontaneous *intracerebral hemorrhages* are in and around the thalamus and basal ganglia. Intracerebral hemorrhages are also common in the brain stem (especially the pons) and the cerebellum. Intracerebral hemorrhages are often associated with elevated blood pressure, but may be spontaneous (having no observable outside cause). Hypertension is present in more than 90% of spontaneous cerebral hemorrhages. Chronic hypertension also leads to degenerative changes in the small penetrating arteries in the brain, weakening arterial walls and creating *microaneurysms.* If a sudden change in blood pressure occurs, a microaneurysm may rupture, with consequent leakage of blood into the brain substance. This leakage often exerts pressure on adjacent vessels, causing them to rupture, and leading to a "snowball" effect, in which the hemorrhage grows by exerting pressure on and displacing adjacent brain tissue, stretching and tearing small blood vessels in the vicinity. Intracerebral hemorrhages dissect brain matter along white matter tracts, but tend not to destroy the tracts themselves. An intracerebral hemorrhage may eventually decompress itself by bleeding into the ventricles or subarachnoid space. Because of their location, usually deep in the brain, most intracerebral hemorrhages are not surgically manageable, and surgery usually is attempted only if the bleeding is life-threatening and the hemorrhage is accessible. Medical management usually includes reduction of blood pressure and treatment to increase the clotting potential of the blood.

(AVM)   *Arteriovenous malformations* are collections of swollen and distended veins connected to a tortuously twisted mass of arteries. When these malformations become large, they may cause headaches and other central nervous system symptoms. As with aneurysms, vessel walls in arteriovenous malformations usually are weak. Consequently, hemorrhages from such malformations often occur, creating subarachnoid hemorrhages. If arteriovenous malformations are identified before massive bleeding occurs, they may be surgically treated.

Recovery From Ischemic and Hemorrhagic Strokes.—Ischemic and hemorrhagic strokes have different courses of recovery. It is difficult to predict a patient's eventual level of neurologic recovery within the first week or two after cerebral injury, because the acute (and transitory) effects of cerebral injury often obscure the effects of the tissue destruction that has occurred. For this reason, one usually has to wait 3 to 4 weeks after onset before attempting to predict, with any assurance, a patient's eventual recovery. When the immediate effects of cerebral injury have dissipated, the relationship between severity of aphasia and the amount of brain damage becomes clearer. The pattern of recovery depends largely on whether the stroke was ischemic or hemorrhagic, and the eventual level of recovery depends largely on the amount of brain tissue destroyed and the location of the destruction.

Recovery from *ischemic strokes* is greatest in the first weeks, with gradual deceleration of the rate of recovery, until stabilization takes place (Fig 3–1). Recovery is greatest for patients in the middle severity ranges. Patients who remain severely aphasic when the acute effects of the stroke have dissipated usually are likely to remain severely impaired. Mildly aphasic patients have little room to recover, because small amounts of improvement bring them back to their premorbid levels. How long it takes for neurologic recovery from ischemic strokes to be completed has not been established. Most recovery takes place within the first 3 months after onset (Culton, 1969; Sarno and Levita, 1971), and recovery almost certainly is complete by 6 months after onset (Basso et al., 1979).

Recovery from *hemorrhagic strokes* usually follows a different course from that of occlusive strokes. Patients with hemorrhagic strokes often show little improvement for the first 4 to 8 weeks after onset, after which there is often a period of rapid recovery (see Figure 3–1). Recovery then slows and stabilizes, usually at a level above that for occlusive stroke patients with equivalent deficits at onset. Patients with hemorrhagic strokes, like those with ischemic strokes, usually have completed their neurologic recovery by 6 months after onset.

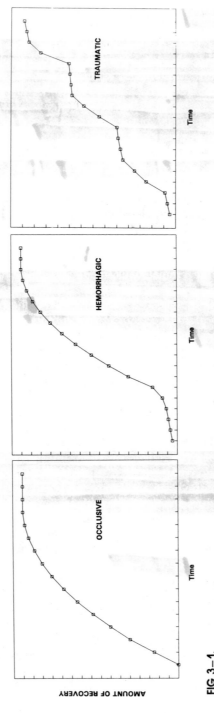

FIG 3–1.

The general course of neurologic recovery according to the etiology of the neurologic disorder. The graphs shown here represent the average course of recovery for groups of patients, and the recovery of individual patients may differ somewhat from the group averages. These curves are based primarily on clinical experience and anecdotal evidence. There is little objective evidence documenting the course of neurologic recovery following strokes or traumatic brain injuries.

INSIDIOUS PROCESSES

Insidious processes make their presence known slowly, over a period of time, rather than all at once. They usually do not have a clearly definable time of onset, and patients often do not see their physician when the first symptoms appear, because the symptoms are mild and appear innocuous. Consequently, the pathology may be advanced when the patient first seeks medical attention. In some cases delay may have no significant consequences, but in other cases (such as intracerebral tumor), it may have serious and sometimes disastrous results.

The major insidious processes that affect the central nervous system are *intracranial tumors, hydrocephalus, infections, progressive diseases, toxicities,* and *metabolic* and *nutritional disorders.* Most of these cause not only aphasia, but may cause dementia, dysarthria, or personality disruptions in addition to language and communicative impairments that would justify the label *aphasia.*

Intracranial Tumors

Tumors growing within the cranial vault may be either *primary* (originating there) or *secondary* (originating elsewhere and migrating to the intracranial regions). The process by which a tumor appears at a secondary site in the body is called *metastasis,* and such tumors are referred to as *metastatic tumors.*

Primary intracranial tumors are most often found in the cerebrum and the cerebellum. They occur at all ages, but are most common in adults from 25 to 50 years old. The causes of most primary intracerebral tumors remain a mystery. Some appear to be related to previous injuries, and there is a tendency for familial incidence of some types of intracranial tumors.

Intracranial tumors, whether primary or secondary, have similar effects on the central nervous system. The tissue around the tumor swells. This swelling is one of the major causes of observable symptoms in cases of cerebral tumor. If the tumor is so located that it exerts pressure on limited areas of the brain or brain stem, then localized symptoms (motor impairments, sensory loss) may be observed. If the tumor causes general swelling of the brain and brain stem, then widespread symptoms of cerebral dysfunction related to pressure and displacement of brain tissue may be observed. It is common to see localized symptoms in the early stages of tumor growth, with increasing and more general dysfunction as intracranial pressure increases as a result of tumor growth and swelling of brain tissue around the tumor. When cerebral swelling is severe, herniation may occur. Large masses in the brain hemispheres (or smaller ones in the brain stem) may force the brain stem downward through the foramen magnum. The consequences of herniations caused by tumors resemble those caused by traumatic brain injuries (see pages 208–209).

The general medical course of cerebral tumor is deterioration. The deterioration may be slow or rapid, depending on the rate at which the tumor grows and on the amount of swelling adjacent to the tumor. If the patient is seen in early stages, when intracranial pressure is low, he or she may complain of nonspecific alterations in mental function—forgetfulness, lack of initiative, and drowsiness. Sometimes the patient will complain of blurred or double vision and of lightheadedness or vertigo. Those around the patient may report that the patient has become more irritable, has undergone personality change, or has lost his or her customary initiative. Headaches are reported by about one third of early tumor patients. These headaches can take several forms, but most are not affected by analgesics, and in many cases they occur during sleep and are present upon awakening. Sometimes they may be severe enough to wake the patient from sleep. Vomiting is sometimes seen in the early stages of tumor growth. When it is seen, it is usually accompanied by headache. Seizures also may be seen in early stages. Usually they are focal, although the focus does not always correspond to the location of the tumor.

Symptoms or Affects of tumors [handwritten margin note]

Tumor patients with elevated intracranial pressure almost always exhibit cognitive impairments, are lethargic, and may be stuporous. In most such cases, the patient reports unremitting bifrontal and bioccipital headache that is not affected by analgesics and that is present day and night. Vomiting frequently is reported. The patient's gait may be unsteady and staggering, and general motor clumsiness may be observed.

The number of symptoms generated by a tumor, and the rate at which symptoms progress, is determined by the *size, rate of growth,* and *location* of the tumor. If the tumor is located in or near areas that serve important functions (sensory and motor cortex, brain stem), a relatively small tumor may quickly generate major symptoms. However, if the tumor is located in a "silent" area of the brain it may grow to surprising volume before generating observable symptoms.

Different kinds of tumors have different rates of growth and differ in malignancy. *Gliomas* are the most common intracerebral tumor. Gliomas can be divided into several subtypes, but the two most frequently observed are *astrocytoma* and *glioblastoma multiforme.* Astrocytomas are the most common and the most benign (nonmalignant) of the gliomas. They usually grow slowly, and symptom development may span 5 or 6 years. Postoperative survival of 10 or more years is common. In some cases, astrocytomas may be completely removed, in which case the patient is considered cured. However, even "benign" astrocytomas can cause substantial neurologic impairments, or even kill the patient, if the tumor is strategically located (e.g., in the brain stem). *Glioblastoma multiforme* is the next most common glioma. It is also one of the most malignant and rapidly growing of all intracranial tumors. Symptoms typically develop during a 3-month to 1-year period, and the average postsurgical survival is only about 6 to 9 months.

Meningiomas are also relatively common tumors that, as the name implies, arise from the meninges. They are among the most benign of all intracranial tumors because they are well-defined and do not usually invade the brain substance. For this reason they often can be completely removed. The symptoms of meningiomas are among the most localizable of intracranial tumors, because they usually generate pressure at specific places on the cortex, and rarely cause general increases in intracranial pressure.

Secondary intracranial tumors (metastatic carcinomas) are tumors that form from cancerous cells that have migrated (usually through the bloodstream) from the primary tumor site to the brain, where they settle and grow. The primary sources for metastatic carcinoma of the brain are, in decreasing order of frequency, the breast, the lungs, and the pharynx and larynx. Metastatic carcinomas of the brain usually are grossly well-defined, but multiple sites of metastasis within the brain are commonly observed. There is usually considerable local swelling around the tumor site. The prognosis for metastatic brain tumor patients usually is poor. The average survival after diagnosis of metastatic brain tumor is 2 to 6 months.

Hydrocephalus

Obstructive hydrocephalus, like brain tumors, generates increased intracranial pressure. Obstructive hydrocephalus is caused by obstruction of interventricular ducts through which cerebrospinal fluid circulates, interrupting the flow of cerebrospinal fluid from the ventricles into the spinal column and meningeal spaces. Sometimes ducts are blocked by material circulating in the cerebrospinal fluid (plugs of bacteria, bits of floating tissue). More often they are closed by swelling of adjacent brain tissue. The most frequent site of obstruction is the *aqueduct of Sylvius,* connecting the third and fourth ventricles. The aqueduct of Sylvius is the longest and narrowest of the interventricular ducts and consequently is the most susceptible to obstruction, usually by swelling of the pons or cerebellum. Because cerebrospinal fluid is formed in the cerebral ventricles, any interruption of its transit from the ventricles causes increased pressure within the ventricles. As the brain is compressed against the skull by the pressure, the patient becomes mentally dulled, lethargic, and hyporesponsive. As intraventricular pressure increases, stupor, unconsiousness, and coma ensue.

The primary medical treatment for obstructive hydrocephalus is an *intraventricular shunt.* A cannula (hollow needle) connected to a small flexible tube is passed through the brain into the ventricles. Excess cerebrospinal fluid is then forced (by intraventricular pressure) through the shunt, decreasing the pressure within the ventricles. The tube may be passed into the neck or the abdominal cavity, where the excess fluid is allowed to drip away. The patient's response to shunt placement usually is dramatic, with few long-term residual deficits, unless intracranial pressure has reached exceptionally high levels or has continued for several weeks.

Nonobstructive hydrocephalus identifies several other conditions causing ventricular enlargement. One of the most common causes of nonobstructive hydrocephalus is cerebral atrophy. Nonobstructive hydrocephalus usually is not accompanied by elevated intracranial pressure.

Infections

Cerebral tissues ordinarily are strongly resistant to infection, but cerebral infections sometimes occur. They may be caused by either bacteria or viruses.

Bacterial Infections.— The major bacterial infections are *bacterial meningitis* and *brain abscess.* In bacterial meningitis, the pia, arachnoid, and the cerebrospinal fluid between them become infected, causing inflammation, swelling, and fluid exudate from the meninges. The patient becomes feverish, chilled, lethargic, and complains of headache, drowsiness, and stiff neck. If the infection is severe, the patient may progress into coma. Bacterial meningitis exacerbates quickly and can be fatal, if treatment is not prompt. The usual treatment is antibiotic medications, which usually cure the infection, although neurologic sequelae may persist.

Brain abscess is caused by introduction of bacteria, fungus, or parasites into brain tissues from a primary infection site elsewhere in the body. Transmission may be through the blood or by migration through tissues. In about 40% of cases, the primary source of infection is the nasal sinuses, middle ear, or mastoid cells. In about 30% of cases the source is the lungs or cardiovascular tissue. Symptom development in brain abscess is slower than that of bacterial meningitis, but the symptoms are similar. The usual treatment is surgical drainage of the abscess in combination with antibiotic medication. Recovery usually is dramatic, although the patient may be left with chronic deficits related to destruction of brain tissue by the abscess.

Viral Infections.—Numerous viruses may infect the central nervous system. The two major sources of central nervous system viral infections are (1) general viral infections, such as mumps or measles; and (2) viruses transmitted by insect or animal bites, such as equine encephalitis or rabies. The course of viral infections depends on the virus involved. In some cases (such as viral meningitis), symptoms develop quickly, followed by gradual improvement. In some cases symptoms develop slowly, followed by gradual improvement. In some cases (such as acquired immunodeficiency syndrome [AIDS]), symptoms develop slowly with continuing worsening, ending in death. In some cases (such as rabies), symptoms develop quickly and dramatically, invariably ending in death. A few antiviral medications that are not toxic to brain tissue have been developed, and may be of benefit. Otherwise, treatment of viral infections is palliative, directed toward maintaining the patient's vital functions, providing adequate nutrition, and regulating fluid balance, hoping that the patient's natural defense mechanisms will rid the body of the infection.

Toxicities

Toxicity is caused by introduction of substances that inflame or poison nerve tissue into the central nervous system. Toxicity may be caused by drug overdoses, drug interactions, bacterial toxins (tetanus, botulism, diphtheria), or heavy metals (lead, mercury). The course of heavy metal or chemical poisoning (such as may occur in occupational exposure to the compounds) is usually one of decreasing mentation and increasing lethargy, with motor or sensory disruptions generally occurring only in advanced stages of poisoning. Poisoning with bacterial toxins usually follows a more acute course with symptoms developing quickly, followed by slow recovery in those patients in whom the poisoning does not lead to death. Treatment is usually directed toward removal of the source of the toxicity, and, sometimes, purging the system of the toxin.

Metabolic Disorders

Metabolic disorders are common causes of central nervous system dysfunction. If severe, hypoglycemia may cause deterioration of cerebral function, leading to confusion, stupor, or coma. Thyroid disorders may generate central nervous system symptoms (apathy, confusion, and intellectual deterioration). Treatment of metabolic disorders usually involves correcting or compensating for the metabolic imbalance, and central nervous system symptoms may regress or resolve when the metabolic disturbance is corrected.

Nutritional Disorders

Nutritional disorders, though rare in the United States, sometimes cause central nervous system dysfunction. One classic central nervous system syndrome caused by nutritional deficiency is *Wernicke's encephalopathy,* which is caused by thiamine deficiency. Other vitamin deficiencies may cause variable neurologic symptoms, including deficiencies in vitamin B12 and nicotinic acid. Neurologic syndromes associated with vitamin excess may also be seen (e.g., overdosage of vitamin A).

Chapter 4 _____

Neurophysiology of Aphasia and Related Disorders

Most neurophysiologic explanations of aphasia and related disorders are based on connectionistic models of brain functions. Connectionist explanations of aphasia have been in the literature since the middle 1800s. They are based on relationships observed between the symptoms exhibited by neurologically impaired patients and the location and size of the brain lesions generating the symptoms. The early years of neurology were dedicated in large part to documenting these relationships. When damage to a given area of the brain regularly produced certain patterns of linguistic impairment, it seemed reasonable to assign the impaired language functions to the damaged part of the brain (*localization of function*).

A strict localizationalist model of the brain and its functions is undoubtedly simplistic. We know that the brain does not operate like a telephone switchboard. Even so, knowledgable clinicians can predict the location of brain damage from the patient's behavioral impairments with reasonable accuracy. The relationships between location and extent of brain damage and behavioral symptoms are imperfect, but they are dependable enough to make localizationalist models of aphasia useful to the clinician who is curious about the location of a patient's brain lesion, given a constellation of behavioral and linguistic symptoms.

LANGUAGE AND CEREBRAL DOMINANCE

Most adults possess brains in which one hemisphere is responsible for most linguistic processes. Almost always the hemisphere dominant for speech and language is contralateral to one's preferred hand. This is nearly always true for right-handers. Over 98% of right-handers will be left-hemisphere dominant for language. Left-handers are not so consistent. In any large group of left-handers about 60% would be left-hemisphere dominant for language, as their right-handed counterparts are. About 30% would be right-hemisphere dominant, and the remaining 10% would have language competence in both hemispheres. Left-handers' brains seem to be somewhat indecisive about which hemisphere is assigned speech and language. This indecisiveness is reflected in the clinical impression that when a left-hander becomes aphasic, the aphasia is less severe and recovery usually is faster for the left-hander than it would be for a right-hander with comparable damage (Glonig et al., 1969; Luria, 1970). However, this impression has not been empirically confirmed.

The question of whether we are born with one hemisphere specialized for language has not been answered, although opinion seems to favor the position that we are not. Studies of children who sustain brain damage suggest that our dependence on the left hemisphere for language develops as we mature, and that hemispheric specialization for language is not complete before adulthood.* The older a child is when he or she sustains brain damage, the more severe and persistent the child's language impairments will be (Lenneberg, 1967; Osgood and Miron, 1963). The brain's ability to compensate for injury by reassigning functions served by damaged tissue diminishes throughout life. This is seen not only during childhood but throughout adulthood. A 30-year-old aphasic stroke patient usually recovers more language than a 50-year-old or 60-year-old patient with equivalent brain damage.

CONNECTIONIST EXPLANATIONS OF APHASIA

Connectionist explanations of aphasia began in the 19th century, and have been expanded and elaborated upon until contemporary times. They are based on the fact that patients with damage in certain regions of the language-dominant hemisphere tend to exhibit similar symptoms, giving rise to aphasia syndromes, in which certain combinations of language impairments are taken as evidence for damage in certain brain regions. The relationship between aphasic symptoms and the location of the brain damage that causes them is imperfect, and becomes less dependable as one moves from global characteristics (such as speech fluency) to more specific aspects of language behavior (such as the nature of word-retrieval failure). The idea that aphasic symptoms tend to cluster into syndromes has been challenged by those who have shown that aphasia test batteries designed to assign patients to aphasic syndromes fail to unambiguously classify from 15% (Poeck, 1983) to 40% of cases (Benson, 1979). Others have argued (Caramazza, 1984) that classical classification schemes are inappropriate for developing theories about normal cognition and brain-behavior relationships. Nevertheless, there are regularities in symptoms among aphasic adults that permit predictions about the location and extent of brain damage, and suggest that certain regions of the brain may have unique responsibilities for some aspects of language. Those who employ connectionistic models will frequently be surprised by patients who do not fit the classical model, but their assumptions will be supported by enough patients who do fit the model to make it a convenient tool

---

*Development of cerebral dominance for language is related to *cerebral plasticity*. Cerebral plasticity relates to the brain's ability to reassign functions served by damaged or destroyed tissue elsewhere. Children's brains are said to be more "plastic" than those of adults, because other parts of their brains can assume responsibility for the functions originally taken care of by the damaged or excised parts.

in clinical care. The connectionistic model may, in some respects, be a fiction, but it is a useful one for the student who wishes to understand the basic relationships between symptoms of aphasia and their causes in the nervous system.

Brain regions involved in aphasia are clustered around the sylvian fissure in the language dominant hemisphere. Cortical areas and nerve fiber tracts with important roles in language are located here. Important perisylvian areas include the following:

1. The *primary auditory cortex* (gyrus of Heschl) on the superior surface of the midtemporal lobe, below the sylvian fissure. The primary auditory cortex is important for perception of auditory stimuli, and it probably plays a role in the discrimination of sounds. The auditory cortices in the left and right hemispheres are bilaterally innervated. Each receives information from both ears. For this reason, destruction of the primary auditory cortex in one hemisphere does not cause deafness. Destruction of the primary auditory cortex in both hemispheres causes *cortical deafness,* in which the patient loses all auditory sensitivity. For some patients, basic hearing sensitivity slowly returns, and his or her pure-tone audiogram may even be normal. However, perception of speech and other more complex auditory stimuli remains profoundly impaired in almost all cases (Jerger et al., 1969).

2. The *auditory association area* or *Wernicke's area* in the midtemporal lobe. Wernicke's area seems to be important for storage and retrieval of auditory and phonologic "images" of words, and for storage and retrieval of word meanings. Wernicke's area also appears to be important in knowledge and use of grammatical and linguistic rules.

3. The *premotor cortex,* just anterior to the primary motor cortex for the speech muscles. The lowest part of the premotor cortex is called *Broca's area* or the *motor speech area.* It seems to be important for planning and organizing motor activities of speech. The premotor cortex for the hand and arm, located just above Broca's area, appears to be important for planning and organizing movements of the (contralateral) hand and arm.

4. The *arcuate fasciculus* is a band of nerve fibers that runs between the midtemporal lobe and the lower portions of the frontal lobe. The arcuate fasciculus is thought to be the primary pathway by which the acoustic-phonemic "patterns" of words are transmitted from Wernicke's area to Broca's area.

SPEECH, LANGUAGE, AND THE BRAIN

In connectionistic explanations of aphasia the neural mechanisms for speech and language are described as a sort of intricate "switchboard" in which neural "codes" and "messages" are transmitted from place to place, much like messages in a telephone system. As was mentioned earlier, a simple connectionistic model cannot explain complex brain functions. Connectionistic models contain many speculations, inferences, and inventions. However, they do provide a convenient summary of the general way in which the brain produces and comprehends speech and language.

Spontaneous Speech.— The connectionist model suggests that, in order for an individual to speak a sentence spontaneously, words are retrieved and encoded in the midtemporal lobe (Wernicke's area). A neurally coded "sentence" that obeys phonologic, grammatical, and semantic rules is also put together by Wernicke's area. The neurally coded sentence is sent forward via the arcuate fasciculus to Broca's area. At Broca's area, the neural "sentence" is translated into a coded sequence of movement "commands" that provides the "pattern" or "template" that subsequently guides the primary motor cortex in producing the sentence.

Repetition.— According to the connectionistic model, repetition of spoken messages tests the entire "circuit" for reception and production of verbal messages, from the primary auditory cortex through the motor cortex for speech. In order for an individual to repeat spoken messages, the message must be perceived (and discriminated) by the primary auditory cortex. The primary auditory cortex translates the message into a neural code, and sends it to Wernicke's area in the midtemporal lobe. In Wernicke's area, the meaning of the message is extracted, the linguistic response to the message is formulated, and the response (in neural code) is sent forward to Broca's area. In Broca's area, the response is transcoded, this time into neural movement instructions, and is sent to the primary motor cortex for execution.

Comprehension of Speech.— In order for the individual to comprehend speech, the spoken message must be perceived by the primary auditory cortex and passed on to Wernicke's area, where word meanings are elicited, and (most likely) the individual's prior knowledge is incorporated into the analysis of the message for its semantic content.

Comprehension of Printed Materials (Reading).— In order to comprehend printed materials, visual information from the printed materials must be received (and probably preprocessed) by the visual cortex and visual association areas in the occipital lobes. The neurally coded "message" that results is then sent to the midtemporal lobe (Wernicke's area), where meaning is extracted in the same manner as for spoken messages. If the individual need only read aloud, and need not understand the printed material, processes similar to those involved in speech repetition probably take place, once the message has reached the midtemporal lobe.

Gestural Responses to Spoken Commands.— In this task, the neural processes are similar to those for speech repetition, except that the neural message from Wernicke's area is directed to the premotor area for the hand and arm, rather than to the premotor area for speech. If the hand and arm response is to be carried out by the limb ipsilateral to the language dominant hemisphere, then the neural message is transmitted to the motor cortex in the nondominant hemisphere via the premotor cortex in the dominant hemisphere. The transmission is from Wernicke's area to the premotor cortex in the dominant hemisphere, then across the corpus callosum to the premotor (or motor) cortex in the nondominant hemisphere.

Writing.—In writing, Wernicke's area participates in elicitation of appropriate words and in construction of a neurally coded grammatic "sentence," as it does in spontaneous speech. This neurally coded sentence is sent forward to the premotor cortex for the hand and arm, which provides the motoric instructions to be followed by the motor cortex.

Connectionistic aphasic syndromes can be divided into *fluent* aphasias (in which speech has essentially normal prosody) and *nonfluent* aphasias (in which speech is nonprosodic). The most frequently occurring nonfluent aphasia is *Broca's aphasia* (also known as *motor aphasia, expressive aphasia,* or *anterior aphasia*). The speech of patients with Broca's aphasia is nonfluent, labored, and halting. Intonation and stress patterns are deficient, and misarticulations are prominent. The speech of patients with Broca's aphasia may be *telegraphic* and *agrammatical.* That is, the "small words" (function words—conjunctions, articles, and prepositions, etc.) are missing. Consequently, grammar is poor and syntax is deficient. Comprehension of language is better than speech production or writing for patients with Broca's aphasia. These patients usually have poor handwriting, and the content of their writing resembles the content of their speech (slow, labored, and distorted). Figure 4–1 shows a transcript of a Broca's aphasic patient describing the "cookie theft" picture from the *Boston Diagnostic Aphasia Examination,* (see Fig 7–5), and a sample of writing from a Broca's aphasic patient.

Broca's aphasia usually is seen following damage to the posterior inferior frontal lobe (the third frontal convolution or the fiber tracts connecting it to the rest of the brain). This area is known as *Broca's area,* after the French neurologist who first identified the area as important to speech. The location of Broca's area is shown in Figure 4–2. Because Broca's area is close to the primary motor cortex for the face, hand, and arm, and because descending pyramidal tract fibers run just beneath Broca's area, *hemiplegia* (paralysis of one side of the body) or *hemiparesis* (weakness of one side of the body) usually accompany Broca's aphasia. For right-handers the paralysis or paresis is almost always on the right, because lesions causing aphasia are almost always left-hemisphere lesions, and motor control is contralateral.

The most frequently described fluent aphasia is *Wernicke's aphasia,* named after the German neurologist who first described the syndrome. Wernicke's aphasia is sometimes called *sensory aphasia, receptive aphasia,* or *posterior aphasia.* The speech of patients with Wernicke's aphasia usually is fluent, except for pauses that may occur when the patient experiences word retrieval difficulty. Such word retrieval failures are common in Wernicke's aphasia. Articulation and prosody (the "rhythm" of speech, including rate, inflection, intonation, and stress) usually are intact, and sentences spoken by Wernicke's aphasic patients usually are grammatical. However, the speech of patients with Wernicke's aphasia may be "empty"—lacking content and meaning. Figure 4–3 shows a transcript of a Wernicke's aphasic patient describing the "cookie theft" picture from the *Boston Diagnostic Aphasia Examination* (see Fig 7–5). Verbal paraphasias (substitution of one word for another, such as "table" for "chair") are common in the speech of patients with Wernicke's aphasia, and literal paraphasias (substitution or transposition of sounds within words, as "velitision"

uh...mother and dad...no...mother...dishes...uh...runnin over...water...and
floor...and they...uh...wipin disses...and...uh...two kids...uh...stool...and
cookie...cookie jar...uh...cabinet and stool...uh...tippin over...and...uh...
that...uh...bad...and somebody...gonna get hurt

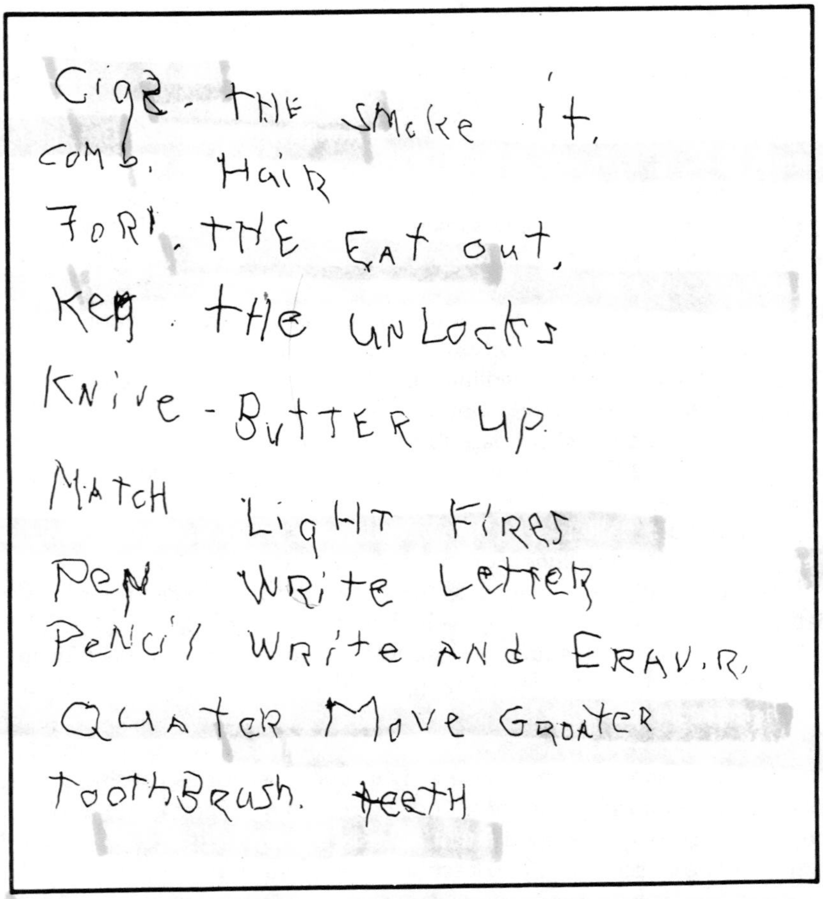

FIG 4–1.
A transcript of a speech sample *(top)* and a writing sample *(bottom)* from a patient with Broca's
aphasia. The speech sample is a description of the "cookie theft" picture from the *Boston Diagnostic Aphasia Examination* (see Figure 7–5). The writing sample is from Subtest A of the *Porch Index of
Communicative Ability*. The patient's speech is nonfluent and telegraphic, containing mostly content words (nouns, verbs, adjectives) with few function words (articles, conjunctions, prepositions).
The patient's writing is mechanically clumsy and telegraphic in content.

for "television") sometimes occur. Neologisms (nonwords such as "carabis") sometimes occur, especially when the patient's aphasia is severe. Auditory comprehension
of patients with Wernicke's aphasia is poor. Their handwriting is mechanically good,
and content usually resembles the content (or lack of content) of their speech (see
Figure 4–3).

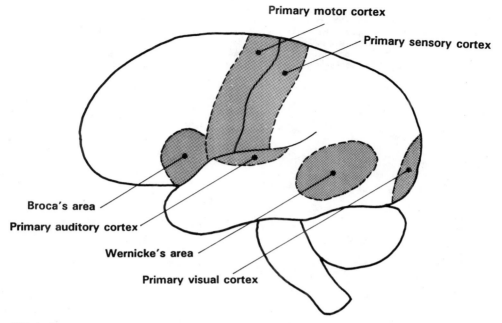

FIG 4–2.
Broca's area and Wernicke's area. Broca's area is adjacent to the primary motor cortex for the face and larynx, suggesting an important role in speech production. Wernicke's area is adjacent to the primary sensory cortex for audition and vision, suggesting an important role in associations involving auditory and visual information. That audition and vision are the two primary language input modalities may account for the importance of Wernicke's area in language comprehension.

Lesions causing Wernicke's aphasia usually occur in the auditory association area of the left temporal lobe (for right handers) or in the fiber tracts connecting it with other areas of the brain. This region is known (not surprisingly) as Wernicke's area, and it lies adjacent to the gyrus of Heschl, which is the primary auditory cortex. Because Wernicke's area is not close to cortical motor areas, hemiparesis and hemiplegia are not usually seen in Wernicke's aphasia, unless the lesion extends into the frontal lobe or descending pyramidal tracts. However, optic nerve fibers pass under Wernicke's area on their way to the visual cortex. Lesions that extend deep into the temporal lobe may interrupt these fibers, causing contralateral visual field blindness.

Conduction aphasia is a fluent aphasia, usually caused by lesions that interrupt the arcuate fasciculus—the primary nerve pathway connecting Wernicke's and Broca's areas. Patients with conduction aphasia usually have good language comprehension, because the primary auditory cortex and the auditory association area (Wernicke's area) are intact. However, because the connections between the auditory and language areas and the area for planning and executing speech (and writing) have been interrupted, conduction aphasic patients are unable to repeat (or write) what they hear. Literal paraphasias are frequent in conduction aphasic patients' speech, and verbal paraphasias sometimes occur. Oral reading, because it

Well, here we have a young boy and a girl. Looks like they're getting into trouble, stealing cookies...cookies from the cookie jar there on the shelf. That stool looks pretty precarious and I'd bet he's gonna fall on his bummer. Mom is standing there at the sink looking out the window at I don't know what. Looks like it might be summer. Mom must be daydreaming, cuz the water's running all over the floor. Looks like there's gonna be trouble when the old man gets home.

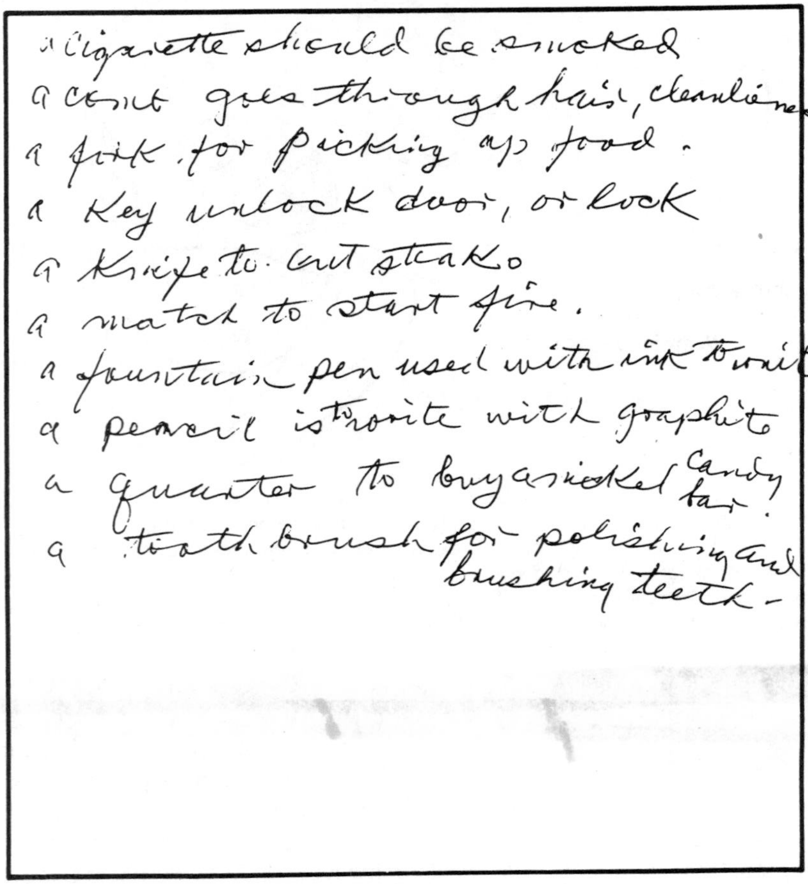

a Cigarette should be smoked
a comb goes through hair, cleanliness
a fork for picking up food .
a Key unlock door, or lock
a Knife to cut steak.
a match to start fire .
a fountain pen used with ink to write
a pencil is to write with graphite
a quarter to buy a nickel Candy bar .
a tooth brush for polishing and
                        brushing teeth —

FIG 4–3.
A transcript of a speech sample *(top)* and a writing sample *(bottom)* from a patient with Wernicke's aphasia. Speech and writing samples are in response to the same stimuli as in Figure 4–7. The patient's speech is fluent and well-formed, but he provides excessive detail.

makes use of the pathway between Wernicke's area and Broca's areas, also is poor, although reading comprehension usually is good.

Whether *anomic aphasia* exists as a separate syndrome is a topic of some disagreement (Albert et al., 1981). The label usually is applied to patients whose major symptom is word retrieval difficulties in spontaneous speech and naming tasks. The spontaneous speech of anomic aphasic patients is fluent and grammatically correct, but it is marked by word retrieval failures. The word retrieval failures generate unusual pauses, circumlocution ("talking around" missing words), and substitution of nonspecific words such as "thing" for missing words. These patients usually have subtle comprehension impairments, and may have other mild language impairments. The anomic aphasia syndrome may be a mild version of Wernicke's aphasia, and Wernicke's aphasia at onset may evolve to anomic aphasia.

Two other aphasic syndromes are caused by damage that isolates perisylvian areas from the rest of the brain. *Transcortical motor aphasia (anterior isolation syndrome)* is caused by damage in the cortical areas around Broca's area, but sparing the arcuate fasciculus and Wernicke's area. Patients with transcortical motor aphasia often exhibit "pathologic inertia" for speech. They tend not to speak spontaneously, and may speak only when given strong urging from those around them. When they do talk, their speech is fluent and well articulated, but sparse. Their utterances tend to be one or two words long, and complete sentences are rare. The paucity of their spontaneous speech is in dramatic contrast to their imitation of spoken sentences. Patients with transcortical motor aphasia can repeat long and complicated sentences with good articulation and prosody.

Transcortical sensory aphasia (posterior isolation syndrome) is caused by damage in the cortical areas around Wernicke's area, but sparing the arcuate fasciculus and Broca's area. Patients with transcortical sensory aphasia produce fluent, empty speech, as patients with Wernicke's aphasia do. Unlike patients with Wernicke's aphasia, those with transcortical sensory aphasia usually can repeat, with little difficulty, what is said to them. Sometimes they may involuntarily repeat virtually everything that is said in their presence (*echolalia*).

MODIFICATIONS TO THE CONNECTIONISTIC MODEL BASED ON CONTEMPORARY FINDINGS

With the advent of computed tomography (CT), it became possible to localize cerebral damage with greater accuracy and in greater detail than before. The capabilities of CT led to renewed interest in the relationships between brain damage and aphasia syndromes. Numerous reports on the relationships between aphasia and lesions defined by CT have appeared in the literature (Mohr et al., 1975; Naeser et al., 1982; Naeser et al., 1981a; Naeser et al., 1981b; Cappa et al., 1983; Cappa et al., 1981; Knopman et al., 1983; Knopman et al., 1984). These reports led to two major modifications in the original conceptualizations of the relationships between brain damage and aphasia syndromes. (1) Aphasia may follow damage deep in the brain, below the perisylvian cortex and its association fibers. (2) Damage confined to Broca's area or Wernicke's area does not usually produce classic Broca's or Wernicke's aphasia.

SUBCORTICAL APHASIA

Studies of patients with subcortical damage have shown that subcortical damage in the vicinity of the left basal ganglia (the internal capsule and putamen) or left thalamus may be accompanied by aphasia (Mohr et al., 1975; Naeser et al., 1982; Ojemann, 1975; Cappa and Vignolo, 1979). Naeser *et al.* (1982) studied nine cases of aphasia caused by damage in and around the basal ganglia, and reported three subcortical aphasia syndromes, based on the front-to-back location of damage. An *anterior syndrome,* caused by capsular-putamenal damage extending into anterior white matter, is characterized by hemiplegia, slow, dysarthric speech with good phrase length and prosody, good comprehension, good repetition, poor oral reading and writing, and poor confrontation naming. A *posterior syndrome,* caused by capsular-putamenal damage extending into posterior white matter, is characterized by hemiplegia, fluent speech without dysarthria, poor comprehension, good single-word repetition but poor sentence repetition, impaired reading and writing, and poor confrontation naming. (This syndrome resembles Wernicke's aphasia except for the presence of hemiplegia in the subcortical syndrome.) An *anterior-posterior syndrome,* caused by capsular-putamenal damage with both anterior and posterior extension, is characterized by a mixture of symptoms consistent with both Broca's and Wernicke's aphasias, "although they did not completely resemble cases of Broca's, Wernicke's, global, or thalamic aphasia in CT scan lesion sites, or language behavior" (Naeser et al., 1982). Cappa et al. (1983) described both an anterior syndrome and a posterior syndrome in patients with capsular-putamenal damage. Their patients had smaller lesions than those of Naeser et al., and their aphasias were milder but resembled those of Naeser's patients. The current evidence suggests that patients with aphasia caused by damage in the basal ganglia exhibit a variety of disruptions in speech and language (Robin and Schienberg, 1990), and that the three syndromes described by Naeser et al. may not completely explain the various aphasias resulting from lesions in the basal ganglia.

Aphasia caused by lesions in the left thalamus also have been described, and the role of the thalamus in language has received attention in recent years (Mohr et al., 1975; Ojemann, 1975; Cappa and Vignolo, 1979). Patients with aphasia caused by thalamic lesions are almost always hemiplegic. They have difficulty initiating spontaneous speech—it is sparse, echolalic, and neologistic. Vocal intensity tends to decrease progressively during utterances. Comprehension and reading usually are good. Writing usually is impaired, and word-finding problems usually are present. These patients tend to be perserverative and their performance tends to fluctuate from task to task and moment to moment. Murdoch (1990) has commented that aphasic syndromes resulting from thalamic lesions resemble transcortical motor aphasia, in that repetition and comprehension tend to be preserved but self-initiated speech tends to be reduced. In general, according to Murdoch, the language problems of patients with left subcortical damage usually are mild, and patients with subcortical aphasia have a better prognosis for recovery than patients with aphasia following cortical damage.

Even though aphasic syndromes follow subcortical damage, it is not clear that the subcortical structures involved directly accomplish language functions. In many of the patients studied, damage was not confined to subcortical structures, but extended to the cortex. Dewitt et al. (1985) reported that magnetic resonance imaging (MRI) scans of patients with subcortical aphasias usually show involvement of cortical tissue not visualized by CT scans. Metter et al. (1983) reported that positron emission tomography (PET) studies of patients with subcortical aphasia almost always revealed decreased cortical metabolism in the left hemisphere, in areas without observable structural damage.

LESION SIZE, LESION LOCATION, AND APHASIA SYNDROME

Several reports have suggested that lesions confined to Broca's or Wernicke's area do not produce persisting Broca's or Wernicke's aphasia. Mohr et al. (1978) studied 22 cases with documented site and extent of lesion and 83 published reports in which autopsy data were given. They concluded that lesions confined to Broca's area produce transitory mutism that is replaced by rapidly improving dysarthric and apraxic speech, with no significant persisting impairments in language. According to Mohr et al., lesions must extend well beyond Broca's area to produce persisting Broca's aphasia. Knopman et al. (1983) also reported that patients with lesions confined to Broca's area exhibit transient nonfluent speech, without persisting nonfluent aphasia. According to Knopman et al., persisting nonfluent aphasia requires a lesion extending from Broca's area into the primary motor cortex or parietal lobe.

Selnes et al. (1983) reported that lesions confined to Wernicke's area do not produce persisting severe deficits in comprehension. Selnes et al. (1985) reported that the most striking persisting consequence of damage confined to Wernicke's area is impaired repetition, and they suggest that persisting severe comprehension deficits require lesions extending beyond Wernicke's area. According to Selnes et al. (1985), patients with lesions confined to Wernicke's area exhibit Wernicke's aphasia at 1 month after onset, but their symptoms evolve to those of conduction aphasia by 6 months after onset.

RELATED DISORDERS

Visual Field Blindness

Patients with damage in the temporal lobe or lower parietal lobe often are blind in parts of their visual fields. The blindness always involves the visual field contralateral to the side of brain damage. This is because of how the human visual system is arranged (Figure 4–4). Optic nerve fibers from the lateral halves of the retinas project to the visual cortex on the same side, while fibers from the nasal halves of the retinas cross (at the *optic chiasm*) and project to the visual cortex in the contralateral hemisphere.

If a lesion destroys the visual fibers posterior to the optic chiasm (as at *C* in Fig 4–5), the patient will be blind in the contralateral visual half-field. Such blindness is called *homonymous hemianopsia* (or *hemianopia*), and occurs following deep lesions in the temporal lobe or lower parietal lobe. (Homonymous = the same part of the visual field in each eye is affected; heteronymous = different parts of the visual field in each eye are affected.) Similarly, if a lesion destroys the visual cortex in one

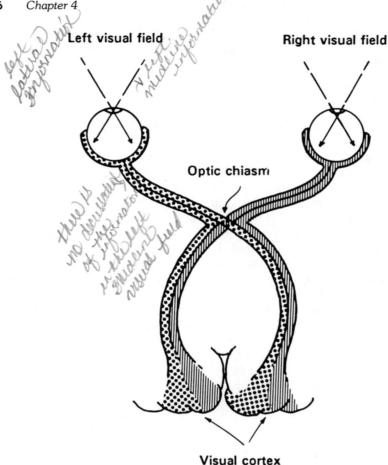

Left visual field   **Right visual field**

Optic chiasm

Visual cortex

FIG 4–4.
The human visual system. Each hemisphere receives visual input only from contralateral visual space. Consequently, lesions that cause aphasia often cause blindness in the visual field opposite to the lesion (the right side for right-handed people).

hemisphere (as at *D* in Fig 4–5), the patient will be blind in the contralateral half of his or her visual space. If the lesion is in the left hemisphere, the patient will be unable to see to the right of the midline (right homonymous hemianopsia), and if the lesion is in the right hemisphere, the patient will be unable to see things to the left of the midline (left homonymous hemianopsia).

If a lesion interrupts one optic nerve (as at *A* in Fig 4–5), the patient will be blind in that eye, and will not see anything when the other eye is occluded. If a lesion destroys the crossing fibers at the optic chiasm (as at *B* in Fig 4–5), the patient will exhibit *bitemporal hemianopsia* (blindness in the lateral visual fields for both eyes), because the fibers that transmit visual information from lateral visual space in both eye fields are gone.

Because aphasia is most often caused by left hemisphere brain lesions, aphasic

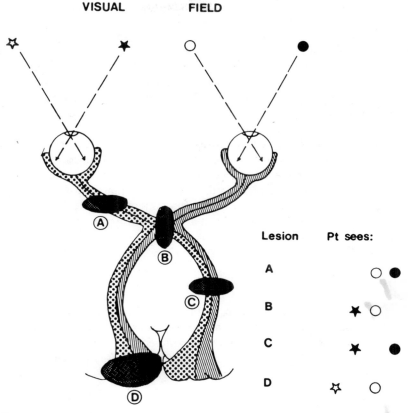

VISUAL   FIELD

Lesion   Pt sees:

A

B

C

D

FIG 4–5.
How damage in various parts of the visual system affect vision. As a general rule, lesions posterior to the optic chiasm cause blindness in the contralateral visual field. *Pt* = patient.

patients who exhibit homonymous hemianopsia usually exhibit right homonymous hemianopsia. Because the visual fibers project to the visual cortex through the lower parietal and the temporal lobes, posterior aphasias (such as Wernicke's and conduction aphasia) are those in which visual field deficits are observed. It is unusual to see anterior aphasia or hemiplegia together with visual field deficits, unless the aphasia is severe and global.

Sometimes visual field blindnesses are observed in which less than half of the visual field is affected. In these cases, only a part of the visual fibers have been destroyed. *Quadrantanopsia* (quadrantic hemianopsia) means that (approximately) one fourth of the visual field is affected. Quadrantanopsias are caused by lesions that interrupt the upper or lower part of the visual fibers within a hemisphere. If the lesion interrupts the upper part of the visual fibers (those in the inferior parietal lobe) then blindness in the lower quadrant of the contralateral visual field follows. If the lesion interrupts the lower part of the visual fibers (those that pass through the temporal lobe), then blindness in the upper quadrant of the contralateral visual field follows.

The general rule is that inferiorly placed lesions posterior to the optic chiasm produce contralateral superior quadrant blindness, and vice versa.

A phenomenon called *macular sparing* often is seen in visual field blindness. The macula of the retina is a small circular area near the center of the retina. This part of the retina is responsible for the center of the visual field, which is the area of greatest visual acuity. In macular sparing, vision in the center of the visual field for the affected eye (that part served by the macula) is spared, so that the hemianopsia or quadrantanopsia is incomplete. If the entire optic tract or the entire visual cortex is destroyed, macular sparing does not occur.

Bilateral destruction of the visual cortex results in a phenomenon called *cortical blindness.* Patients who are cortically blind have great difficulty discriminating visual shapes and patterns, but remain sensitive to light and dark. In some cases perception of simple visual stimuli may be preserved, although the patient usually has difficulty reporting them or incorporating them into other mental activity. Occasionally patients with cortical blindness may deny that they cannot see, producing elaborate confabulations when asked to describe their surroundings. This condition is called *Anton's syndrome,* or *visual anosognosia.*

Apraxia

Apraxia is a label for several different syndromes characterized by deficiencies in volitional movement sequences, in the absence of sensory loss or paralysis sufficient to explain the deficiencies. Apraxia often accompanies aphasia, especially aphasia caused by damage in the frontal or anterior parietal lobes. Apraxia is discussed in Chapter 12.

Agnosia

Agnosia means the inability to recognize, through an intact sensory modality, stimuli that are recognized in other modalities. The incidence of true modality-specific agnosias is extremely low, and some may not exist, in spite of descriptions in the literature. Many cases of "agnosia" reported in the literature appear not to be true agnosias, but perceptual or sensory discrimination deficiencies, general comprehension or cognitive disorders, psychogenic symptoms, or multiple-modality recognition disorders. Many diagnoses of "agnosia" seem to be the result of incomplete testing. Therefore, the examiner must be careful to exclude all other possible explanations for the patient's deficit before assigning the label "agnosia."

The three major types of agnosia described in the literature are *visual, auditory,* and *tactile* agnosia. *Visual agnosia* is a perceptual disorder in which patients are unable to recognize objects visually, although they can prove that they can see by matching identical objects or forms, and can prove that they are familiar with the visually unrecognized objects by recognizing them when they are allowed to feel them with their hands or when they hear the sounds that the objects make. Visual agnosias usually occur after damage (usually bilateral) to the visual association areas in the occipital lobes, to the posterior parietal lobes, or to fiber tracts that connect the visual cortex to other areas in the brain. Visual agnosias usually are incomplete, intermittent, and inconsistent. Patients with visual agnosias usually function adequately in their environment. They do not behave as if they are blind, bumping into things and groping their way about. They usually recognize and respond appropriately to at least some visually sensed objects in their environment, especially familiar ones. Sometimes they recognize objects that they have failed to recognize in the past and will fail to recognize in the future. A few cases of *visual-verbal agnosia* have been reported. These patients usually have lesions that isolate the cortical language areas from the visual cortex. The patient's deficit is limited to printed symbolic materials (letters, words, numbers), while visual recognition of nonlinguistic stimuli is unimpaired. The patient's major deficiency is inability to read or to do printed calculation problems. The examiner must be cautious that such cases of "visual-verbal agnosia" are actually agnosia, and do not represent reading disabilities or general language problems.

Auditory agnosia is a syndrome in which a patient is unable to recognize sounds, even though hearing acuity is adequate. Such patients can hear—they respond to sound by turning toward sound sources, and they usually exhibit startle or withdrawal responses to loud sounds—but they appear not to attach meanings to the sounds that they hear. Visual or tactile recognition of objects that make sounds is intact, but the patient usually cannot match an object with the sound that it makes. As in the case of visual agnosia, auditory agnosia frequently is incomplete or intermittent—the patient sometimes responds appropriately to sounds, or may respond appropriately to certain sounds or categories of sounds. A number of cases of *auditory-verbal agnosia* have been reported, usually in patients who have brain damage that separates Wernicke's area from the primary auditory cortex in both hemispheres. The patient exhibits agnosia only for spoken words, while responding appropriately to nonverbal sounds. This syndrome has sometimes been called *pure word deafness*. Patients with auditory-verbal agnosia are said to perceive spoken words, but are unable to understand their meaning, even though reading comprehension is intact. They often behave as if their native language has become a foreign language, but their speech usually is appropriate both in content and form. Patients with "word deafness" must be carefully examined to ensure that their "word deafness" is not an auditory perceptual or auditory discrimination deficit, a general language comprehension deficit, or a psychogenic manifestation. A patient with "auditory-verbal agnosia" must have functional hearing for nonverbal sounds, and must also have unimpaired (or minimally impaired) recognition and comprehension of verbal material presented visually. Unless this discrepancy between auditory and visual modalities exists, the patient does not have "auditory-visual agnosia."

Tactile agnosia is a syndrome in which patients are unable to recognize objects by touch and palpation, in the absence of tactile sensory deficit, and in which the objects are recognized if they are presented in other sensory modalities. Tactile agnosia usually occurs with damage in the parietal lobes that isolates tactile sensory areas from other parts of the brain. A patient with tactile agnosia can report touch, pinprick, and other stimulation of the cutaneous receptors, but he or she cannot name, describe, talk about, or demonstrate the use of objects palpated with the hands. The diagnosis of tactile agnosia must exclude sensory deficiencies and cognitive, language, or response impairments that might account for the deficient performance. The term *astereognosis* is sometimes used in a broader sense than the term "tactile agnosia" as a label for the inability to recognize objects by touch or palpation even when the deficit is secondary to sensory impairment. In its more limited sense, it refers to disruption of the ability to recognize objects by touch or palpation *in the absence of sensory disruption*. This latter definition appears to be analogous to the definition of tactile agnosia. Tactile agnosia (or astereognosis in its more limited sense) can be identified by the fact that the patient with tactile agnosia often can draw or demonstrate the shape and size of objects with the affected hand, and usually can choose matching objects from a group of objects with the affected hand when vision is blocked. Once again, the problem is not one of perception, but of recognition.

Because of the rarity of "pure" forms of agnosia, the examiner must be certain that alternative explanations for the disorder have been excluded before calling the disorder "agnosia." In arriving at the diagnosis of agnosia, one must exclude a number of alternative explanations, including the following:

1. *Sensory deficits in the affected modality.* Agnosias can only be diagnosed when sensory function in the modality of the agnosia is adequate for perception of the stimuli that are not recognized by the patient.

2. *Comprehension disorders.* Comprehension disorders that prevent the patient from understanding what is required in the test for agnosia must be ruled out.

3. *Expressive disturbances.* Asking the patient to name a stimulus item, describe it, tell its function, or write its name or function are not good ways to test for agnosias, because failure may result from a patient's inability to produce verbal responses, rather than from failure to recognize the stimuli. Another method of testing, which does not require verbal responses from the patient, is preferable. Allowing a patient to match identical test items in the affected modality would be a reasonable alternative.

4. *Unfamiliarity with the test stimulus.* One must be certain that the patient has had experience with the tested items, so that "agnosia" is not simply a failure to recognize objects that the patient has never encountered before. If the patient recognizes the stimulus in another modality, one can probably conclude that unfamiliarity is not a likely explanation for the "agnosia."

Disconnection Syndromes

Disconnection syndromes occur following interruption of the nerve fibers crossing between the hemispheres. Complete disconnection of the hemispheres as a result of vascular or traumatic events is rare. Surgical disconnection of the hemispheres occasionally is done, usually to control otherwise uncontrollable epileptic seizures. Patients with *commissurotomy* (cutting of the commissures) appear to the casual observer not to exhibit any great changes in abilities as a result of the surgery. However, formal testing demonstrates that these patients possess unusual and striking deficits, which are caused by isolation of the nonverbal right hemisphere from the language competent left hemisphere. These patients are unable to name common objects held, out of sight, in the left hand, because the sensory input from the hand goes into the mute right hemisphere, which has no way of transferring the information to the verbal left hemisphere. These same patients name objects held in the right hand with facility. They will be able to choose a palpated object from a group of objects with the same hand used to palpate, but not with the contralateral hand, and they will be able to demonstrate the use of a palpated, but unseen, object with the hand used to palpate the object, but not with the contralateral hand. If pictures of common objects are flashed in such a way that the visual information goes into the right hemisphere, the patient will be unable to name them or to talk about them, but, if given a choice among several objects, the patient will be able to choose the pictured item with the left hand. In general, patients with disconnection syndrome can verbalize about stimuli that are presented to the left hemisphere, but not when they are presented to the right hemisphere. Patients with commissurotomy do not frequently encounter situations in their daily environment that restrict stimulus input to one hemisphere. Consequently, these individuals may function normally in daily life.

There are two incomplete disconnection syndromes that may be caused by surgery, tumors, vascular events, or traumatic events. *Anterior disconnection syndrome* is caused by interruption of the anterior corpus callosum. Anterior cerebral artery infarctions are the most frequent cause of anterior disconnection syndrome. Patients with anterior disconnection syndrome cannot follow verbal commands requesting responses with the left hand (unilateral apraxia of the left hand), and are unable to talk about or to name objects held in the left hand, although they usually can draw the item, demonstrate its function, or choose the item from a group, if they use their left hand. These symptoms are generated by disconnection of the sensory areas for the left hand (in the right hemisphere) from the verbally competent left hemisphere.

Posterior disconnection syndrome is caused by disconnection of the posterior corpus callosum. The most frequent causes of such interruption are tumors and cerebral infarctions. Patients with posterior disconnection syndrome generally complain of nonspecific visual disturbances. (In fact, many patients with posterior disconnection syndrome go to their ophthalmologist or optometrist, rather than to a neurologist, because they believe that the problem is in their eyes, rather than in their brain.) If the left visual cortex is destroyed and the posterior corpus callosum is severed, the patient will exhibit alexia without agraphia.

Alexia without agraphia is a rare disability in which there is severe impairment of reading along with intact or nearly intact writing. Patients exhibiting alexia without agraphia cannot read aloud and do not comprehend printed materials, but can write spontaneously and copy printed material. However, they cannot then read aloud what they have written. Alexia without agraphia is caused by a complex lesion (or combination of lesions) that destroy the left visual cortex and the connections between the right visual cortex and the left hemisphere (Fig 4–6). As a consequence, visual information from the language incompetent right hemisphere cannot reach the language competent left hemisphere, and the patient cannot deduce the meaning of printed materials. The patient can still write, because the connections between Wer-

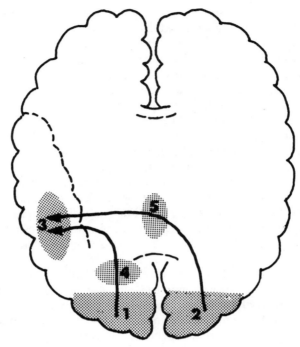

FIG 4–6.
A diagram representing how damage in the brain produces alexia without agraphia. The visual cortex in the left and right hemispheres *(1,2)* is isolated from the language area *(3)* by one lesion *(4)* that disconnects the left visual cortex from the language area *(3)*, and another lesion *(5)* that interrupts the crossing fibers from the right visual cortex.

nicke's area (which formulates the messages) and anterior motor planning and execution regions are intact. Another syndrome, *alexia with agraphia*, is caused by lesions in the region of the angular gyrus, at the posterior end of the Sylvian fissure. These lesions disconnect the visual association areas from Broca's and Wernicke's areas, so that visual information from printed materials cannot be communicated either to Wernicke's area or to anterior motor planning and execution regions.

Chapter 5 _____

Assessing Aphasia and Related Impairments

PRELIMINARIES TO FORMAL TESTING

Assessment of patients with neurogenic communication disorders, whether aphasia, dysarthria, right hemisphere syndrome, or any other neurogenic communication disorder, does not begin with testing. Most clinicians spend some time acquiring background information about the patient before testing begins. This information provides a context from which the clinician can make predictions about the nature and severity of the patient's disabilities and decide which tests are likely to be most appropriate. The information for this context comes from three sources—*the referral, the patient's medical record,* and *the interview.*

The Referral

The clinician begins the assessment when the referral is received. The first impressions of the patient come from the referral, which usually contains a short description of the patient, together with the reasons for referral, as in:

> Sixty-one-year-old right-handed male with posterior left-hemisphere stroke 4 days ago. Please evaluate and make recommendations regarding treatment.

After reading this referral the clinician knows the patient's age, the reason he is hospitalized, that he probably is aphasic, and that he is in the early stages of neurologic recovery. The clinician might expect that the patient will exhibit a fluent aphasia with impaired language comprehension and that his aphasia may spontaneously improve during the next few weeks, because he is in the early stages of recovery. The clinician then goes to the patient's medical record, to get more detailed information about the patient and his or her problems.

Medical Record Review

Medical records are divided into sections. Each section contains different kinds of information. How medical records are divided depends to some extent on the medical facility in which the record is located, but most will resemble the arrangement described herein. Knowing what these sections are and what kinds of information can be found in them is important if the review is to be fast, efficient, and thorough.

Patient Identification.—Every page in the medical record is labeled with the patient's name and other identifying information in a space at the bottom of each page. This information usually includes the patient's name, address, date of birth, Social Security number, and ward. It may also contain other information, such as home telephone number, next of kin, religion, and diagnostic or other codes.

Personal History.—The patient's personal history contains information about the patient's age, education, occupation, marital status, number of children and their ages, where the patient lives and with whom, vocation, and work history. Information about the patient's emotional and social history may also appear here—the presence of previous or current emotional or personal problems, the nature of the patient's relationships with others, and whether there is a history of alcoholism or other substance abuse.

Medical History.—The patient's medical history contains information about the patient's past illnesses, injuries, or medical conditions, and his or her current disabilities and complaints. It usually is obtained by means of an interview by a physician. Sometimes the interview is supplemented by previous medical records. The medical history contains information about the patient's general physical condition—height, weight, temperature, blood pressure, respiration, strength, stamina, and ambulation—together with information about the patient's previous and current medical conditions and complaints. Past cerebrovascular disorders, disorientation, confusion, slurred speech, loss of consciousness, or seizures are noted, as are chronic medical conditions such as diabetes, vascular disease, heart disease, pulmonary disease, hearing loss, or visual problems. The patient's current symptoms and complaints are usually summarized in a *problem list,* which lists both preexisting and current medical problems in the order of their perceived importance. The medical history contains information about the time of onset of problems on the list, their nature and severity at onset, and their evolution from onset to the time at which the history was obtained.

Progress notes are written by physicians, nurses, and other patient care personnel. They are a chronologic record of the patient's physical, behavioral, and mental status during his or her hospitalization. Entries in the progress notes provide information about the patient's general orientation to time and place, emotional state, social behavior, and his or her reactions to physical and medical problems. Day-to-day changes in the patient's behavior or physical condition are routinely described in progress notes by those involved in the patient's care. If the patient is seen by other services, such as occupational therapy, physical therapy, psychology, vocational counseling, or social work, their comments also may be found in the progress notes. The physician's interpretations of laboratory tests sometimes are found in the progress notes.

The *doctor's orders* section of the medical record contains the physician's orders for the patient's care, including medications, special tests, special diets, monitoring of fluid or caloric intake, and rehabilitation services.

Most medical records have a separate section for *laboratory test reports*. Results of tests such as glucose tolerance tests, computed tomography (CT) scans, and electroencephalograms (EEGs) are found in this section of the medical record. In some cases, other kinds of reports, such as reports of surgical procedures, may be found in this section.

Examples of Medical Record Reviews

To illustrate the amount and variety of information that can be gotten from medical records, the following examples of medical record reviews are provided. They are based on patients referred to a speech pathology service for evaluation and treatment.

Mr. Brown

Mr. Brown was referred to speech pathology by his physician about 1 week postadmission because he was "dysarthric." Mr. Brown's *personal history* was provided by his wife, who accompanied him to the medical center. She reported that he was 55 years old, and had been a foreman in a small manufacturing plant prior to his admission to the hospital. They had been married for 19 years and had a son and a daughter, both of high-school age. His wife had at one time worked as a registered nurse, but had not worked for the past 10 years to stay at home and care for the children. Mrs. Brown reported no significant family problems, but expressed great concern about her husband's recovery and about the emotional and economic effects of his medical problems on the family.

Mr. Brown's *medical history* began with his wife's report that he had been in good health until the afternoon of his admission to the hospital. He had just come up the stairs from the basement when his speech suddenly became slurred, and his right arm became paralyzed. He also complained of numbness in the right side of his face. Mrs. Brown called an ambulance and he was taken to the hospital. The medical examination performed on admission revealed an alert, cooperative, well-nourished male, "in no apparent physical distress." Blood pressure and pulse rate were within normal limits. Mr. Brown complained of weakness and numbness on the right side of his face and in his right hand, arm, and leg, difficulty speaking, and chest pains. Neurologic examination revealed dense right hemiplegia and decreased sensation on the right side of Mr. Brown's face and body. Hyperreflexia was observed in both right extremities, and a Babinski reflex was elicited in his right foot. Testing also revealed a right central VIIth (facial) nerve paralysis. Visual acuity, visual fields, and auditory acuity appeared to be within normal limits.

Laboratory reports indicated the presence of mild diabetes mellitus. Mr. Brown's electrocardiogram (ECG) suggested "mild coronary artery disease." Blood chemistry, except for serum glucose levels, was within normal limits. A CT scan suggested "a recent infarct in the anterior distribution of the left middle cerebral artery."

The *doctor's orders* contained orders for referrals to occupational therapy, physical therapy, and speech pathology, a request that social work be contacted, and an order that the patient be placed on anticoagulants.

An entry by the physician in the *progress notes* stated that Mr. Brown could write words with his left hand, and could also say "a few words, but with difficulty." The notes also contained reference to what the physician believed to be "buccofacial apraxia." Three days after admission, the physician wrote the following note: "the patient's language-handling problems appear to be more dysarthric than receptive or expressive in nature. This implicates the rolandic branch of the left middle cerebral artery." During the following week Mr. Brown's paralyzed leg regained some motor function, but his arm remained paralyzed. Ward nurses had made several entries in the progress notes: "The patient appears to be alert and well motivated. He can understand and write, but cannot talk." "Today the patient asked me to write down the letters of the alphabet so that he can sound them out. He thinks that this will help him talk." "Patient indicates numbness on right side of face and down right side. Appears to be in no discomfort." "Patient is cheerful and likes to run errands."

Summary.—The review of Mr. Brown's medical record suggests that he has had a cerebrovascular accident in the anterior left hemisphere. The presence of right hemiplegia, right central VIIth nerve paralysis, hyperreflexia and a Babinski reflex on the right side all suggest anterior left hemisphere damage. The clinician might question the physician's diagnosis of "dysarthria" in this case, because persisting dysarthrias rarely occur following unilateral upper motor neuron damage. However, transitory dysarthrias sometimes follow such damage, and this may be what the physician is describing. The physician's order for anticoagulant medication suggests an occlusive cerebrovascular accident, probably embolic, based on the time of day that it happened and the patient's history of cardiac problems. The absence of pronounced hemiplegia and Mr. Brown's ability to communicate by speech and writing in rudimentary fashion soon after onset suggests that the lesion is probably not massive, and that Mr. Brown's residual aphasia may not be severe. The hypothesis of an anterior lesion is supported by Mr. Brown's apparently good comprehension. He seems able to follow spoken directions well enough to run errands for ward personnel. One would expect Mr. Brown to exhibit speech and language disabilities consistent with those of Broca's aphasia or "apraxia of speech." One would not expect persisting dysarthria because of what seems to be a unilateral lesion at or near the cortex. The presence of diabetes mellitus and atherosclerotic heart disease are negative prognostic indicators. However, both are described as "mild," so that with proper medical supervision their effects may be minimized. Evidence that the infarct is small in size and the fact that Mr. Brown has already recovered some speech and language are positive signs. That he is eager to run errands for ward personnel and his request for help in improving his speech suggest that he is motivated to recover. His wife's concern about his condition and his recovery is also a positive sign. However, Mr. Brown was the only source of financial support for his family before his accident. This suggests that his wife may need vocational counseling and perhaps retraining if it becomes necessary for her to return to work. This may create stress for Mr. Brown and his family. Finally, the doctor's orders suggest that the speech-language pathologist will be coordinating his or her evaluation and treatment with physical therapy, occupational therapy, and social work.

Mr. Green

Mr. Green was a 61-year-old man who had a stroke about 4 months before his referral to speech pathology. After his stroke, he had been hospitalized in a private hospital in his home town, which was in a rural area. He was discharged to his home. After several months at home, he came to Minneapolis Veterans Affairs Medical Center with his wife, complaining of transient periods of confusion and memory loss. He was admitted for neurologic evaluation to determine the cause of his complaints. Shortly after his admission, he was referred to speech pathology for evaluation of his speech and language.

Mr. Green's *personal history* was obtained from his wife by the admitting neurologist. Mr. Green had three children, all grown and living independently. He had worked in a middle-level managerial position for a railroad for 15 years until his medical retirement at the age of 59 following a heart attack. His medical retirement was based on the presence of chronic hypertensive vascular disease and congestive heart disease. Since his retirement he had been living at home with no notable medical problems until his stroke 4 months earlier.

Mr. Green's *medical history* was also obtained from Mrs. Green, who reported that, at the time of his stroke 3 months earlier, Mr. Green had awakened in the morning to discover that his right arm was numb. He woke his wife, and, according to her, "was very upset and made no sense when he talked." Mrs. Green took him to their local hospital, where he was admitted, stayed for 9 days, and then was discharged to his home. The diagnosis upon admission to his local hospital was "probable left hemisphere stroke." Upon admission there, he exhibited weakness in his right arm and leg, right homonymous hemianopsia, exaggerated reflexes on his right side, and a right-sided Babinski. Mr. Green's symptoms gradually worsened during the next 2 hours, then stabilized. During the remainder of his hospitalization the right-sided weakness cleared and the exaggerated reflexes diminished. However, the homonymous hemianopsia persisted. Mr. Green had been seen briefly by physical therapy, but had not been referred to speech pathology. During his hospitalization he was given medications to reduce his blood pressure. Then anticoagulants were added, and he was discharged on those medications.

The medical examination upon admission to Minneapolis Veterans Affairs Medical Center revealed a thin, somewhat agitated white male, who complained that he "forgot where he put things and sometimes wasn't sure where he was at." Mr. Green's right side was weak but not paralyzed, and a right homonymous hemianopsia was present. Blood pressure and pulse rate were above normal. The admitting neurologist noted the presence of "severe receptive aphasia" and "confusion as to time and place." The remainder of the examination was unremarkable.

The *doctor's orders* contained orders for continuation of antihypertensive and anticoagulant medications, a CT scan, and routine urinalysis and blood work. An ECG (electrocardiogram) was also requested. Requests for evaluation of Mr. Green by speech pathology and dentistry were also contained in the orders, the latter because Mr. Green had dentures "that no longer fit." The doctor's orders later contained a request for evaluation of Mr. Green's nutritional needs by dietetic service, and preparation of a "diabetic diet" for him.

The *laboratory reports* of urine and blood analyses showed that Mr. Green had elevated blood sugar, consistent with diabetes mellitus. A subsequent glucose tolerance test confirmed the diagnosis. Mr. Green's blood coagulation time was decreased, suggesting that he might be at risk for the occurrence of thrombi. The ECG revealed irregularities "consistent with atherosclerotic heart disease of long-standing origin," suggesting that emboli might be a concern. The CT scan showed a "clearly demarcated large infarct in the left temporal lobe, with extension into the midparietal lobe."

An entry in the *progress notes* by the physician 3 days after admission stated that "the patient's mentation appears to be clearing. Suspect transient ischemic attack as the reason for his complaints." The progress notes subsequently contained a series of notes from the physician indicating that Mr. Green's blood pressure was decreasing in response to medication, and that coagulation time had increased to normal limits.

Progress notes made by nursing staff during the first few days after admission suggested that Mr. Green was confused and disoriented. "He tends to wander away from the ward if not watched closely." "Today he asked me if I was Mrs. Nelson. When I asked him who Mrs. Nelson was, he said, 'you're my eighth grade teacher, aren't you?'" By the third day postadmission, the character of the entries began to change. "He seems much more alert today." "He has begun to socialize with the other patients on the ward." "He seems better, but he still has trouble saying what he wants to say. This makes him frustrated." "He still seems easily confused by what you say to him." A note by the physician on the fifth day after admission stated that "patient's diabetes appears to be responding to diet. Blood sugar approaching normal limits."

Summary.—The results of the CT scan show that Mr. Green has a large lesion in the left temporal lobe. Other observations are consistent with this finding. Mr. Green is not hemiparetic. He has right-sided visual field blindness. His speech and language disabilities are consistent with left temporal lobe damage. There is no mention of struggle or distortions in speech, but there are reports of word-finding problems, and Mr. Green's speech does not always make sense. His "confusion" appears to be clearing, and it is likely that Mr. Green's major continuing problems will be those caused by his stroke 3 months previously. (One sometimes finds that older patients become "confused" when they are suddenly placed in a new and unfamiliar environment, even when nothing neurologic has happened to them. It is sometimes difficult to separate this "situational" confusion from that attributable to organic causes. However, Mr. Green's confusion began at home, in a familiar environment. Consequently, it appears unlikely to be situational.)

Mr. Green's cardiovascular disease, high blood pressure, and diabetes mellitus cloud the prognosis. However, the fact that medications and diet appear to control both blood pressure and diabetes suggests that their effects can be minimized with appropriate medical care. However, Mr. Green remains at risk for another stroke or heart attack.

There is little direct mention of Mr. Green's speech and language in the medical record. However, based on the site and extent of his brain lesion, we can expect that he will have problems comprehending spoken and written language, and that he will have word-retrieval problems when speaking or writing. The fact that he is more than 3 months postonset of aphasia with no treatment for his speech and language problems suggests that he may have potential for improvement, given an appropriate treatment program. His awareness of his problems and his dissatisfaction with them also suggest a positive response to treatment. His medical problems seem to be clearing rapidly. Consequently, he is likely to be discharged soon, making inpatient treatment of his linguistic deficits unlikely. Mr. Brown lives in a rural area, so that it may be difficult to find a suitable outpatient treatment program for him, if he returns to his home.

Mr. Blue

Mr. Blue came to the medical center after a 3-week period of fever, chills, and increasingly severe headaches. During the week before admission his right hand and arm became moderately weak. He was brought to the hospital by a friend, who provided a fragmentary history. A more complete history was available from medical records related to a previous hospitalization for a fracture.

Mr. Blue's *personal history,* obtained from the friend and the old medical records, showed that he was a 58-year-old retired military officer. He was unmarried and lived alone in an apartment house. His nearest relatives were his mother, who lived in a small town about 200 miles away, and two brothers who lived in distant cities. He had been living an active and independent life until his admission.

According to the *medical history,* Mr. Blue had "caught a cold" about 3 weeks before admission. His symptoms became gradually more severe, with increasing fever, chills, headache, and muscle soreness. About 1 week before admission Mr. Blue began complaining of weakness on the right side of his body. He eventually requested that his friend take him to the hospital.

The medical examination conducted upon admission revealed a "drowsy but easily aroused aphasic male" who complained of headache, sore throat, weakness, and chills. Mr. Blue's temperature, pulse, and respiration were elevated, and his blood pressure was in the high normal range. He was oriented to time and place, and could answer questions. Neurologic evaluation revealed moderate weakness in Mr. Blue's right hand and arm, a positive Babinski reflex on the right, and right homonymous hemianopsia. The admitting neurologist also noted that Mr. Blue was unable to follow complex spoken directions.

The *doctor's orders* contained requests for routine blood chemistry, urinalysis, an EEG, a CT scan, cerebrospinal fluid cultures, and evaluations of Mr. Blue by neuropsychology and speech pathology. Administration of a regimen of broad-spectrum antibiotics was also ordered.

Several *laboratory reports* were in Mr. Blue's medical record. The EEG, performed within a few hours of admission, showed general diffuse slowing, consistent with generalized cerebral impairment. A spinal tap revealed cloudy cerebrospinal fluid. A CT scan done a day after admission revealed a large area of abnormality deep in the temporal lobe, consistent with brain abscess. Cerebrospinal fluid cultures grew a strain of *Streptococcus* bacteria.

The *progress notes* indicated that Mr. Blue was admitted to the ward on a litter, in a drowsy state. They noted that he talked freely but inappropriately, and that he did not always make sense. A number of entries indicated that his condition was slowly deteriorating, with increasing lethargy, drowsiness, confusion, and euphoria. He became incontinent of urine shortly after admission.

Summary.—Examination of Mr. Blue's records suggests that there is general involvement of cerebral processes, and that his condition is slowly worsening. The laboratory reports suggest that he has a brain abscess in the temporal lobe. Behavioral observations are consistent with this diagnosis—Mr. Blue's increasing lethargy and generally worsening condition are consistent with increasing pressure generated by a growing abscess. The presence of homonymous hemianopsia, fluent speech that does not always make sense, and problems with comprehension of spoken language are consistent with temporal lobe involvement. His increasing lethargy and euphoria suggest that evaluation of his speech and language will be difficult. Because of the seriousness of his medical problems, comprehensive assessment of speech and language was not attempted. The assessment was delayed until Mr. Blue's medical problems were dealt with.

Mr. Blue was taken to surgery 3 days after admission, and an abscess in the left temporal lobe was drained. His condition immediately began to improve. The speech and language pathologist administered a short speech and language test battery at 1 week postsurgery and at weekly intervals thereafter. One month after surgery, the speech and language pathologist observed a sudden decrement in Mr. Blue's test performance. Nurses' progress notes also suggested that Mr. Blue's speech, language, and cognition were deteriorating. His physician was notified. A CT scan was ordered. The scan revealed enlarged ventricles, and a diagnosis of obstructive hydrocephalus was made. Mr. Blue was taken to surgery where a ventriculoperitoneal shunt was installed to relieve ventricular pressure. Installation of the shunt was followed by gradual improvement in his condition. The speech-language pathologist continued to monitor Mr. Blue's speech and language until his medical condition had improved enough that he could begin daily language treatment sessions, at which time he was enrolled in a treatment program to improve listening and reading comprehension. His listening comprehension improved markedly, but reading comprehension remained essentially unchanged, because of persisting visual perceptual impairments.

Mr. White

Mr. White was a 23-year-old male who, about 1 year before admission, had been struck on the head by a fire hose nozzle while fighting a fire in the Air Force. He came to the medical center complaining of "memory difficulties."

Mr. White's *personal history* indicated that he had graduated from high school, worked as an automobile mechanic in his hometown, and then enlisted in the Air Force. During the subsequent 3 years he had been a fireman at an air base. Both parents were alive and living in Mr. White's home town in rural Wisconsin. Mr. White had two older brothers and a younger sister, all married and living in Wisconsin. He apparently had been an "average" student, and had completed high school in his home town.

The *medical history* indicated that at the time of his injury, Mr. White had been on duty and fighting a fire when a fire hose broke loose and struck him on the left side of his head. He sustained a skull fracture and was unconscious for a week following the incident, at which time a left parietal subdural hematoma was surgically removed. Mr. White regained consciousness that evening. His subsequent recovery was uneventful, except that about 2 weeks after surgery he experienced a grand mal seizure. He was placed on seizure control medication and no more seizures occurred. During his convalescence from surgery, he complained of frequent occipital and left temporal headaches. About 6 months later, he was hospitalized in a military hospital and taken off seizure medication. Four days later, he experienced a grand mal seizure. Seizure control medications were reinstated and he was discharged from the hospital a week later. No additional medical problems were reported prior to his current admission.

The medical examination on admission revealed an alert, oriented, well-nourished male in no apparent distress, but complaining of "memory problems." He had a circular (diameter = 2 cm) skull defect in the left temporal area. Neurologic examination was generally unremarkable, except for moderate bilateral weakness in both arms and shoulders.

The *doctor's orders* contained requests for routine blood work and continuation of seizure control medication. An electroencephalogram and CT scans were ordered. Evaluation of Mr. White by neuropsychology and speech pathology was requested. An ophthalmologic evaluation was also requested, based on his complaints of "problems with my eyes."

Several *laboratory reports* were in Mr. White's medical record. Mr. White's EEG record demonstrated "asymmetric electrical activity, localized primarily over temporal regions, bilaterally." The CT scan showed asymmetric ventricles with the left lateral ventricle larger than the right, a bony defect in the left temporal area of the skull, and surgical clips in place beneath the skull defect. These findings were said to be "consistent with previous surgical procedures in the left temporal area." A report from ophthalmology service indicated that Mr. White was "mildly myopic with some difficulty with focus, possibly secondary to his old brain injury."

Progress notes were generally unremarkable, and suggested that Mr. White had no obvious medical problems. Nursing notes suggested that he was alert, friendly, and cooperative. A progress note by the physician commented that "there appears to be no evidence of severe memory loss about matters concerning his hospitalization."

Summary.—The nature of Mr. White's medical problem is obvious from the history and laboratory reports. However, the effects of his injury on his mental abilities are not, at this point, clear. Mr. White complains of memory problems and difficulty with vision. Both complaints are consistent with injury to the temporal lobe, and perhaps to the occipital lobe. Mr. White's report of occipital headaches also suggests occipital lobe involvement, as does his report of visual problems. There is no mention of aphasia in Mr. White's medical records. However, the fact that Mr. White's left temporal lobe has been damaged makes the existence of aphasia likely, because damage to the temporal lobe in the language-dominant hemisphere almost always causes problems with language comprehension and word retrieval. Evaluation of Mr. White by speech pathology and neuropsychology is appropriate. The speech and language pathologist might expect subtle language comprehension deficits, verbal formulation problems, and verbal memory problems, because of Mr. White's temporal lobe involvement. His reading should be tested in case his visual problems interfere with reading. The neuropsychologist might expect problems with attention and memory, and perhaps subtle cognitive impairments.

This concludes the examples of medical record review. In addition to showing what kinds of information may be found in a patient's medical records, the examples show how the speech-language pathologist functions as a part of a larger group of professionals, each responsible for certain aspects of a patient's overall program of care.

The Interview

The clinician's assessment of the patient continues with an *interview*. It is carried out in a quiet place, free from intrusions and distractions. If a "significant other" (spouse, another family member, or a close friend) is available, they should be invited to join the interview. If the patient's aphasia is mild or moderate, the significant other may corroborate the information given by the patient and help the patient if he or she has difficulty remembering or producing information. If the patient's aphasia is severe, the significant other may be the primary source of information, and the patient's role may be one of confirmation and corroboration. During the interview the clinician asks questions about the patient's previous history, current complaints, family history, and educational and work background; observes how the patient communicates; and makes preliminary decisions about the focus of testing.

Information from the interview may confirm, supplement, or elaborate on information from the medical record. The interview also allows the patient and the clinician to become comfortable with each other and permits the patient to adjust to the surroundings in which testing will be carried out. By the end of the interview the clinician usually has a good idea of the tests that he or she will begin with and the approximate level of difficulty at which the examination will be carried out. Information from the referral, the patient's medical records, and the interview determines which tests are selected. The clinician's experiences with the patient during the interview largely determine the level of difficulty at which the examination will be conducted.

Toward the end of the interview the clinician spends some time discussing with the patient (and family members or caregivers, if present) the testing that is likely to follow and what the purposes of the testing are. According to Lezak (1983) the clinician should always address the following topics in the interview:

1. The purpose of testing.
2. The nature of the tests likely to be given.
3. How the information from the tests will be used.
4. What will be done to protect the patient's privacy and the confidentiality of test results.
5. Who will report test results to the patient and family, and when they will be reported.
6. A brief explanation of test procedures.
7. How the patient feels about taking the tests.

According to Lezak, patients who have severe disabilities may not appreciate everything in the above list, but the clinician should make an effort to see that every topic is covered within the limits of the patient's comprehension, and that the patient has had an opportunity to communicate his or her feelings about the tests and to ask questions about them. When the clinician finds that the patient does not comprehend well enough to appreciate the information given, the information should be conveyed to the patient's spouse or another person who is close to the patient.

HOW THE CLINICIAN DECIDES WHAT TO TEST

The clinician rarely knows exactly what tests are to be given before testing begins. Most begin with a basic test or set of tests that are likely to address key behaviors or abilities. These initial tests are selected based on the referral, the patient's medical history, and the initial interview with the patient. The patient's performance on these initial tests govern how the clinician proceeds.

Lezak (1983) describes this stage of assessment as a period of *hypothesis testing*. The hypothesis testing begins as the results of the first tests answer the clinician's initial questions, suggest new ones, or shift the focus of attention to a different set of questions. The clinician may continue to change procedures and alter the focus of testing throughout the examination until he or she is satisfied that the nature and severity of the patient's disabilities have been adequately described. An important part of this process is what Lezak calls *testing the limits*. Clinicians test the limits by going beyond the limits set by standard procedures for administering a given test.

For example, a patient who fails a standard test of written spelling might be allowed to spell the same words orally. Normal performance on the latter would prove that the deficient performance on the standard test was not because the patient could not spell, but perhaps because he or she could not write. If the patient were to fail the oral spelling test, the clinician might proceed to a test in which the patient chooses correctly spelled words from sets of printed words in which the correctly spelled word is shown with incorrectly spelled foils. According to Lezak, "The examiner should test the limits whenever he suspects that an impairment of some function other than the one under consideration is interfering with an adequate demonstration of that function."

During the examination the clinician monitors the patient's performance to determine whether some tasks are either easier or more difficult than the patient's overall performance suggests that they should be. The clinician watches for signs of complicating conditions such as deficient visual acuity or hearing loss. If the patient's performance shows islands of either preserved or impaired functions relative to his or her overall performance, or if there are signs of complicating conditions, then these areas are tested in greater detail.

The foregoing may make it appear that assessment begins with the referral and ends when treatment begins. Assessment is hardly ever compartmentalized so neatly. The clinician's assessment of the patient almost always continues throughout treatment as the patient's performance changes and as the clinician gains new insights into the nature of the patient's disabilities. The ability to detect and capitalize on sometimes subtle changes in performance over time or from task to task is an important part of clinical expertise, and should be cultivated by clinicians.

COMPREHENSIVE APHASIA TESTS

Comprehensive aphasia tests provide an overall description of a patient's communicative ability across stimulus and response modalities, and at various levels of difficulty within modalities or combinations of modalities. All are designed to identify communicative disabilities, to estimate their severity, and to describe their nature. Some permit clinicians to assign patients to diagnostic categories. Some permit clinicians to predict the eventual level of a patient's recovery of communicative ability. Some are useful in differential diagnosis. When a potentially aphasic patient is referred, a comprehensive aphasia test usually is administered to get an overview of the patient's impairments. Follow-up testing with more specialized tests may further define the nature and severity of the patient's disabilities.

Most comprehensive aphasia tests include combinations of some or all of the following subtests.

1. Reciting days of the week, months of the year, and counting aloud.
2. Naming objects indicated by the examiner.
3. Naming pictures indicated by the examiner.
4. Matching pictures or geometric forms.

5. Matching printed words to pictures.
6. Repeating words, phrases, and sentences spoken by the examiner.
7. Answering printed or spoken questions.
8. Pointing to objects named by the examiner.
9. Pointing to pictures named by the examiner.
10. Carrying out spoken directions.
11. Reading aloud printed numerals, letters, words, and phrases.
12. Silently reading sentences and paragraphs and answering questions about them.
13. Writing letters, words, and sentences spoken by the examiner.
14. Performing arithmetic computations.

Most comprehensive aphasia tests permit clinicians to score the quality of patients' responses as well as their correctness or incorrectness. This is accomplished either by means of a scoring system that allows the examiner to show the quality of responses as well as their correctness or by means of longhand notes about a patient's performance. Many permit clinicians to summarize a patient's performance in a profile. Some provide normative information that allows a clinician to compare the performance of a given patient with the performance of groups of aphasic persons who have certain characteristics in common. Profiles and norms may be useful in predicting the course and extent of a patient's recovery, and in designing a treatment program.

Weisenberg and McBride (1935), Schuell (1965), and Porch (1967) have each discussed the characteristics that comprehensive aphasia tests should have. The following list summarizes the ideas of the three authors.

1. The test should sample a large number of performances at different levels of difficulty in each modality, so that all potentially disturbed performances are evaluated.
2. The test should sample in a consistent manner the input modality through which the test instructions are delivered, the input modality used while the task is performed, and the output modality necessary for carrying out the task.
3. The test should be standardized so that results are reliable from test to test and examiner to examiner. It should provide for control of relevant variables such as method of stimulus presentation, instructions to the patient, and response scoring.
4. The test should record patient performance in such a way that the quality of responses, as well as their correctness, is recorded.
5. The test should include a sufficient number of items within each subtest to permit the user to reliably determine average performance on each subtest.
6. The test should include a variety of nonlanguage tests, to measure processes that may underlie language.
7. The test should minimize the effects of intelligence and education on the estimates of communicative ability obtained.

8. The test should suggest the reasons for a patient's deficient performance on test items.
9. The test should permit predictions regarding aphasic persons' eventual recovery of speech and language.

Aphasia Severity and Test Sensitivity

Most comprehensive aphasia tests are most sensitive when used to test patients who fall somewhere near the middle of the severity continuum. They contain subtests that are of moderate difficulty for most aphasic patients, with some tasks on which a moderately aphasic person will make no errors, and some on which a moderately aphasic person will make nothing but errors. If one attempts to use such an examination to evaluate a severely aphasic person, one is likely to find that there are few, if any, tasks in which the patient makes no errors, and that most of the tasks generate nothing but error responses. If one uses such an examination to evaluate a mildly aphasic person, one is likely to find that the patient makes no errors on most test items, and that there are no subtests that are completely failed. In the case of the severely aphasic person, one has failed to identify a level at which he or she can perform without error, and in the case of the mildly aphasic person, one has failed to identify a level at which performance breaks down completely. Both levels are important for understanding a patient's abilities and disabilities, and for planning treatment programs that take these abilities and disabilities into consideration.

In the case of a *severely aphasic* patient, the clinician may be tempted to forego formal testing with standard test instruments in order not to subject the aphasic person to the frustration and emotional stress that are likely to accompany experiences in which failure is the most prominent occurrence. Such a decision, while sparing the aphasic person's feelings, usually is not therapeutically wise, for two reasons. First, the clinician remains ignorant about the nature and extent of the patient's disabilities. The clinician may then overlook areas in which the patient's abilities might be better than one might predict, leading to poorly advised decisions about the feasibility of treatment and the patient's potential for recovery. Second, the clinician has no way of documenting the patient's change in communicative abilities over time, either as the result of treatment or of neurologic recovery.

In order to obtain a more useful sample of behavior from severely aphasic patients, the clinician may devise a nonstandard set of tasks that samples behavior at a lower level of complexity than is tested by standard aphasia examinations. It is not too difficult to devise tasks that give reasonably accurate estimates of such patients' speaking and writing abilities. However, assessing severely aphasic patients' comprehension of spoken and written language usually is more difficult, because their response repertoire usually is so limited that they cannot reliably indicate to the examiner whether they have comprehended the materials. Unless a patient can generate consistent, interpretable responses to at least some auditory or visual stimuli, the clinician can make few inferences about the state of the patient's comprehension (except that the patient's comprehension cannot reliably be assessed).

When a patient is severely aphasic, the comprehensive aphasia test may be replaced by a test such as the *Boston Assessment of Severe Aphasia (BASA)* (Helm-Estabrooks et al., 1989). The BASA is a short (61 items) examination for assessing severely aphasic adults. It provides for assessment of spoken, gestural, and written responses, and of comprehension of spoken, printed, and gestural messages. Some behavioral aspects of responses also are assessed (emotional state, perseveration).

If a comprehensive aphasia test is used to evaluate severely aphasic persons, at least the first few items in each subtest should be attempted, even if the examiner thinks the patient is likely to fail them. If the patient fails to make a reasonable response to, say, the first three items in a subtest, the examiner may choose not to administer the rest of the subtest. However, if the patient makes a reasonable response to one of the items, or if his performance appears to be improving across the first few items, the examiner may choose to continue the subtest.

Because the severely aphasic patient is likely to be experiencing substantial amounts of failure during the examination, the examiner should provide continual support and reassurance. It is important that this support and reassurance be honest. Most patients are quick to recognize the falsity of clinicians who say "you're doing fine!" when they are not. Supporting and encouraging remarks should be general, and not contingent on the patient's responses to individual test items. The clinician who says "right" after correct responses and "wrong" after errors is providing reinforcement (or feedback), rather than general encouragement, and may be treating, rather than testing the patient.

If it is not prohibited by the test procedures, the examiner may choose to intersperse tasks in which the patient has success among tasks in which he or she has substantial amounts of failure. It may be necessary in some cases to administer small sections of the examination on several successive days, in order to minimize the patient's fatigue and stress.

Evaluation of *moderately aphasic* patients is likely to present fewer problems than evaluation of severely aphasic patients. Comprehensive aphasia tests usually provide the clinician with information regarding the levels at which the patient's performance is error-free, the levels at which no correct responses are made, and the levels between, where the patient's performance contains both correct and error responses.

Evaluation of *mildly aphasic* patients is likely to be complicated by the fact that most comprehensive aphasia tests do not contain enough difficult items. Such patients may have little or no difficulty with most items on standard aphasia examinations, but may still possess impairments that interfere with their social, vocational, and educational activities. Such patients usually benefit from treatment. For this reason, the clinician should examine the upper limits of mildly aphasic patients' abilities. The clinician may construct tests to assess specific socially, academically, or vocationally useful abilities. Sometimes commercially available tests designed to measure normal persons' abilities (such as reading, spelling, and arithmetic) are appropriate. Standard achievement tests often are useful for assessing the capabilities and deficits of persons with mild aphasia.

During assessment, the clinician should observe the patient's general responses to the test situation and test stimuli to determine whether some tasks are easier or more difficult than the patient's overall performance suggests that they should be. The clinician should be particularly alert for signs suggesting the presence of complicating conditions, such as deficient visual acuity, visual field deficits, hearing loss, and so forth. If the patient's performance on a standard test battery suggests that there are areas in which the patient performs better or worse than his or her overall performance would suggest, or if the clinician observes signs of complicating conditions, then the areas of unusual performance should be investigated in greater detail, either by means of standard tests or tests devised by the clinician.

DESCRIPTIONS OF MAJOR COMPREHENSIVE APHASIA TESTS

In the following section, I will describe seven aphasia tests that may be used to obtain an overall view of an aphasic person's communicative abilities and impairments. These seven represent, in my opinion, the seven most widely used general aphasia tests, and their descriptions should give the reader a sense of the commonalities and differences among such tests in scope, complexity, standardization, administration time, and cost. I have not included descriptions of short screening examinations or of tests that are designed for evaluating subsets of the aphasic population. Exclusion of a test does not imply that it is not meritorious. The information given in this section was correct at the time this section was written, but may, of course, change as time passes.

Title: Aphasia Language Performance Scales (ALPS)
Authors: Joseph S. Keenan, Eleanor G. Brassel
Publisher: Pinnacle Press, PO Box 1122, Murfreesboro, TN 37130
Cost: Complete test kit: $23.00
Latest revision: 1975
Administration time: 20–45 min
Norms available: Mean scores and correlations between ALPS scores and other measures are given in a technical manual. However, neither the characteristics of the aphasic population upon which the test was standardized or the distribution of scores for that population are provided.
Scoring method: Three-category scoring system: "correct," "prompted," and "incorrect."
Method of summarizing data: Test results are summarized by writing each item score and totals for each subtest on a score sheet. Space is provided on the score sheet for listing *indicators of improvement, patient's chief communicative interests,* and *patient's apparent communicative needs. Cumulative record* sheets are provided, on which a patient's scores for *listening, talking, reading,* and *writing* can be plotted over time. Severity ratings can be made, based on scores on the listening, talking, reading, and writing subtests. Subtest scores of 0 to 1 are labeled *profound aphasia,* scores from 1.5 to 3.0 are labeled *severe aphasia,* scores from 3.5 to 5.0 are labeled *moderate-severe aphasia,* scores from 5.5 to 7.0 are labeled *mild-moderate aphasia,* scores from 7.5 to 9.0 are labeled *mild aphasia,* and scores from 9.5 to 10.0 are labeled *insignificant aphasia.*
Prognostic capability: General guidelines for prognosis, based on test results and medical history, are offered. No test-based prognostic procedures that consider time postonset and patterns of test performance are offered.

Other: According to the authors, the ALPS is intended to be a short examination that avoids several of what the authors believe are "unsatisfactory features" of other standard aphasia examinations: (1) other tests are too time-consuming; (2) other tests are limited by space and environmental restrictions (the need for electric power, a quiet room with a table, or the need for "considerable paraphernalia"); (3) other tests are so formal that they interfere with rapport between the clinician and patient; and (4) other tests give too little help in planning treatment.

The test contains 40 items, 10 in each of four subtests: *Listening, Talking, Reading,* and *Writing.* Items within subtests are heterogeneous and in general order of increasing difficulty within subtests. Responses are scored as "correct," "prompted," or "incorrect." The examiner is encouraged to intersperse praise, encouragement, and reassurance among presentation of test items. The examiner also is allowed to delete test items that, in the examiner's judgment, the patient would easily pass, as well as those items that, in the examiner's judgment, the patient would certainly fail. General principles governing prediction and treatment planning using the ALPS are included in the technical manual. Several examples of the use of the ALPS in testing and treating aphasic patients also are included in the manual.

The technical manual contains an extensive section on the reliability and validity of the ALPS. The data in this section consist of test-retest and split-half reliability scores on the ALPS, correlations between ALPS scores and scores on the *Porch Index of Communicative Ability,* and correlations between ALPS scores and scores on IQ and achievement tests. Little information is provided about the characteristics of the standardization sample of aphasic patients, or the distribution and range of test scores within the sample.

Title: The Boston Diagnostic Aphasia Examination (BDAE)
Authors: Harold Goodglass, Edith Kaplan
Publisher: Lea and Febiger, 200 Chesterfield Parkway, Malvern, PA 19355-9725
Cost: Complete test set: $32.50 (includes BDAE stimulus cards and the *Boston Naming Test*)
Latest revision: 1983
Administration time: 1–4 hrs
Norms available: Normative data are presented for both the (original) 1972 version and the 1983 revision. The data for the 1972 version were acquired from 207 aphasic patients, and those for the 1983 revision were acquired from 242 patients. Percentile ranks for a patient's performance on each subtest of the BDAE are obtained from the Subtest Summary Profile. Data obtained from intercorrelation analyses, factor analyses, and reliability coefficients among subtests are provided in the test manual.
Scoring method: Plus-minus coded scores, category system rating scale, written notes.
Method of summarizing data: Overall severity of aphasia is rated on a 6-point scale. *Speech characteristics* can be described using seven descriptors. Subtest summary profiles can be plotted for any patient. "Characteristic" patterns of performance that would be expected for Broca's aphasia, Wernicke's aphasia, anomic aphasia, conduction aphasia, and transcortical sensory aphasia are described in the test manual.
Prognostic capabilities: None claimed.
Other: The purposes of the *BDAE* are said by the authors to be (1) "diagnosis of presence and type of aphasic syndrome, leading to inferences concerning cerebral localization"; (2) "measurement of the level of performance over a wide range, for both initial determination and detection of change over time"; and (3) "comprehensive assessment of the assets and liabilities of the patient in all language areas as a guide to therapy." The examination is based on an assumption that the nature of the aphasic deficit is deter-

mined by (1) organization of language in the brain; (2) the location of the lesion causing the aphasia; and (3) interactions among parts of the language system. The examination provides materials and procedures to evaluate the following aspects of speech and language: (1) articulation, (2) fluency, (3) word-finding ability, (4) repetition, (5) serial speech, (6) grammar and syntax, (7) paraphasias, (8) auditory comprehension, (9) reading, and (10) writing.

The results of four factor analyses of the normative group's performance on the BDAE are included in the test manual. The results of two discriminant analyses are also reported, along with procedures by which patients can be assigned to one of four diagnostic categories (Broca's, Wernicke's, conduction, other) based on their performance on the BDAE. Suggestions for administering, scoring, and interpreting performance on subtests in the BDAE are given in the test manual, as well as directions for plotting and interpreting patient profiles. Sections on supplementary language and nonlanguage tests describe a number of supplementary tests, their scoring and interpretation, and their uses.

Title: Examining for Aphasia
Author: Jon Eisenson
Publisher: The Psychological Corporation, PO Box 839954, San Antonio, TX 78283-3954
Cost: Complete test set: $77.50
Latest revision: 1954
Administration time: 30 min.–2 hr
Norms available: None.
Scoring method: Plus-minus with written notes.
Method of summarizing data: Rates modalities and levels according to amount of deficit: complete, severe, moderate, little, or none.
Prognostic capabilities: None claimed.
Other: Two shorter versions of the test are suggested. The screening version consists of the first item from each subtest, and the short version consists of every other test item.

The author defines aphasia as "impairment in the ability of the individual to behave appropriately in situations which involve a significant amount of symbolization. . . . Aphasia may be considered defective symbol behavior." The aphasic patient's deficits are said to be manifest in internal symbolic processes (thinking) as well as in external symbolic processes. Eisenson (1990) considers *Examining for Aphasia* "an inventory of language and related materials that provide experienced clinicians with a basis for arriving at a clinical judgment about the nature and approximate degree of impairment of persons who by virtue of medical history are likely to be aphasic." The test attempts to provide a means for identifying both the area and the level of any patient's symbolic dysfunction. The levels of potential dysfunction are (1) subsymbolic, (2) low symbolic, and (3) high symbolic. Subsymbolic behaviors include agnosias, apraxias, automatic responses, and copying. High symbolic behaviors include naming, oral propositional language, reading, spelling, writing, and calculation. The test divides abilities into two major categories: "predominantly receptive" and "predominantly expressive." The purpose of *Examining for Aphasia* is to determine the patient's maximum performance under optimum conditions. To maximize the probability of correct responses by the patient, the examiner is permitted considerable latitude in presentation of test items and instructions. A variety of responses to any given test item may be acceptable, if the examiner believes that the response signifies that the patient understood the item. Responses are scored plus-minus. Any deviations from the "standard" manner of presenting test stimuli are noted by the examiner, and patient responses not matching the "standard" response to a test item are transcribed verbatim by the examiner. No scales to measure severity of aphasia are provided. An estimate of the patient's degree of impairment in each category of symbol function tested is made in terms of whether the impairment appears to be "complete," "severe," "moderate," "little," or "none." The test items in the examination are said to be "relatively easy for a person with a grammar school education." Some of the verbal materials are said to be "sufficiently difficult so that non-brain-injured persons who are average or below in functional mental capacity or achievement would fail them." The examination is not standardized, either in terms of providing normative information against which to compare an individual's performance, or in terms of standardized procedures for presenting test items and scoring patients' responses.

Title: The Minnesota Test for Differential Diagnosis of Aphasia (MTDDA)
Author: Hildred Schuell
Publisher: The University of Minnesota Press, University of Minnesota, Minneapolis, MN 55455; also available from The Psychological Corporation, PO Box 839954, San Antonio, TX 78283-3954
Cost: Complete test set: $77.50
Latest revision: 1972
Administration time: 2–6 hr (average, 3 hr)
Norms available: Standardized on 157 aphasic subjects. Mean scores, standard deviations, median scores, and percentage of subjects making errors are provided for each subtest.
Scoring method: Plus-minus, with written transcription of some responses.
Method of summarizing data: Test scores are summarized by number of errors on the face sheet of the record form. The test manual provides a list of "signs" and "most discriminating tests" that enable the user to assign tested patients to one of five major and two minor categories of aphasia. Patients are assigned to categories according to pattern of impairment, rather than severity of impairment.
Prognostic capabilities: The test manual provides prognoses for recovery for each of five major and two minor categories of aphasia.
Other: A short version of the MTDDA has been described (Schuell, 1957). Schuell subsequently disavowed the short version, and instead suggested a "baseline-ceiling" procedure for shortening the test. The procedure is described in the test manual.

Schuell defines aphasia as a "reduction of available language that crosses all language modalities and may or may not be complicated by perceptual or sensorimotor involvement, by various forms of dysarthria, or by other sequelae of brain damage." According to Schuell, the "overall pattern" of impairment differs from patient to patient, making differential diagnosis possible. Schuell maintains that differential diagnosis is the basis for both description and prediction in aphasia, and adds that careful description provides a guide for treatment, because treatment must deal with the disabilities that are identified by the description. Schuell believes that "well studied patterns of aphasia should be expected to carry reliable prognoses for recovery of language functions." Schuell emphasizes that predictions will not be accurate unless the tests upon which predictions are based are accomplished when the patient is "neurologically stable." She offers 3 months as the "consensus" period of "spontaneous recovery." She also emphasizes that it is necessary to ask not only *how* but *why* the patient makes errors. According to Schuell, "it is possible to describe patterns of aphasic impairment in terms of test profiles that reflect quantitative errors, but it is more meaningful to describe the performance of an individual patient in terms of the kinds of errors he makes, or clinical signs." Schuell rejected standard scores as "meaningless when dealing with aphasic populations which are heterogeneous in age, intelligence, cultural milieu, medical history, locus and extent of brain damage, and severity and duration of aphasia." Schuell maintained that "the most effective way of interpreting test data is in terms of clinical signs and total test pattern."

The five major patient categories in Schuell's classification system are:

Group 1: Simple aphasia.
Group 2: Aphasia with visual involvement.
Group 3: Aphasia with sensorimotor involvement.
Group 4: Aphasia with scattered findings compatible with generalized brain damage.
Group 5: Irreversible aphasic syndrome.

The two minor categories are:

Minor Syndrome A: Aphasia with partial auditory imperception.
Minor Syndrome B: Aphasia with persisting dysarthria.

The MTDDA is divided into five sections, each section containing several subtests. The sections are:

1. Auditory disturbances.
2. Visual and reading disturbances.
3. Speech and language disturbances.
4. Visuomotor and writing disturbances.
5. Disturbances of numerical relations and arithmetic processes.

Directions for administering test items include the verbal instructions to be given by the examiner, and directions for scoring patients' responses. Several subtests require relatively long verbal instructions by the examiner, so that patients with auditory comprehension disabilities might have difficulty with these tests because of problems in understanding the instructions, rather than because of inability to deal with the test items themselves.

Title: The Neurosensory Center Comprehensive Examination for Aphasia (NCCEA)
Authors: Ottfried Spreen, Arthur L. Benton
Publisher: Neuropsychology Laboratory, Department of Psychology, University of Victoria, Victoria, British Columbia, Canada V8W2Y2
Cost: Contact publisher for current cost.
Latest revision: 1977
Administration time: 1–2 hr
Norms available: Percentile scores for each of the 20 language tests in the NCCEA are provided in profile sheet form for a group of 210 aphasic persons, 86 right-hemisphere-damaged persons, and a normative group of non-brain-damaged persons.
Scoring method: Weighted plus-minus scoring, plus written notes. A five-category qualitative scoring system is provided for naming subtests.
Method of summarizing data: Total score for each subtest is recorded in an answer booklet and entered on a profile sheet.
Prognostic capabilities: None claimed.
Other: The NCCEA was originally an experimental aphasia test. It is available as part of the *Compendium of Neuropsychological Tests* by O. Spreen and E. Strauss (Oxford

University Press, 1991). It has been in use at the University of Iowa and the University of Victoria since 1967. The NCCEA contains 20 subtests, which assess language production and understanding, retention of verbal material, reading, and writing. The test manual is composed primarily of instructions for administration of test items and scoring of patient responses. The test manual includes profile sheets that give percentile ranks for scores on each of the 20 subtests for aphasic, nonaphasic brain-damaged, and non-brain-damaged persons.

The NCCEA contains several subtests that are not found in most other aphasia tests—tactile naming with right and left hands, repetition of digits (forward and backward), word fluency, sentence construction, and tactile-to-visual matching. Normative data for children tested with the NCCEA also are available.

Title: The Porch Index of Communicative Ability (PICA)
Author: Bruce E. Porch
Publisher: Consulting Psychologists Press, 3803 East Bayshore Road, PO Box 10096, Palo Alto, CA 94303
Cost: Complete test set: $140.00
Latest revision: 1981
Administration time: 30 min–2 hr (Average, 60 min)
Norms available: The PICA is standardized on 357 left-hemisphere-damaged patients, 96 right-hemisphere-damaged patients, and 100 bilaterally damaged patients. Volume 1 of the test manual contains information about the development of the battery, interscorer and test-retest reliability, and internal consistency. Volume 2 contains percentiles for the overall score, for each subtest, and for various combinations of subtest scores under each modality. Recovery curves are provided, from which the examiner can predict a patient's expected recovery based on his or her current PICA scores.
Scoring method: Each response is scored according to a 16-category, binary-choice system, on the basis of accuracy, responsiveness, completeness, promptness, and efficiency. A system of diacritic marking can augment the 16-category system to increase the descriptiveness of response scoring.
Method of summarizing data: Each response is scored using the 16-category scoring system and the score is written on the score sheet. A mean score for the entire test (overall score) is calculated, as well as modality mean scores for writing, copying, reading, pantomime, verbal, auditory, and visual subtests. Profiles may be plotted on a *rating of Communicative Ability* sheet that groups subtests according to each of the modalities, or on a *ranked response summary* graph that plots subtest scores in order of decreasing subtest difficulty across the page. Changes in a patient's performance over time can be recorded on an *aphasia recovery curve* sheet, on which the overall percentile score and the peak-mean difference score, a measure of intrasubtest variability, can be plotted.
Prognostic capabilities: The PICA provides procedures for predicting the recovery of any given patient by plotting a recovery curve, which allows predictions about eventual recovery of communicative ability based on the patient's performance 1 month or more after onset of aphasia. Recovery is predicted by reference to a family of recovery curves generated by the sample of 280 patients. Treatment is said to raise the end point of the recovery curve and to reduce intrasubtest variability.
Other: The PICA defines aphasia as a deficit in language processing rather than as a deficit in language itself. The test manual describes several deficits in processing that can be observed in patients' performance on the PICA ("slow rise time," "noise buildup," "difficulty in switching tasks").

The test manual contains sections on general PICA theory, profile pattern analysis, localization, estimating a future recovery level, and treatment principles based on PICA theory. It also contains descriptions of patient test patterns that may be encountered in any sample of brain damaged patients, including (1) left hemisphere patterns divided into seven subgroups; (2) right hemisphere patterns; (3) bilateral and diffuse damage patterns; and (4) nonaphasic patterns related to psychologic problems.

Title: The Western Aphasia Battery (WAB)
Author: Andrew Kertesz
Publisher: The Psychological Corporation, PO Box 839954, San Antonio, TX 78283-3954
Cost: Complete test kit: $85.00
Latest revision: 1982
Administration time: 1–4 hr

Norms available: No normative information is provided in the test manual. The reader is referred to Kertesz (1979) and Shewan and Kertesz (1980) for information on standardization of the 1977 version of the WAB. Subtest mean scores and their standard deviations are reported in Kertesz (1979) for 365 aphasic and 162 nonaphasic persons from two standardizations of the WAB. The first, in 1974, included 150 aphasic and 59 control subjects. The second, in 1979, added 215 aphasic and 63 control subjects. Information on the reliability of the WAB and on correlations between the WAB and the NCCEA are provided in Kertesz (1979). To support the validity of the 1982 version of the WAB, correlations between subjects' performance on the 1979 and 1982 versions of the test are reported in the test manual. Twenty "consecutively seen" patients were tested with both the 1979 and 1982 versions of the WAB, and correlations between subtest scores on the two test occasions were calculated. These correlations, together with subtest mean scores on the two versions, are reported in the manual. Correlations ranged from .54 to .99. The author concludes that "there is no substantial difference between this new version and the previously standardized version of the test."

Scoring method: The scoring method used depends on which subtest is scored. For example, spontaneous speech is rated for "information content" using a ten-category system, and for "fluency, grammatical content, and paraphasias" with a different ten-category system. Other subtests are scored with a plus-minus system in which points are awarded for "correct" responses to various aspects of test items. The manner in which points are awarded and the number of points possible differ from subtest to subtest.

Method of summarizing data: A patient's scores on each subtest are entered on a score sheet, which is the last page in the test booklet. These subtest scores can be used to calculate an *aphasia quotient* and a *cortical quotient.* The oral language subtest scores are used to calculate the aphasia quotient, and both language and nonlanguage subtest scores are used to calculate the cortical quotient. The aphasia quotient is said by the author to be "a reliable measure of the severity of language impairment." The cortical quotient is intended to be a measure of "cognitive functions." Shewan and Kertesz (1984) described an additional summary score, the *language quotient.* The language quotient includes scores from reading and writing subtests as well as the oral language subtest scores that are included in the aphasia quotient.

Prognostic capabilities: None claimed in the test manual. A table in the test manual provides score ranges on the characteristics of "fluency," "comprehension," "repetition," and "naming" for eight traditional aphasia types (Broca's, Wernicke's, etc.). Patients can be assigned to type categories based on their performance on the WAB. Category membership could presumably carry prognostic significance, although the test manual does not claim this. Extensive discussion of the relationships between aphasia type and severity, as measured by the WAB, and recovery is provided in Kertesz (1979).

Other: The WAB employs what Kertesz calls a "taxonomic" approach to classifying patients, in which patients are assigned to diagnostic categories (Broca's, Wernicke's, etc.) according to their scores on WAB subtests.

The WAB includes tests of nonlanguage abilities (apraxia, figure drawing, calculation, and block design.) The score from Raven's *Coloured Progressive Matrices* is included as part of the patient's "construction" score. The WAB requires the manipulation of a large number of materials in order to administer the test. This may pose problems for untrained examiners.

The WAB has been standardized on a sample of dementia patients (Appell et al., 1982) and according to Kertesz (1990) it is appropriate for testing and follow-up of patients with Alzheimer's disease and vascular dementia.

ASSESSMENTS OF FUNCTIONAL COMMUNICATION

Comprehensive aphasia tests provide the clinician with a general sense of the nature and severity of a patient's linguistic and communicative disabilities. They do not always provide dependable estimates of how well a patient will communicate in daily life situations. Two instruments designed to estimate aphasic adults' functional daily life communication have been published: *The Functional Communication Profile* (Sarno, 1969), and *Communicative Abilities in Daily Living* (Holland, 1980).

Title: The Functional Communication Profile (FCP)
Author: Martha Taylor Sarno
Publisher: Institute of Rehabilitation Medicine, New York University Medical Center, Monograph Department, 400 E. 34th St., New York, NY 10016
Cost: Complete test kit: $9.00
Latest revision: 1969
Administration time: 30 min–1 hr
Norms available: No normative information is provided. Examples of "typical" profiles of left and right hemiplegic patients are given in the manual.
Scoring method: Rates behaviors on a nine-point scale, from zero to normal (100%). Converts these ratings into a percentage that reflects a person's remaining communicative function, expressed as a percentage of their presumed premorbid communication function. Sarno (1969) reported reliability coefficients greater than .87 for the five categories of behavior sampled by the FCP (see below).
Method of summarizing data: Forty-five items are listed on the record form. Each is rated on the nine-point scale, resulting in a "profile" of the patient's "functional" communication abilities.
Prognostic capabilities: None claimed. The FCP is intended to provide an index of a patient's current functional communication abilities.
Other: The FCP is designed to "quantify the communication behaviors which a patient actually uses in the course of interaction with others," in contrast with language elicited in structured test settings. It assesses 45 communication behaviors considered "common functions of everyday urban life," and rates each on a nine-point scale of current ability as a proportion of the patient's estimated premorbid ability. The profile divides be-

haviors into five major categories: *movement* (gestural communication); *speaking* (saying name, giving directions, etc.); *understanding* (verbal and gestural directions, television, etc.); *reading* (signs, newspapers, letters, etc.); *miscellaneous* (time orientation, handling money, etc.). Sarno suggests that the ideal way to measure an individual's communicative function would be to follow the individual for a time in the course of his or her everyday life. However, a nonstructured interview is suggested as the most practical method for observing the patient's natural communication behavior. During this interview the clinician makes no notes; the profile is filled out after the interview. Reports of the patient and those around the patient are also used to fill out parts of the profile, if necessary.

Directions for rating behaviors, computing percentage of premorbid ability, and construction of the profile are included in the monograph. A short section on interpretation of profiles is included. Sections on reliability and validity also are included.

Title: Communicative Abilities in Daily Living (CADL)
Author: Audrey L. Holland
Publisher: Pro-Ed, 8700 Shoal Creek Blvd., Austin, TX 78758-9965
Cost: Complete test kit: $79.00
Latest revision: 1980
Administration time: 30 min–1 hr
Norms available: Normative information is provided for a group of 130 aphasic adults ranging in age from below 46 to over 65, and a matched group of 130 nonaphasic adults. Half the subjects in each group were living in institutional environments and half were not. Extensive descriptions of the characteristics of the normative groups are provided, and performance of each group on CADL according to various characteristics such as age and living environment is described in the CADL manual. Cutoff scores for aphasic subjects' performance according to age and living environment are provided, and an item analysis of CADL performance of aphasic subjects is included in the manual.

Scoring method: Three category system: 0 = "wrong," 1 = "adequate," 2 = "correct." Responses are scored on their communicative adequacy, rather than on their grammatical or linguistic correctness. Training materials to teach examiners how to score each CADL item are provided. Two completed CADL test forms and an audiotape containing verbal responses made by aphasic patients are included. These materials can be used to learn administration and scoring techniques for CADL.

Method of summarizing data: None. Total score is used to compare tested patients with the normative group. In the test manual Holland describes ten categories of behavior that are sampled by CADL: (1) reading, writing, and using numbers; (2) speech acts (explaining, correcting, requesting, etc.); (3) using verbal and nonverbal context; (4) role playing; (5) sequenced and relationship-dependent communicative behavior (dialing a telephone, etc.); (6) social conventions; (7) divergences (generating logical possibilities); (8) nonverbal symbolic communication; (9) deixis (movement-related or movement-dependent communicative behavior); and (10) humor, absurdity, metaphor. An analysis of test items according to these ten categories is provided in the manual.

Prognostic capabilities: None claimed.

Other: The emphasis in CADL is on measuring the *functional adequacy* of communication behaviors rather than their grammatical or linguistic correctness. Patients' communicative behaviors are sampled (1) in role-playing activities that mimic daily life situations such as keeping an appointment at a doctor's office, and (2) in traditional interview or examination format. As part of the standardization of CADL, Holland compared aphasic persons' CADL performance with their actual communication behaviors in daily life (as measured by observers in daily life environments). These comparisons appear to confirm CADL's validity for estimating daily life communicative competence. Information about CADL reliability and correlations of CADL performance with performance on other aphasia tests is provided in the manual. The results of studies of the performance of mentally retarded persons and hearing aid users on CADL also are reported there. Recent studies have demonstrated that CADL is useful in measuring communicative deficits in individuals with Alzheimer's disease.

OTHER TESTS OF SPEECH AND LANGUAGE

Assessment of aphasic adults rarely ends with a comprehensive aphasia test. The results of a comprehensive aphasia test almost always lead to other tests, which assess in greater detail areas of disability identified by the comprehensive aphasia test. Which follow-up tests are administered depends on the nature and severity of the patient's impairments. When impairments are identified by the comprehensive aphasia test, follow-up testing provides a more detailed analysis of the extent and nature of a patient's impairments. The following section contains descriptions of supplemental tests that may be administered to supplement a comprehensive aphasia test. This section, like the preceding one, is intended to provide a representative sample of the many tests that are available, and exclusion of a test does not imply that it is not meritorious.

Tests of Auditory Comprehension

The Token Test.—The *Token Test* and its variants (DeRenzi and Vignolo, 1962) are probably the most widely used tests for assessing auditory comprehension in aphasia. The DeRenzi and Vignolo version contains 62 spoken commands, which request the patient to touch or manipulate large and small circles and squares of various colors. There are five parts in the Token Test. (The original version used circles and rectangles, but most current versions substitute squares for rectangles.) Table 5–1 gives examples of commands from each of the five parts. Responses are scored

TABLE 5–1.

Examples of Commands From Each of the Five Parts of the Token Test (DeRenzi and Vignolo, 1962).

Test Part	Command
Part 1	Touch the red circle.
Part 2	Touch the large blue square.
Part 3	Touch the red square and the blue circle.
Part 4	Touch the large white circle and the small green square.
Part 5	When I touch the green circle, you take the white square.

correct or incorrect for each test command—the maximum score is 62. No norms are provided in DeRenzi and Vignolo (1962), although norms can be found elsewhere (Wertz et al., 1971).

Several modified versions of the *Token Test* have been published. The Spreen and Benton version (1977) is a subtest of the *Neurosensory Center Comprehensive Examination for Aphasia*. It contains 39 test commands equivalent to those in the original *Token Test*. Instead of scoring each sentence as correct or incorrect, the Spreen and Benton version scores each critical element in test commands. Thus, the command "point to the *small white circle*" would be worth 3 points, 1 for each critical element. There are 163 possible points in this version of the test. Normative information is provided for aphasic and nonaphasic persons.

The Revised Token Test.—The *Revised Token Test* (RTT) (McNeil and Prescott, 1978), is a longer and more elaborate version of DeRenzi and Vignolo's test. The RTT contains ten subtests; each contains ten homogeneous test commands. The first four subtests are similar to the first four parts of the original *Token Test*. Tests 5 and 6 each contain ten items that test position (e.g., in front of, behind, above, below). Tests 7 and 8 also test position (right, left). Tests 9 and 10 contain conditionals (e.g., instead of, if). Patients' responses are scored with a multidimensional system similar to that for the *PICA* (Porch, 1981a). Five profiles for "auditory processing deficits" (fatigue, cumulative noise, specific linguistic deficit, etc.) are provided in the test manual. An assortment of procedures for scoring and analyzing patients' responses are provided.

The Auditory Comprehension Test for Sentences.—The *Auditory Comprehension Test for Sentences* (ACTS) (Shewan, 1979) manipulates the length, vocabulary difficulty, and syntax of spoken sentences. Sentences are spoken to the patient, and the patient points to one of four pictures on a page to show comprehension of the sentences. There are 21 sentences in the test. Patients' responses can be scored either plus-minus or with a five-point category system. Additional qualitative analyses of patients' responses can be accomplished by means of a "qualitative analysis error form." This form allows the examiner to record (1) the position of errors (first or second part of sentence); (2) the grammatical form of errors (noun, verb, adjective, pronoun); (3) syntactic errors (negation); and (4) linguistic constituent errors (noun phrase, verb phrase, prepositional phrase). Mean scores and standard deviations are provided for 30 normal and 90 aphasic persons (30 Broca's, 30 Wernicke's, 30 amnesic aphasic).

The Northwestern Syntax Screening Test.—The *Northwestern Syntax Screening Test* (NSST) (Lee, 1971) is a screening test of sentence comprehension for use with children. The test consists of 20 sentences and 10 four-choice picture pages. The 20 sentences evaluate comprehension of various syntactic structures (locational prepositions, negation, subject-verb agreement, tense, etc.). Responses are scored plus-minus. Norms for children are given.

The Test for Auditory Comprehension of Langauge.—The *Test for Auditory Comprehension of Language* (TACL) (Carrow, 1973; Carrow, 1984) is a sentence comprehension test designed for use with children, although the 1984 version contains guidelines for use with adults. The TACL-R (the 1984 revision) contains 120 plates, each with three line drawings. Words, phrases, and sentences are spoken to the examinee, and the examinee points to the appropriate picture for each spoken stimulus. The test assesses three categories of materials; (1) word classes and relations (nouns, verbs, adjectives, adverbs); (2) grammatical morphemes (noun-verb agreement, number, tense, and case); and (3) complex sentence constructions (embedded sentences, partially connected sentences). Extensive normative information on children is provided.

Comprehension of Yes-No Questions.—Being able to answer yes-no questions is important for patients who cannot speak or write well enough to express their needs. Communication with such patients often involves asking the patient yes-no questions in order to find out what it is they wish to communicate. Unfortunately, there are no standard tests of yes-no question comprehension available, although some aphasia test batteries contain subtests with yes-no questions. However, the questions in these subtests do not take into account the effects of topic on the difficulty of yes-no questions. Questions that test personal information are almost always easier for brain-damaged patients than questions that test nonpersonal information. This effect will be discussed at greater length subsequently.

Commentary on Single-Sentence Tests of Auditory Comprehension

Token Tests.—The *Token Test* and its variants appear to be sensitive measures of comprehension disabilities. Even patients with very mild aphasia are likely to have difficulty with some elements of the token tests. However, this sensitivity makes the tests quite difficult for persons with severe aphasia. There is some question regarding the degree to which a patient's score on a token test predicts his or her comprehension in daily life. Although token test scores and scores on other sentence-level tests of comprehension are moderately correlated, several investigators have reported that token test scores do not predict performance on multiple-sentence spoken discourse (Stachowiak et al., 1977; Brookshire and Nicholas, 1984a; Wegner et al., 1984).

Some patients with poor comprehension may improve their performance on token tests by visually fixating the tokens named in the command. The performance of these patients deteriorates if the tokens are covered while the commands are spoken. If one wishes to be certain that one is testing auditory comprehension and retention, and not visual strategies, test tokens probably should be covered while test commands are being spoken.

The rate at which token test commands are spoken may influence aphasic patients' performance on the tests (Parkhurst, 1970; Liles and Brookshire, 1975). Slowing the rate at which commands are spoken or placing pauses in test commands apparently facilitates the performance of a significant proportion of aphasic patients.

Unfortunately, we do not know who is likely to be affected by rate manipulations, and we cannot be certain that the effects will be consistent from test to test, even for the same patient (Brookshire and Nicholas, 1984b). It is also possible that the intonation and stress patterns employed by the speaker may affect patients' performance. Pashek and Brookshire (1982) found that placing emphatic stress on crucial elements of token test commands improved patients' performance at slow speech rate, but not at fast speech rate. For these reasons, it may be worthwhile for the clinician who plans to use a token test to record the test commands with uniform speech rate and consistent intonation, stress, and pauses. By using such a recording, the clinician can limit response variability caused by changes in rate and prosody as commands are spoken.

The difficulty of token tests can be increased by interposing a delay interval between commands and the opportunity for the patient to respond. A 10- or 20-second delay interval may help to identify even very subtle deficiencies in auditory retention.

A few patients do poorly on token tests even though their performance on other tests of auditory comprehension suggests that their comprehension is quite good. The reasons for these discrepancies appear to include (1) specific difficulty in comprehension of color or shape words; (2) the unnaturalness of token test commands; (3) temporal sequencing difficulties, so that errors are made in the order of responses in commands; and (4) limb apraxias, which interfere with the pointing responses required by the test. The latter seems to be very rare. Few patients have limb apraxia severe enough to compromise their ability to point to test tokens.

In order to rule out problems with comprehension of color, shape, and size, one should pretest patients by asking them to point to "a red one," "a circle," "a small one," and so forth. A pretest is included in the Spreen and Benton version (1977) and the *Revised Token Test* (McNeil and Prescott, 1978). If such a pretest is not given, then deficits in color, shape, or size recognition could masquerade as deficits in auditory comprehension. If one is concerned that the patient may have problems in executing pointing responses, one can pretest the patient by asking him or her to imitate sequences of pointing responses modeled by the clinician. If the patient can imitate sequences of pointing responses, then it is unlikely that inability to point to test tokens causes deficient test performance.

Shortcomings of Single-Sentence Comprehension Tests.—Single-sentence tests of comprehension place heavy emphasis on short-term auditory memory. A string of information new to the patient is presented, and the patient is expected to retain the information verbatim for a few seconds—long enough to point to tokens or a picture, at which time the information can be forgotten. The situation is similar to tests for immediate memory in which lists of numbers or words are presented and the person being tested is expected to recognize or reproduce them after a few seconds delay. It would be unusual, in real life, to encounter spoken messages which (1) challenge short-term memory capacity, and (2) need not be remembered by the listener for more than a few seconds.

Existing tests of sentence comprehension present stimuli that usually are not connected in any straightforward way with the patient's experience. Rarely in real life do listeners encounter sentences such as "the spotted dog is under the small table" in isolation and without preceding material leading up to the assertion about the dog. Furthermore, in real life, speakers usually relate new information to what they assume the listener already knows about the situation being talked about.

In daily life, spoken messages almost always occur in situational and verbal contexts. Existing tests of sentence comprehension eliminate that context. This may be unwise when aphasic persons are being tested, because there is evidence that aphasic listeners rely on context to help them comprehend what they hear (Stachowiak et al., 1977; Waller and Darley, 1978). We have mentioned earlier that token test scores do not usually correlate very strongly with comprehension of paragraph-length spoken materials. This is probably also true for other tests of comprehension in which isolated sentences are presented (Brookshire and Nicholas, 1984a).

There is another problem with sentence comprehension tests in which the examinee is asked to choose from a set of pictures the one that best expresses the meaning of a heard sentence. In some cases, the correct picture choice can be made without hearing the sentence that describes it.

Figure 5–1 contains four line drawings resembling those found in several sentence comprehension tests. In many cases, once one knows the form of the target

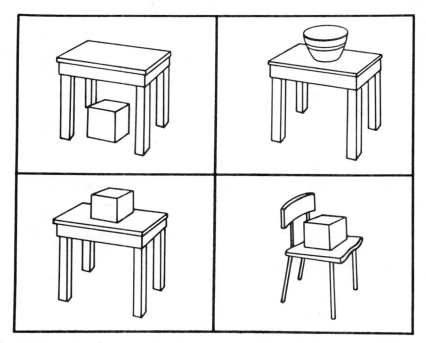

FIG 5–1.
A test plate that resembles those found in many sentence comprehension tests. Deducing the relationships between foils and the target picture may allow correct responses without comprehension of the target sentence, in this example, "The box is on the table."

sentence, the content of the target sentence can be deduced, because foils contrast with the target picture in certain predictable ways, and each foil differs from the target in one characteristic. The easiest way to locate the target picture is to count which characteristics are most often represented in the four choices. In Figure 5–1, "box" is represented three of four times, "on" is represented three of four times, and "table" is represented three of four times. Putting the three words together generates the target sentence "The box is on the table." With a little practice, one can quickly identify the target pictures in items such as these, without ever hearing the target sentences. We do not know whether or not aphasic persons take advantage of this phenomenon, but its existence should cause the user of such comprehension tests to be cautious when interpreting aphasic patients' performance on the tests.

Comprehension of Spoken Discourse

No standardized tests for assessing adults' comprehension of spoken discourse have been published. The BDAE (Goodglass and Kaplan, 1983b) tests comprehension of four short paragraphs and the MTDDA (Schuell, 1972) tests comprehension of one 175-word paragraph. Neither constitutes an adequate test of discourse comprehension. A test of discourse comprehension should test comprehension of several samples of discourse, and it should control or manipulate variables that are known to affect comprehension of normal listeners. The primary determinants of how well non-brain-damaged listeners will comprehend and remember information from spoken discourse are (1) the importance of the information to the overall theme or topic of the discourse, and (2) how explicitly the information is stated. More important information (the *main ideas*) is almost always comprehended and remembered better by non-brain-damaged listeners than less important information (the *details*) (Meyer, 1975; Kintsch, 1974; and others). The importance of information in discourse seems to depend on (1) how often it is embellished by other statements; (2) the extent to which the information relates to other information in the discourse; and (3) the length, complexity, or completeness of the information. Several studies have shown that aphasic listeners usually comprehend and remember main ideas from discourse better than they remember details (see pages 166–167) (Brookshire and Nicholas, 1984a; Wegner et al., 1984; Nicholas and Brookshire, 1986).

Normal speakers do not always specify all the information needed for listeners to understand the meaning and intent of the speaker's utterances (Clark and Haviland, 1977). They often leave informational gaps in what they say, expecting the listener to make inferences and assumptions to fill in the gaps. Consider the following segment of discourse:

> The expensive vase lay on the floor, broken into a thousand fragments. The boy was crying. The red-faced man was shouting angrily at him.

Most normal listeners (or readers) would assume that (1) the boy broke the vase, and (2) the vase belonged to the man. (They would also assume that "him" refers to the boy.) Most normal listeners routinely make such inferences, usually without realizing it (Clark and Haviland, 1977; Kintsch, 1974). However, non-brain-damaged and aphasic listeners usually comprehend and remember explicitly stated information better than implicitly stated information (Brookshire and Nicholas, 1984a; Nicholas and Brookshire, 1986.

OTHER TESTS OF COMMUNICATIVE FUNCTIONS

Auditory Discrimination

Aphasic adults are no more likely to to have auditory discrimination problems than nonaphasic adults of similar age. However, clinicians may encounter a patient whose performance on other tests suggests that they have problems in auditory discrimination. Several tests for assessing auditory discrimination are available (see Darley, 1979, for descriptions of the better-known ones). Most are designed for use with children, and probably are not suitable for use with aphasic adults. Two appear appropriate for aphasic adults: the *Auditory Discrimination Test* and the *Goldman-Fristoe-Woodcock Test of Auditory Discrimination.*

The *Auditory Discrimination Test* (Wepman, 1978) contains 40 pairs of words. They are spoken, 1 pair at a time, by the examiner, and the patient indicates whether each pair contains words that are "same" or "different." Thirty of the pairs contain words that differ by a single phoneme. Ten pairs contain words that do not differ. The test was designed for use with children, who were expected to say "same" or "different" for each pair. For use with aphasic patients, it may be necessary to modify the test procedures so that patients can indicate nonverbally whether the words in pairs are same or different. It may be difficult to administer the test to some aphasic patients who have comprehension problems, because the format of the test is not one that makes sense without verbal instruction. Consequently, repeated instruction and demonstration may be necessary for some aphasic patients to understand what they are to do. Unfortunately, the test procedures are not easily explained nonverbally. An additional difficulty for some aphasic persons will be the concepts "same" and "different," which may prove difficult.

In the *Goldman-Fristoe-Woodcock Test of Auditory Discrimination* (Goldman et al., 1970) the examiner says a one-syllable word and the examinee points to a picture representing the word from a set of four pictures. The test is unique in three respects: (1) it provides procedures for training examinees; (2) test stimuli are presented from a standard audiotape recording, rather than live-voice; and (3) test stimuli are presented both in quiet and in competing noise. The test manual reports that the test was standardized on a sample of 745 persons ranging in age from 3 years to 84 years. Means, standard deviations, and sample sizes are provided for ages 3 years 5 months to 86 years. The *Goldman-Fristoe-Woodcock Test of Auditory Discrimination* appears to be better controlled and to have better norms than the *Auditory Discrimination Test,* although it takes somewhat longer to administer.

An audiometric examination should be performed on all patients whose test performance suggests the presence of auditory perceptual or discrimination deficiencies, in order to determine whether hearing acuity is sufficient for the patient's needs, and if a hearing loss is present, whether a hearing aid or aural rehabilitation might be of value.

Vocabulary

Tests to measure listening or reading vocabulary come in a variety of formats. Most reading tests contain tests of reading vocabulary. Reading vocabulary tests will be discussed later. Picture vocabulary tests, in which the examiner says a test word and the patient chooses, from a set of pictures, the picture that best fits the word, can be useful in evaluating aphasic patients' listening vocabulary. The *Peabody Picture Vocabulary Test* (PPVT) (Dunn, 1965) is the best-known picture vocabulary test in use today. The PPVT is administered by placing a card containing four pictures in front of the patient, saying a stimulus word, and allowing the patient to choose the picture that best matches the word. We have found it useful to present the PPVT in auditory and visual versions. The auditory version is administered in the traditional fashion. In the visual version, instead of saying the stimulus word, the examiner shows the patient a card upon which the word is printed in large black letters.

If a patient does less well on the visual test than on the auditory test, we might suspect the presence of deficiencies in visual perception or visual discrimination. (However, one would first wish to verify that the patient could read before his aphasia. Illiterate aphasic adults occasionally are encountered.) If a patient's performance on the visual version of the test suggests visual perceptual or discrimination anomalies, then the clinician may wish to determine whether the patient can match identical pictures, shapes, symbols, numbers, letters, and words. Efficient matching performance with a given set of printed stimuli would suggest that the patient's visual perception and discrimination are functional. Even though the patient may match identical forms and letters, the patient's ability to match capital letters to small letters and to match block letters to cursive letters should be evaluated if performance on the visual version of the picture vocabulary test is deficient. One may occasionally see patients who do well when matching identical visual stimuli, but perform poorly when they are required to match nonidentical forms or letters, such as matching capital to small letters or block to cursive letters. In these cases, the problem is not likely to be a simple visual perceptual or discrimination problem, but may represent inability to categorize visual symbols on the basis of similarity, or inability to attach meaning to the visual symbols perceived.

If a patient does markedly less well on the auditory version than on the visual version of the test, then the clinician might suspect the presence of auditory perceptual or discrimination anomalies. Tests in which the patient is required to indicate whether pairs of either verbal or nonverbal sounds presented at comfortable listening levels are "same" or "different" are the most convenient method for evaluating a patient's auditory perception and discrimination, although the cautions mentioned in connection with the *Auditory Discrimination Test* and the *Goldman-Fristoe-Woodcock Test of Auditory Discrimination* should be observed.

The standard procedure for administering the PPVT is to establish "basal" and "ceiling" levels. The "basal" is the examinee's last eight consecutive correct responses. The "ceiling" is the point at which the examinee has made six errors in any eight consecutive items. The assumption is that the examinee would not make a significant number of errors on items below the basal, and would miss almost all the items above the ceiling. Many aphasic patients exhibit intermittent patterns of deficit when dealing with language materials. (These patterns will be discussed subsequently.) Because of this intermittency, aphasic patients may make occasional errors on test items that they ordinarily would not miss, and some patients may generate strings of errors that have more to do with the current state of their language processing system than with the actual difficulty of the test items presented. For these reasons, it is probably wise to begin testing aphasic patients with the first item in the test, and to continue testing at least until the point at which nonaphasic adults would be expected to ceiling, or until the examiner is satisfied that the patient is unlikely to respond correctly to a significant number of remaining items.

Reading

A large number of standardized reading examinations are on the market. Most are designed to measure the reading abilities of normal children and adults. Consequently, many are unsatisfactory for testing aphasic persons who may have retention problems or difficulties in following instructions. Therefore, the clinician should select reading tests for aphasic patients with several criteria in mind.

The test should measure both *reading vocabulary* and *reading comprehension*. Reading vocabulary can (loosely) be defined as the number of words that the patient can read and understand. Reading vocabulary usually is measured in one of two ways. The more common way is by means of sentences such as the following, in which the examinee circles, underlines, or points to his choice, as in:

The bell *chimed.*

A. fell B. rang C. rested D. turned

A *strange* person is one who is

A. frightening B. odd C. powerful D. ugly

(From the Nelson Reading Skills Test (Hanna et al., 1977).

Some reading tests, especially those intended for use with primary grade children, assess vocabulary by presenting the individual with pictures and printed words. The examinee circles, underlines, or points to the word that best identifies the picture.

Reading comprehension usually is measured by presenting printed paragraphs together with sets of questions that sample information from each paragraph. The examinee reads each paragraph and answers questions about it. Paragraphs in most reading comprehension tests increase in length and complexity as the test progresses. Some tests (usually those designed for primary grades) employ a picture-to-sentence matching format. The examinee is shown a set of pictures (usually four), along with a question or sentence that identifies one of the pictures. The examinee marks or points to the picture that best represents the sentence or answers the question.

Most reading vocabulary and paragraph comprehension tests are administered with a time limit, and norms are based on test scores obtained under the time limit. In assessing reading abilities of aphasic persons, it is important to know how much the patient can accomplish within the specified time interval, in order to compare the patient's performance with the performance of the group on which test norms are based. However, it is also useful to know how much the patient can accomplish if he or she is permitted to work without time constraints. Therefore, we customarily allow the patient to work at the test for the prescribed time interval. At the end of that interval, the last item completed by the patient is marked, and the patient is permitted to continue until he or she finishes the examination or can go no farther. The time at which the patient stops is then recorded, and the last item completed is marked. By testing in this way, the clinician can obtain estimates of the patient's *reading rate* and *reading capacity*. The former tells us how much the patient can read and understand under normal time constraints, while the latter tells us how much he or she can read under ideal conditions. Most aphasic patients' reading rates are slower than their premorbid rate, even when their vocabulary, word recognition, and word understanding are intact. Therefore, we need to know the patient's ultimate "capacity" in terms of what he or she can read or understand in an ideal situation, with no time pressure. This information is important in planning treatment programs, in counseling the patient and family about what the patient's daily-life capabilities and limitations are likely to be, and in speculating about the eventual recovery of reading abilities.

Reading tests that assess aphasic persons' reading abilities should cover a reasonable range of reading levels. Aphasic patients' reading abilities are distributed across a wide range, from inability to read single words to college-level reading proficiency. Reading examinations for evaluating aphasic persons should measure across this range. However, tests designed to measure primary-grade reading abilities should be chosen carefully, because these tests often contain juvenile themes and artwork that aphasic adults may resent.

The responses required by the reading test should be simple and straightforward if the test is to be used with aphasic patients. Reading tests for use with aphasic persons should not require that answers be written, but should allow the examinee to respond by checking, marking, underlining, or pointing to the correct item chosen from a group of foils.

The test arrangement should be straightforward and unambiguous. Text and response choices should be arranged so that the patient can easily perceive what he or she is to do, without a great deal of instruction from the examiner. Tests that depend heavily on printed or spoken instructions usually are not good choices for evaluating aphasic persons. Ideally, reading tests for aphasic patients should be constructed and arranged so that moderately aphasic patients know what they are to do without verbal instruction. The spatial arrangement of test materials within the test booklet is an important determiner of how easy it will be for aphasic patients to understand what they are to do. Tests in which stimulus items are adjacent to their response choices or questions are better than tests in which a series of test stimuli are given in succession, with response choices presented in a group at the bottom of the page or on a following page.

The test content should be such that it tests reading vocabulary and comprehension, and does not make disproportionate demands on memory, problem-solving strategies, or manual dexterity. For this reason, tests that use machine-scorable answer sheets, in which the patient must read a stimulus item, choose the correct answer from a group of possible answers, remember the number of the test item and the number or letter of the correct choice, find the corresponding test item and choice number or letter on the answer sheet, and blacken the appropriate area on the answer sheet, are inappropriate for use with aphasic patients. Examinations that contain machine-scorable answer sheets often generate transcription and bookkeeping errors, even by nonaphasic persons. Such tests usually can be modified for aphasic individuals so that they do not test memory, bookkeeping, and manual dexterity in addition to reading.

Reading comprehension tests for adults usually make no attempt to measure component skills that underlie comprehension of printed materials. The examiner usually has only a test score, perhaps a percentile rank, and a reading grade level after administering most adult reading comprehension tests. There is disagreement about which "basic skills" are crucial to reading, but we have found that the categories of skills suggested by the *Specific Skills Series* of remedial reading materials (Boning, 1976) offer a useful mechanism for analyzing aphasic patients' reading disabilities. The *Specific Skills Series* divides reading into eight basic skills: (1) matching sounds to symbols, (2) following directions, (3) using context, (4) locating answers, (5) getting facts, (6) getting main ideas, (7) drawing conclusions, and (8) recognizing sequences. Materials are available at several levels of difficulty within each skill. We have found it useful to use samples from appropriate levels within the various skill categories as informal diagnostic tests to assess aphasic patients' reading disabilities and to construct reading treatment programs for them.

The *Nelson Reading Skills Test* (Hanna et al., 1977), an updated version of the *Nelson Reading Test* (Nelson, 1962), is suitable for testing word and paragraph reading for adults with mild to moderate aphasia. The test contains a vocabulary section and a paragraph comprehension section. The vocabulary section of the *Nelson Reading Skills Test* contains items such as:

Strange

    A. frightening
    B. odd
    C. powerful
    D. ugly

The paragraph comprehension section contains paragraphs, followed by multiple-choice questions about the paragraph. The examinee indicates his or her answers by circling or making check marks by choices. Both sections are timed. Eight minutes are allowed for the vocabulary section and 25 minutes are allowed for the paragraph comprehension section. In order to estimate aphasic patients' reading capacity one can mark the last item completed when the prescribed time interval has elapsed, and then allow the patient to proceed until he or she either finishes the section or indicates that he or she can do no more. Reading grade levels and percentile ranks can then be calculated for both timed and untimed performance. (Vocabulary grade levels are higher than paragraph reading grade levels for most aphasic patients.)

The *Nelson Reading Skills Test* measures reading grade levels from grade 3 to grade 9. Many aphasic patients are reading at the lowest levels measured by the *Nelson Reading Skills Test*. Primary grade level reading tests may be useful for assessing these patients' reading abilities. The *Gates-MacGinitie Reading Tests* (primary A and primary C) are appropriate for this purpose. The *Gates-MacGinitie Reading Tests* contain vocabulary and comprehension sections. The *primary A* test measures reading at approximately grade 2. The vocabulary section of the primary A test contains 45 test items, each consisting of a picture and four words, one of which names or describes the picture (Fig 5–2). The examinee marks his choice for each item. The comprehension section contains 40 test items, each consisting of four pictures and a sentence or short paragraph that defines or describes one of the pictures. The examinee marks the picture that best matches the sentence. The *primary C* test measures reading at approximately grade 3. The vocabulary section of the primary C test contains 45 items consisting of a stimulus word and four words or phrases, one of which is synonymous with the stimulus word. The examinee marks the word or phrase that

B

A

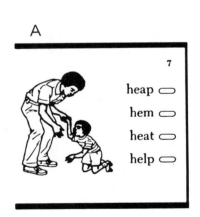

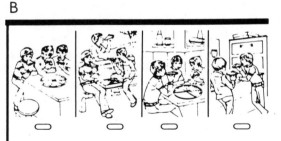

FIG 5–2.
A vocabulary test item **(A)** and a comprehension test item **(B)**. (From the *Gates-MacGinitie Reading Test* (Primary C). Copyright 1978 by Riverside Publishing Company. Used by permission of Houghton-Mifflin Co.)

best defines the stimulus word. The comprehension section of the primary C version contains 22 short paragraphs, each followed by two multiple-choice questions about the paragraph. The examinee marks the word or phrase that best answers each question.

The reading comprehension subtest of the *Peabody Individual Achievement Test* (PIAT) (Dunn and Markwardt, 1970) is appropriate for use with patients representing a range of aphasia severity. In this test, a printed sentence is shown to the patient, then covered by a page containing four pictures, one of which represents the meaning of the sentence. Sentences increase in length (from 5 to 30 words) and difficulty of vocabulary as the test progresses. Norms (grade equivalents and percentiles) are provided for "normal" persons to age 18 years. Most aphasic patients will complete the test in less than 30 minutes, making the test useful for patients with moderate to severe aphasia who might not tolerate longer tests.

The *Reading Comprehension Battery for Aphasia* (RCBA) (LaPointe and Horner, 1979) is the only currently published test designed specifically for evaluating aphasic persons' reading abilities. The RCBA contains ten subtests. Subtests 1, 2, and 3 assess single-word reading. These subtests are designed to detect visual confusions, auditory confusions, and semantic confusions, respectively. Subtest 4 tests "functional reading" of signs, calendars, recipes, and so forth. Subtest 5 requires the examinee to choose synonyms for printed words. Subtest 6 presents single sentences and the examinee is required to choose, from sets of three pictures, the one that best illustrates the meaning of each sentence. Subtest 7 contains two-sentence paragraphs. For each paragraph the examinee chooses, from a set of three pictures, the one identified by the paragraph. Subtests 8 and 9 present 52-word paragraphs and require examinees to demonstrate comprehension of stated and implied information from the paragraphs by selecting a phrase (from three choices) to complete open-ended test sentences. Subtest 10 is a sentence-to-picture matching task in which the subject chooses (from three sentences) the one that best describes a picture. The choice sentences differ in morphology and syntax.

The test manual contains information about test construction and instructions for test administration, response scoring, and test interpretation, together with a short list of references on reading disabilities in aphasia. The test manual contains no documentation of the RCBA's reliability and validity. Some normative information is available elsewhere (VanDemark et al., 1982; Pasternack and LaPointe, 1982).

Most multiple-sentence reading tests intended for use with aphasic persons (reading subtests from aphasia test batteries and the RCBA) are compromised by what is known as the "text independence" of response choices. Text independence means that items testing the information content of paragraphs can be answered without reading the material to which test items refer. Nicholas and Brookshire (1986) evaluated the text independence of multiple-sentence reading subtests from several aphasia test batteries and from the RCBA and found that more than half of the test items in those tests could be answered correctly beyond chance levels by aphasic and non-brain-damaged subjects who had not read the paragraphs to which test items referred. When test items are text independent, one is more likely to be testing general knowledge and cognitive skills than reading comprehension. The test items in the *Nelson Reading Skills Test* have acceptable passage dependence, so this test would probably be a better choice for testing aphasic patients' reading comprehension than multiple-sentence reading tests designed for use with aphasic adults.

Word Retrieval, Formulation

Word Retrieval.—Tests that require the examinee to retrieve and produce words under controlled conditions often are administered to aphasic patients. The *Word Fluency Measure* (Borkowski et al., 1967) is a subtest of the NCCEA (Spreen and Benton, 1977). In the *Word Fluency Measure,* the patient is asked to say, in 1 minute, as many words that begin with a specified letter of the alphabet as he or she can think of. The letter (either F, A, or S) is specified by the examiner. The patient's score is the total of all appropriate words spoken within the 1-minute interval. (Proper names and repetition of the same word with different endings are not accepted.) Norms are provided for aphasic and nonaphasic adults. The *Word Fluency Measure* appears to be a sensitive indicator of brain injury, but it does not discriminate well between aphasic and nonaphasic persons with brain injury. It appears to be of limited usefulness in planning treatment, because the task is an unusual one, with little relationship to daily-life communication.

The *Boston Naming Test* (Kaplan et al., 1983) assesses naming abilities of children, aphasic adults, and normal adults. The test consists of 60 line drawings. The drawings are shown to the examinee one at a time, and the examinee is asked to name each of them. Familiarity (frequency of occurrence of target names) decreases as the test progresses. Responses are scored for latency and correctness. When the examinee misses an item, two kinds of cues may be given. A "stimulus cue" is a short phrase that gives additional information about the target item (e.g., "something to eat"). A "phonetic cue" is the first sound of the target word. Scores are summarized according to (1) number of spontaneously given correct responses, (2) number of correct responses following stimulus cues, and (3) number of correct responses following phonetic cues. The number of stimulus cues and the number of phonetic cues given by the examiner also are recorded. Norms (means, standard deviations, and range of scores) are provided for 30 children (K–5), 84 normal adults (ages 18–59), and 82 aphasic persons (at six levels of aphasia severity).

Sentence Production.—The *Reporter's Test* (DeRenzi and Ferrari, 1978) is a modification of the *Token Test* (DeRenzi and Vignolo, 1962), in which the examiner points to or manipulates tokens in various sequences, and the patient is asked to describe what the examiner does. The *Reporter's Test* has five parts that are analagous to the five parts of the *Token Test.* There are four test items in each of the first four parts and ten in the fifth part. Scoring of responses is either plus-minus or a three-category system in which errors receive 0 points, correct responses receive 1 point, and correct responses following prompts receive 0.5 point. Mean scores and standard deviations are presented for normal and (Italian) aphasic adults. Wener and Duffy (1983) compared the *Reporter's Test* with other measures of speech production and comprehension for English-speaking aphasic persons.

Speech Fluency.—Several methods for assessing speech fluency of patients with neurogenic communication disorders have appeared in the literature. None have been standardized, and their reliability remains to be documented, but they do provide procedures with which patients' speech fluency can be assessed in more or less systematic fashion.

Wagenaar et al. (1975) attempted to construct procedures by which the type and severity of any patient's aphasia could be determined on the basis of the patient's speech. They carried out a factor analysis on the speech production of 156 Dutch aphasic patients. They evaluated 30 factors and concluded that:

(1) The primary dimension for classifying aphasia patients on the basis of their spontaneous speech production is a fluency scale. (2) Telegraphic speech and empty speech exist as identifiable syndromes, and represent two separate scales, not opposite ends of a single 'semantic density' scale. (3) Grammatical mistakes and articulatory difficulties are separate factors in the speech of aphasics, [sic] not directly related to the fluency dimension. (4) Patients can be classified as fluent or nonfluent on the basis of two variables, speech tempo and mean length of utterance.

"Speech tempo," according to Wagenaar et al., is the number of words produced in 6 minutes. The authors reported that they were developing a shortened version of their procedures for clinical use. The procedures described in their 1975 report are too cumbersome for routine clinical use, but their list of variables and their results may be useful for the clinician who wishes to develop a systematic procedure for analyzing aphasic patients' spontaneous speech.

The BDAE (Goodglass and Kaplan, 1972; Goodglass and Kaplan, 1983) includes a "rating scale profile of speech characteristics" with which a patient's spontaneous speech (elicited during the conversational and expository speech section of the BDAE) is rated on melodic line, phrase length, articulatory agility, grammatical form, paraphasia, repetition, and word finding. Volume (voice intensity), voice quality, and speech rate can also be rated. The rating scale is relatively subjective, but can be used to construct a speech profile that can be compared with profiles for major aphasia syndromes. The scale also is useful as a general description of the characteristics of a given patient's speech.

The WAB (Kertesz, 1982) includes several speech production subtests, and patients' speech is scored for both form and content, using an 11-point (0–10) scale for each dimension. Speech fluency is important in Kertesz's "taxonomic" approach, in which patients may be assigned to diagnostic categories (Broca's, Wernicke's, etc.) according to their performance on the WAB. Trupe (1984) has questioned the reliability of the WAB's procedures for scoring spontaneous speech, as well as the validity of assigning patients to diagnostic categories based on those scores.

Intelligibility.—The major standardized measure of speech intelligibility for use with brain-injured adults is *Assessing Intelligibility of Dysarthric Speech* (AIDS) (Yorkston and Beukelman, 1981). Speech intelligibility is more often of concern with dysarthric than with aphasic speakers. The AIDS test is discussed in that context (see pages 258–259).

Paraphasia.—Description of what are called "paraphasic" speech errors can be useful in assigning aphasic patients to diagnostic categories, and the occurrence of paraphasic errors in the speech of an aphasic patient can give clues to the nature of the patient's word retrieval, encoding, and production problems. A *paraphasia* is an error in speaking. Two kinds of paraphasias have been described in the literature, although there is some confusion about which speech errors qualify as paraphasias. *Literal paraphasias* (sometimes called phonemic paraphasias) are errors in which some of the sounds in a word are incorrectly produced or in the wrong place ("pote" for "coat", or "tevelision" for "television"). Literal paraphasias consist of syllable transpositions, intrusions of extraneous sounds, or substitutions of one correctly articulated phoneme for another. *Verbal paraphasias* (sometimes called semantic paraphasias) are errors in which a complete word is substituted for the intended word ("chair" for "table", or "socks" for "shoes"). Verbal paraphasias usually have some semantic relationship to the intended word, but this is not always the case. Literal paraphasias are associated with parietal or temporal lobe lesions, and verbal paraphasias are associated with temporal lobe lesions.

It is important to differentiate between literal paraphasia and the "phonetic disintegration" that occurs with lesions in the posterior inferior frontal lobe (causing Broca's aphasia, or "apraxia of speech"). Literal paraphasias occur in a context of otherwise fluent and effortless speech, with essentially normal rate, intonation, and inflection, although some struggle may be seen when the patient attempts to correct an incorrectly produced word or phrase. "Phonetic disintegration" occurs in a context of effortful and nonfluent speech, in which rate, intonation, and inflection are diminished, and effortful articulatory posturing is present, both on the original attempt and on attempts at correction.

Canter (1973) has suggested that the term "literal paraphasia" should refer to a *pattern* of articulatory errors that are made by aphasic persons, and that the term should not be used to describe individual articulatory errors, especially those committed by patients who are dysarthric rather than aphasic. For this reason, it is not sufficient to tabulate only the frequency and kinds of articulatory errors that occur in the speech of those with central nervous system injuries. One must also consider the context in which the articulatory errors occur. Articulatory errors by aphasic persons that occur in a context of fluent, effortless speech may be labeled "paraphasias"—those that occur in a context of nonfluent, effortful articulatory posturing cannot be so labeled.

Spelling

The spelling subtest of the *Wide Range Achievement Test* (WRAT) (Jastak and Wilkinson, 1984) can provide information about aphasic patients' spelling abilities. The spelling subtest has three parts—copying marks that resemble printed letters, writing one's name, and writing single words to dictation. Norms are available for normal adults through 64 years of age. We have found it useful to give the test in three versions: (1) the examiner says the word and the patient writes it (the standard procedure); (2) the examiner says the word and the patient spells it aloud; and (3) the examiner spells the word aloud and the patient names the word. The latter two versions are only partially a test of spelling ability, because they place demands on patients' auditory memory and sequencing abilities, especially as words become longer. Aphasic patients with posterior cerebral injuries and impaired language comprehension do especially poorly on the latter two versions, even when their written spelling is relatively good.

The spelling subtest of the PIAT (Dunn and Markwardt, 1970) may also be useful in evaluating aphasic patients' spelling, especially when the clinician suspects that production problems may interfere with the patient's ability to produce words that he or she knows how to spell. The test requires that the patient recognize and point to the correctly spelled word when it is shown on a card along with three misspelled versions of the word. The test begins with a 14-item training set, in which the patient is trained, by successive approximations, how to do the test. (This section may be useful when a severely aphasic patient is tested.) The spelling test itself contains 70 words with frequency of occurrence gradually decreasing as the test progresses. Norms (grade equivalents and percentiles) are given for persons 5 to 18 years of age. For aphasic patients, recognition of correctly spelled words is almost always better than correct written production of the same words. Consequently, most aphasic patients will get higher scores (and higher grade levels) on recognition spelling tests (such as the PIAT) than on tests in which they must produce the words (such as the WRAT).

Although some aphasia test batteries include tests of spelling in which patients write words to dictation, the results of these spelling tests do not allow one to compare the patient with nonaphasic persons of equivalent age. Tests such as the spelling subtests of the WRAT and the PIAT allow one to transform a patient's score into a spelling grade level or a percentile rank that allows one to estimate how the patient's spelling compares with "normal" spelling. Such estimates may be meaningful to family members, physicians, and others who may not be trained in interpretation of the tests administered to the patient. Furthermore, knowing a patient's spelling grade level allows us to estimate his or her functional spelling ability in daily-life environments with somewhat more assurance than if we have only a score, with no conversion to grade equivalents or percentiles for a normal population.

Arithmetic, Mathematics

In many cases, the clinician may wish to assess an aphasic patient's arithmetic ability. This is more likely to be the case with patients whose aphasia is moderate or mild and who are functioning independently or semi-independently in daily life than it is for patients with severe aphasia who do not have functional communicative abilities. In those cases in which the clinician simply wishes to determine whether the patient can perform basic arithmetic operations (addition, subtraction, multiplication, division) in order to carry out daily-life activities such as making change, balancing a checkbook, and so forth, the arithmetic subtest of an aphasia test battery such as the MTDDA (Schuell, 1972) or the supplemental arithmetic subtest from the BDAE (Goodglass and Kaplan, 1983) may be sufficient. In those cases in which the clinician wishes a more extensive analysis of a patient's mathematical abilities, or wishes to compare the patient's mathematical abilities with those of nonaphasic persons, a standardized arithmetic examination should be administered. We have found the arithmetic subtest of the WRAT (Jastak and Wilkinson, 1984) useful for these latter purposes. The WRAT arithmetic subtest has two levels. Level 1 is less difficult than Level 2, and is more appropriate for aphasic patients. The problems in Level 1 range in difficulty from simple addition and subtraction to finding square root and solving simple equations.

The PIAT (Dunn and Markwardt, 1970) also contains a mathematics subtest, in which the examiner reads aloud a problem and the examinee selects the correct answer from a plate of four answers. Because of the demands that this format places on auditory comprehension, this mathematics test may not be satisfactory for many aphasic patients. However, if a patient could not write numbers but had good auditory comprehension, the mathematics test from the PIAT might be useful.

TESTS OF INTELLECT AND COGNITION

In addition to tests of communicative function, the clinician may administer other tests that are designed to evaluate a patient's verbal and nonverbal intelligence, attention, memory, and perception. Many of these tests are also administered by neuropsychologists as part of their assessment battery for brain-injured patients. If neuropsychologic services are available, the speech-language pathologist and the neuropsychologist may divide the responsibilities for assessment, with the speech-language pathologist concentrating on the patient's communicative abilities and the neuropsychologist assessing other aspects of the patient's intellectual and cognitive abilities.

Verbal and Nonverbal Intelligence

Aphasic patients' scores on *verbal intelligence tests* are almost always depressed because of their problems with comprehension and production of verbal materials. Even so, the results of testing verbal intelligence can be of value if the effects of aphasia on the scores obtained are considered, and if the results are used to deduce the nature of the patient's problems with verbal material rather than as an estimate of his or her intelligence.

Estimates of an aphasic patient's *nonverbal intelligence* are of great importance in assessment of the patient's deficits, and in planning treatment for the patient's aphasia. In most cases of aphasia caused by unilateral lesions, we expect that the patient's nonverbal intelligence should be at or near premorbid levels. If an aphasic patient's nonverbal intelligence is abnormally depressed, the prognosis for recovery is more pessimistic, and the objectives of treatment may be modified to account for the patient's intellectual limitations.

Note: In order to protect the integrity of the tests described in the following section, the examples given are similar to, but not identical with, actual items in the tests.

The Wechsler Adult Intelligence Scale

The most widely used measure of adult intelligence is the *Wechsler Adult Intelligence Scale* (WAIS) (Wechsler, 1955), and its revised version, the *Wechsler Adult Intelligence Scale–Revised* (WAIS-R) (Wechsler, 1981). The WAIS-R is divided into two sections—a *verbal scale* and a *nonverbal (performance) scale.* Verbal and nonverbal subtests alternate when the WAIS-R is administered.

The Verbal Scale.—There are six subtests in the verbal scale. The *information* subtest tests general knowledge that could be acquired by anyone growing up in the United States. The questions range in difficulty from those that only retarded persons would fail (e.g., "How many days are there in a week?") to those that only a few "normal" persons would answer correctly (e.g., "Who wrote *The Republic?*").

The second subtest in the verbal scale is the *digit span* subtest, containing *digits forward* and *digits backward.* In *digits forward,* the examiner reads a random number sequence aloud at a rate of one number per second and the patient is asked to repeat the sequence back to the examiner. Sequences range in length from three to nine numbers. In *digits backward,* the examiner reads the number sequences aloud and the patient is asked to repeat them back in reverse order. Sequences range in length from two to eight numbers.

The third subtest in the verbal scale is the *vocabulary* subtest. It contains 35 words, arranged in increasing order of difficulty. The examiner says each word aloud in the carrier phrase "what does _____ mean?" Test items range from easy ("What does *window* mean?") to difficult ("What does *ostentatious* mean?").

The fourth subtest in the verbal scale is the *arithmetic* subtest. Problems range from simple calculations to complex word problems. In the standard administration of this subtest, problems are given orally and oral responses are required.

The fifth subtest in the verbal scale is the *comprehension* subtest. It includes two kinds of open-ended questions. Most assess common sense, judgment, and reasoning ("Why do children attend school?"). A few ask the patient to give the meaning of proverbs ("What does this saying mean? 'Still waters run deep.'"). Some of the questions are long ("What is the thing to do if you are in a grocery store and you see a broken jar of jelly on the floor?"). Patients with decreased short-term verbal memory may fail these questions for that reason.

The sixth subtest in the verbal scale is the *similarities* subtest. In this subtest the examiner says pairs of words to the patient and the patient is asked to tell what the words have in common. The pairs range from easy (carrot-potato) to difficult (bird-violin).

The Performance Scale.—There are five subtests in the performance scale. The first is *picture completion.* A series of pictures that contain missing elements is shown to the patient, and the patient is asked to tell the examiner what is missing (or point to the location of the missing element). Picture completion seems to be sensitive to general intellectual ability, and to visual-spatial ability.

The second performance scale subtest is *picture arrangement.* In this subtest several sets of cartoon-like pictures are shown to the patient. Each set can make a chronologically organized story. Pictures within each set are presented in scrambled order, and the patient is asked to arrange the pictures in the set so that they tell a story. Each set is timed, and there is a time limit for each set. The picture arrangement subtest appears to be sensitive to brain damage in general. Patients who have difficulties with temporal order will have deficient performance on this subtest, and there appears to be an element of "social sophistication" operating in performance on this subtest (Lezak, 1983).

The third performance scale subtest is the *block design* subtest. The patient is given either four (initially) or nine (later) red and white blocks and asked to construct reproductions of patterns constructed by the examiner or depicted on cards. The test is timed, and the way in which the patient goes about the task may be recorded and analyzed. Block design appears to be sensitive to general intellectual abilities, visual-spatial abilities, and constructional abilities. Left hemisphere lesions are less likely than right hemisphere lesions to cause deficient block design performance, although patients with left parietal damage usually show deficient performance on this subtest.

The fourth subtest in the performance scale is the *object assembly* subtest. In this test, four cut-up pressboard figures of common objects are presented, one at a time, to the patient, and the patient is asked to assemble each of them. There is a time limit for each item. The object assembly subtest appears to be sensitive to visual-spatial reasoning abilities and attention.

The fifth subtest in the performance scale is the *digit symbol* subtest (Fig 5–3). In the test, the patient is given a sheet of paper on which there are 100 blank boxes, each with a randomly assigned number from 1 to 9 printed above it. A key, which is printed at the beginning of the subtest, assigns a simple graphic nonsense symbol to each number (1–9). The patient's task is to write, in each blank box, the symbol

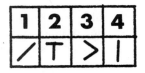

FIG 5–3.
An example of a digit symbol subtest task. A key assigns symbols to numbers *(top)*. The examinee fills in the blank boxes *(bottom)* according to the key.

that goes with the number just above the box. The test is timed (90 sec). The digit symbol test requires attention, visual-spatial ability, and motor coordination, and appears to be a sensitive indicator of even minimal brain damage.

We usually expect that aphasic patients without other complicating mental conditions will do much better on the performance scale of the WAIS than they will do on the verbal scale. In fact, many aphasic patients may score within normal limits on the performance scale, although few would achieve such scores on the verbal scale. Test items in the verbal scale are said aloud by the examiner, and many are relatively long. Consequently, deficiencies in auditory memory and auditory comprehension may cause aphasic patients to have problems understanding the stimuli in the verbal subtests. Items in the verbal subtests also require spoken responses. Aphasic patients who have production and formulation difficulties will have difficulty with these subtests. For aphasic patients, the verbal scale subtests are more likely to be a measure of aphasia than intelligence.

Raven's Progressive Matrices

Raven's *Standard Progressive Matrices* (Raven, 1960), and *Coloured Progressive Matrices* (Raven, 1965) are tests of intelligence and reasoning ability with low verbal loadings. Consequently, they are useful in estimating the intellectual and reasoning abilities of aphasic patients. Both tests are multiple-choice tests in which the patient is shown visual patterns in which a part is missing. The patient is asked to choose from a set of six or eight choices the one that completes the stimulus (Fig 5–4). The *Standard Progressive Matrices* consists of 60 items, divided into five sets of 12 items each. The *Coloured Progressive Matrices* consists of 36 items, is easier, and is for testing children and for testing adults 65 years old and up. The *Standard Progressive Matrices* has numerous difficult items that may require verbal reasoning for their solution. For most aphasic patients, the *Coloured Progressive Matrices* are appropriate. However, for the aphasic patient with mild aphasia, the standard (more difficult) version may be appropriate.

Other Measures

A number of other measures often are useful in understanding the nature of aphasic patients' problems, and in planning their treatment. These measures allow us to estimate the patient's intellectual and cognitive abilities, memory, planning abilities, and perceptual abilities. All are important in management of the patient and his or her treatment program.

Sustained Attention, Set-Shifting

The *Wisconsin Card Sorting Test* (Grant and Berg, 1948) has limited verbal loading and may be useful in evaluating aphasic patients' sustained attention and cognitive flexibility. The patient is given a pack of cards. On each card is printed one or more colored symbols (triangle, star, circle, cross). The patient is asked to sort the cards into groups having a common characteristic. The patient is not told the characteristic, but must deduce it from the examiner's feedback as the patient sorts the

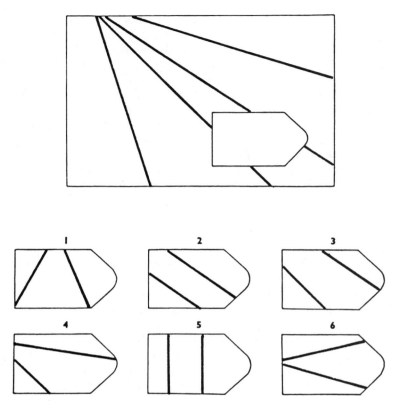

FIG 5–4.
An example of the Progressive Matrices task. The examinee chooses the pattern segment at the bottom that best completes the overall pattern at the top.

cards. The examiner tells the patient "right" or "wrong" after each card placement. The first relevant dimension is color, and the patient is reinforced for sorting the cards into groups in which all cards have the same color. When the patient makes ten consecutive correct sorting responses with color as the relevant dimension, the examiner changes (without announcing it to the patient) the relevant dimension to form. When the patient makes ten consecutive correct sorting responses using form as the relevant dimension, the examiner changes the relevant dimension to number, without telling the patient. When the patient makes ten consecutive correct responses using number as the relevant dimension, the examiner changes the relevant dimension to color, and testing continues until color, form, and number have been used twice each. The *Wisconsin Card Sorting Test* appears to measure patients' ability to change "set" within a task. The test appears to be sensitive to frontal lobe damage, especially damage to the left frontal lobe.

The *Trail-Making Test* (War Department, 1944) measures sustained attention and visual-motor coordination. In part A of the test, the patient is given a pencil and a paper on which an array of circled numerals is printed. The patient is instructed to draw a line that connects the circles, starting at 1 and going to 2, and so forth. When the patient has finished part A, he or she is given part B, which assesses the patients's ability to shift mental set, in addition to the skills mentioned above. In part B, the patient is given a page on which is printed an array of circled numerals and letters. The patient is instructed to draw a line that connects the numerals and letters in sequence (e.g., 1−A−2−B, and so forth). The *Trail-Making Test* is sensitive to brain injury, and it has been suggested that patients with left hemisphere injuries do strikingly less well on the numeral-letter version than on the numeral only version (Reitan and Tarshes, 1959). The *Trail-Making Test* appears to be strongly correlated with general intellectual ability. Because of its low verbal loading, it may give useful estimates of aphasic patients' cognitive functioning, and observation of how the patient goes about the task may provide useful information about his or her general approach to solving such problems.

Memory

The *Wechsler Memory Scale* (WMS) (Stone et al., 1946) is a well-known memory test battery. It contains seven subtests. The *personal and current information* subtest asks for information about contemporary government officials ("Who is President of the United States?"). The *orientation* subtest asks questions about the patient's current surroundings ("What day is today?"). The *mental control* subtest asks the patient to recite automatized sequences (the alphabet) and to count (by either threes or fours). In the *logical memory* subtest, two paragraphs are read to the patient and the patient is asked to retell each of them. The *digit span* subtest is similar to the digit span subtest in the WAIS. In the *visual reproduction* subtest, the patient is shown line drawings of geometric figures and is asked to draw them from memory. In the *associate learning* subtest, the patient hears ten pairs of words read aloud (six are "easy," four are "difficult"), and is asked to retell all the pairs that he or she remembers. The list is presented three times, with a recall trial after each presentation.

A number of shortcomings of the WMS have been pointed out (Lezak, 1983). One of the more important, with respect to aphasic patients, is that six of the seven subtests require relatively good comprehension of verbal materials or the ability to produce verbal responses. Consequently, the WMS may be inappropriate for use with many aphasic patients.

Russell (1975) developed the *Revised Wechsler Memory Scale,* (RWMS), which includes the *logical memory* and *visual reproduction* subtests from the WMS (Wechsler, 1945). Memory is tested immediately after test items are presented and after 30 minutes of intervening activity. The *Revised Wechsler Memory Scale,* like the original, may be inappropriate for many, if not most, aphasic patients because of the high verbal loading on the logical memory test. In addition, there is some evidence that verbal skills may participate in delayed recall of visual figures such as those in the visual reproduction test (Lezak, 1983).

Verbal Memory.— Digits forward and digits backward subtests are administered as part of the WAIS (Wechsler, 1955; Wechsler, 1981) or the WMS (Wechsler, 1945; Wechsler, 1987). The two tests also can be administered by themselves. The results give an estimate of the patient's immediate verbal memory. Immediate memory appears to be important in oral repetition, in some kinds of comprehension tasks (such as the *Token Test*), in some arithmetic tasks, and in some spelling tasks.

Nonverbal Memory.—Tests of nonverbal memory usually require recognition or reproduction of geometric designs or sequences of nonverbal symbols. In the *Visual Retention Test* (Warrington and James, 1967), a series of 25-cell arrays with 5 black cells in each array are presented, 1 at a time, and the patient is asked to choose the figure from a set of 4 (Fig 5–5).

The *Memory for Designs Test* (Graham and Kendall, 1960), and the *Revised Benton Visual Retention Test* (Benton, 1974) present visual designs and ask the patient to draw the designs from memory (Fig 5–6). (There is also a multiple-choice version of the *Revised Benton Visual Retention Test.*) Tests that allow the patient to choose "just-seen" stimuli from a group appear to be somewhat more clearly related to visual memory than tests that require the patient to draw the designs, because the latter require manual dexterity and visual-spatial abilities for successful performance.

"Functional" Memory

The *Rivermead Behavioral Memory Test* (Wilson et al., 1985) is a short test of "everyday memory functioning" that tests a patient's ability to remember in ana-

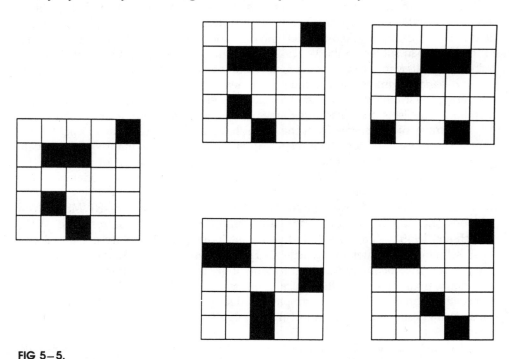

FIG 5–5.
A visual retention test task. The stimulus at the *left* is shown and removed, and the examinee chooses the stimulus array from a set of four *(right)*.

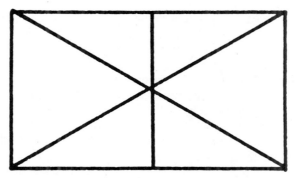

FIG 5—6.
A memory for designs test task. The examinee is shown a design such as the one shown here and draws it from memory.

logues of daily life situations that, in the authors' experience, are difficult for patients with brain injuries. The test assesses (1) remembering a name (first and second) of a person in a photograph; (2) remembering where the examiner has hidden one of the patient's belongings; (3) remembering an appointment; (4) immediate memory for pictures of common objects; (5) memory for a short narrative passage that the examiner has read aloud; (6) delayed memory for pictures of common objects; (7) face recognition; (8) remembering a short route demonstrated by the examiner; and (9) orientation to time, place, and person. The maximum score possible is 12 points. A score of 9 or lower is considered "impaired."

Planning and Foresight

One of the most popular tests of planning and foresight is the *Porteus Maze Test* (Porteus, 1959). The test has minimal verbal loading, and can be a useful indicator of an aphasic patient's ability to plan and carry out alternative courses of action. The test consists of a series of printed mazes of increasing difficulty. The patient is given a pencil and is instructed to trace a path through each maze without entering any blind alleys. The test is not timed, and may be performed with either hand. A patient's "quantitative" score is based on the number of times blind alleys are entered. A patient's "qualitative" score is affected by crossing lines or leaving gaps in the traced line. The test is sensitive to brain damage, particularly damage to the right frontal lobe, but it appears not to be particularly sensitive to aphasia—many aphasic patients will score within the normal range on this test.

Visual Perception

Aphasic patients sometimes exhibit visual perceptual anomalies that may influence testing and treatment. The most frequently seen anomalies in visual perception in aphasia are *visual organization* disorders. Tests of visual organization often present *incomplete visual stimuli, fragmented visual stimuli,* or *figure-ground discrimination* (Lezak, 1983). According to Lezak (1983), tests involving incomplete visual stimuli are not very sensitive to perceptual problems and will identify only relatively severe problems. Tests with fragmented visual stimuli appear sensitive to problems of visual organization. The *object assembly* subtest of the WAIS (Wechsler, 1955; Wechsler, 1981) presents fragmented visual stimuli. The *Hooper Visual Organization Test* (Hooper, 1958) is a relatively popular test of visual organization that tests perception of fragmented stimuli. The patient is presented with a series of pictures depicting cut-up line drawings of common objects and is asked to say or write the name of the object depicted in each picture (Fig 5–7). Because of the verbal nature of the responses required, this test may not be appropriate for aphasic patients who have difficulty writing or speaking. However, the test could be modified to allow aphasic patients to point to their choice from a set of foils.

Visual figure-ground tests usually involve (1) stimuli in which test figures are embedded in more complex figures, as in the *Hidden Figures Test* (Thurstone, 1944); (2) stimuli in which test figures overlap (Fig 5–8) (Poppelreuter, 1917); or (3) stimuli in which lines are drawn over test figures (Luria, 1965). In most of these tests the patient is expected to name the test stimuli (the *Hidden Figures Test* is an exception). Consequently, these tests may not be appropiate for many aphasic patients, unless the response format is changed to eliminate the possibility that naming problems may affect test results.

Tests of visual perception are often important in assessing patients with nondominant-hemisphere damage who often exhibit striking anomalies in visual perception and organization. One of the most striking of these anomalies is *visual neglect*, or inattention to visual stimuli on the side contralateral to the brain damage. Tests for visual neglect are discussed as part of assessment procedures for patients with nondominant-hemisphere damage (see Chapter 8), but the reader should remember that other tests of visual perception are also important in assessing patients with nondominant-hemisphere pathology.

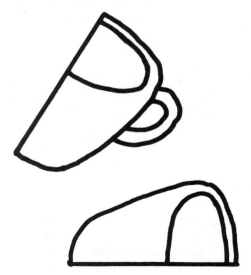

FIG 5–7.
An example of a fragmented stimulus test item. The examinee names the object depicted.

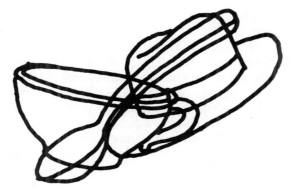

FIG 5–8.
An example of an overlapping figures test item. The examinee names all the items that he or she can identify.

TEST INTERPRETATION

Differential Diagnosis

In differential diagnosis of neurogenic communication disorders one identifies a given patient's speech and language disabilities, and affixes a label to the patient's condition. The label may have several implications, including (1) the location of the lesion(s) causing the patient's symptoms; (2) the nature of the patient's communicative disabilities; and (3) the patient's probable course of recovery.

Labels are convenient devices for describing a given patient in terms of the characteristics that generally are seen in the population of patients bearing that particular label. However, there are dangers associated with labeling. If a patient differs in some respects from the general characteristics of the diagnostic group (and most aphasic patients do), then these differences may be obscured, lost, or forgotten, and it will (incorrectly) be assumed that the patient has only those characteristics implied by the label. Another danger is that when a label is affixed to a patient, the clinician may assume that further exploration of the patient's disabilities is not needed. As a consequence, the patient's deficits may be inaccurately or incompletely described and treatment may be inefficient or ineffective. It is true that one treats patients and not diagnostic labels. However, this truth may be violated in the rush to affix a diagnostic label to the patient's condition.

Affixing a diagnostic label to a patient has an all-or-none character that may not match reality. Concluding that a patient is aphasic implies that there are two mutually exclusive and exhaustive categories of persons—"aphasic" and "not aphasic." No such dichotomy exists. Any demarcation point that separates individuals into "aphasic" and "nonaphasic" groups must be established arbitrarily. No matter where the demarcation point is, there will be an area around it containing individuals who are similar in their communication abilities. Yet some would be labeled "aphasic," while others would be labeled "not aphasic." Similar problems exist no matter what label is affixed. However, the advantages of labeling—a convenient shorthand for communicating about patients—are sufficient to justify it, as long as one recognizes the problems of labeling.

Differential diagnosis in aphasia usually means determining whether a given patient is aphasic, and then deciding what "kind" of aphasia is present. Sometimes clinicians are asked to determine whether a patient's condition represents aphasia or some other disorder of language or cognition. Questions of differential diagnosis most frequently involve differentiating aphasia from confusion, dementia, nondominant hemisphere pathology, psychiatric states, or malingering. Assessment of dementia and nondominant hemisphere pathology will be discussed subsequently. Confusion, psychologic disturbances, and malingering are discussed below.

Confusion

"Language of confusion" has been described by Halpern et al., (1973), who reported that patients with language of confusion exhibit mild overall impairments in language functions, with moderate impairments in arithmetic, reading comprehension, writing to dictation, and semantic relevance of speech output. According to Halpern et al. confused patients usually exhibit subtle impairments in auditory comprehension and short-term auditory memory, speech fluency and syntax, naming, and the correctness and elaborateness of responses. According to Wertz (1978) confused patients have difficulty recognizing and understanding their surroundings, and exhibit faulty memory, muddled thinking, and disorientation to time and place. Confused patients' vocabulary and syntax usually are within normal limits, but spontaneous speech may be confabulatory and not relevant to the situation. The onset of confusion usually is abrupt, and confusion sometimes follows physical or medical mishaps. Traumatic head injuries, metabolic or chemical disruptions, intoxication, withdrawal, infections, and central nervous system disease or pathology can cause confusion. At other times confusion appears without observable cause, and confusion is an important symptom of dementia (to be discussed later). Confused patients usually have relatively good comprehension, vocabulary, and syntax. This helps to differentiate confused patients from those who are aphasic. The irrelevant, confabulatory, and sometimes bizarre spontaneous speech of confused patients also helps to differentiate them from patients who are aphasic, although the spontaneous speech of patients with severe Wernicke's aphasia may sometimes resemble that of confused patients. However, the confused and confabulating patient's comprehension is likely to be far superior to that of a patient with severe Wernicke's aphasia. Most confused patients are unaware of the aberrant quality of their speech. This helps to differentiate them from most aphasic patients (patients with severe Wernicke's aphasia are the exception).

Psychologic Disturbances

Some psychologic disturbances may generate speech and language anomalies and make one wonder if the patient might be aphasic. However, in most cases of psychopathology, patients' auditory comprehension, reading comprehension, and syntax are normal. In most psychologic disorders, the abnormalities are in the content of spoken and written language. These abnormalities usually relate to the appropriateness, relevance, and cohesion of ideas, rather than to problems in word selection, word retrieval, and sentence formulation such as one sees in aphasia. Patients with psychologic disorders usually exhibit disruptions of affect and lucidity, and may report hallucinations. Psychologic disorders usually are gradual in onset, and there may be a family history of psychologic problems. The course of the disorder may be one of exacerbation and remission, with symptoms advancing and retreating in cyclic fashion. None of these characteristics are commonly associated with aphasia.

Malingering

Occasionally one sees a patient who is suspected of malingering (purposely exhibiting aphasic symptoms in the absence of organic pathology). Porec and Porch (1977) have described several signs of malingering. The most consistent sign is equivalent performance across subtests, regardless of the linguistic difficulty of the subtests. That is, malingerers tend to make too many errors on subtests that would be easy for aphasic persons, and not enough errors on subtests that would be difficult for aphasic persons. According to Porec and Porch, malingering patients have a tendency to focus on speech—they often present severe speech impairments with little or no impairment of comprehension. Another sign of nonorganicity is inconsistency in test performance on successive test occasions. If the same tests are repeated several times, a few days to a week apart, the performance of many "malingering" patients changes unpredictably from test to test. Finally, one can sometimes find a "payoff" for being aphasic in the lives of malingering patients, although it is by no means always the case. We once saw a patient who had developed severe expressive aphasia and dense hemiplegia three times several months apart, with a "miraculous" cure and complete recovery each time. Each time he was cured, his church had a service of thanksgiving for him, in which he was the center of attention. We suspected that the attention may have helped to precipitate his bouts of "aphasia."

Chapter 6

The Context for Treatment of Neurogenic Communication Disorders

In spite of more than a century of concern about treatment of adults with neurogenic communication disorders, it remains as much art as science. Of the thousands of data-based studies of neurogenic communication disorders, only a small proportion are directly relevant to remediation. Of the many published reports of treatment procedures, most are simply descriptions of the procedures, with anecdotes or the author's opinions substituting for empirical evidence concerning their efficacy. Consequently, decisions about how to approach a given patient's communicative impairments usually rely more on experience and intuition than on empirical evidence. There are regularities in how adults with neurogenic communication disorders respond to manipulations of the clinical environment, and patients with certain characteristics tend to respond to those manipulations in predictable ways, although idiosyncratic responses are common. In this chapter I will discuss the context in which treatment of neurogenic communication impairments takes place. I will describe how brain damage may affect general processes and create behavioral predispositions that affect how treatment progresses and what the outcome will be, how clinicians decide *who* and *what* to treat, and some general characteristics of treatment for patients with neurogenic communication disorders.

GENERAL EFFECTS OF BRAIN DAMAGE ON BEHAVIOR

In addition to creating specific impairments in reading, writing, speaking, and listening, brain damage often alters the way patients approach tasks, solve problems, respond to stimuli, and monitor their performance. These alterations are not task-specific, although they usually are exacerbated when the patient is having difficulty.

116

Although they are not in themselves communicative impairments, they often interfere with communication, and modifying them often makes the patient a better communicator.

Diminished Response Flexibility

Most brain-damaged patients have difficulty adjusting their behavior when tasks or response requirements change. Their performance tends to deteriorate when new tasks are introduced, or when stimuli or response requirements change within tasks. A patient who has been naming objects may continue to name when the task changes to description of function, and may periodically revert to naming thereafter. For most patients, this initial worsening of performance is followed by gradual recovery as long as the new conditions continue unchanged.

Task-Related Anomalies

Impulsiveness.—Some brain-damaged patients are unusually impulsive. They respond quickly to questions, assertions, problems, and situations on the basis of their initial impressions, without taking time to deduce the actual meaning of stimuli, events, or situations. This causes them to miss implications, inferences, and nuances of meaning. Impulsiveness is common after traumatic brain injuries, and many right-hemisphere-damaged patients are impulsive. Impulsiveness is less common in aphasic patients, although patients with fluent aphasia and posterior lesions sometimes are impulsive.

Excessive Caution.—Some brain-damaged patients are excessively cautious and reluctant to respond whenever they are uncertain about a situation or their performance. These patients mistrust their own perceptions of stimuli, events, and situations and their ability to judge the adequacy of their responses. This mistrust makes them hesitate to "take a chance" in challenging, threatening, and unpredictable situations, and they sometimes become excessively cautious and reluctant to respond. Excessive caution is relatively common in patients with mild focal impairments, in high-level patients with traumatic brain injuries, and in patients with mild dementia.

Horner and LaPointe (1979) characterized brain-damaged persons' impulsiveness and cautiousness as variations in *cognitive style*. Patients with *reflective style* proceed through tasks slowly, take a long time to respond, and (usually) make few errors. Patients with *impulsive style* proceed through tasks quickly, respond quickly, and (usually) make many errors. They suggested that treatment should take a patient's cognitive style into account. According to Horner and LaPointe, patients who go slowly but make many errors need training in or revision of the task to make it easier. Patients who proceed through a task slowly and make no errors may be speeded up, as long as speeding them up does not generate errors. Patients who respond quickly and make many errors may be helped by slowing them down. Patients who respond quickly but make no errors in a task probably need a more difficult task (Fig 6–1).

Perseveration.— Many brain-damaged persons exhibit perseveration. Perseveration refers to the repetition of responses when they are no longer appropriate, such as when a patient who has correctly named a pencil calls the next several objects pencils, or when a patient who has correctly given his name in response to the examiner's request continues to give his name in response to the examiner's questions about his address and vocation. The frequency and persistence of perseverative responses seems to be related to the severity of the patient's brain damage, although the relationship is far from perfect. Perseverative behaviors are seen after unilateral damage in either brain hemisphere, after generalized damage caused by traumatic injuries, and in the middle to late stages of dementia. The neurophysiologic causes of perseveration are not known, although it is likely that perseveration may arise from a number of neurologic or cognitive anomalies.

Deficient Self-Monitoring.— A patient's ability to monitor his or her performance and his or her awareness of errors is an important indicator of the potential success of treatment. Patients who are unaware of errors usually do poorly in treatment until they learn to monitor their performance. Patients who are unaware of errors and also deny them usually are questionable candidates for treatment until they begin to recognize deficient performance. Some patients are aware of their errors but appear unconcerned about them. These patients are not necessarily bad candidates for treatment, if their overt lack of concern does not actually represent their true attitude toward errors. Deficient self-monitoring is often seen in patients with posterior (fluent) aphasia, in patients with right-hemisphere brain damage, in patients in late stages of dementia, and in some traumatically brain-injured patients.

Inability to Anticipate Errors.— Many brain-damaged patients recognize errors when they occur, but cannot anticipate them—they must see or hear the error before they recognize it as an error. These patients do a lot of self-correcting. Self-corrections are a favorable sign, because they show that the patient is aware of errors and can do something about them. If patients' attempts at self-correction are successful, their communicative efficiency often can be improved by helping them to anticipate errors and teaching them strategies for modifying their response before an overt error occurs.

| | ERROR RATE | |
RESPONSE RATE	Low	High
Slow	Make task more difficult	Slow patient down
Fast	Speed patient up	Make task easier

FIG 6–1.
Treatment manipulations that might be made in response to a patient's cognitive style.

Information Processing Deficits.—Brain-damaged patients often exhibit what appear to be general anomalies in dealing with incoming information. Several patterns of deficient processing have been described. They include *slow rise time, noise buildup, retention deficit,* and *intermittent imperception.* Porch (1967) described slow rise time and noise buildup, Brookshire (1979) first described retention deficit, and Schuell et al. (1965) were the first to describe intermittent imperception. They were describing aphasic patients, but patients with neurogenic communication disorders other than aphasia often exhibit similar processing anomalies.

Patients exhibiting *slow rise time* require longer than normal to focus their attention on incoming information. Consequently they tend to miss the first part of the information, and they may have difficulty when the nature of a treatment task changes without warning. When these patients are asked to repeat sentences spoken by the clinician, they may repeat only the last parts of the sentences. When responding to spoken instructions they tend to miss information in the first part of the instructions, and may completely miss short instructions. For example, a patient with slow rise time when asked to "point to the large green circle and the small yellow square" may point only to the small yellow square.

Patients with *noise buildup* get worse the longer they work at difficult tasks. These patients typically respond appropriately to the first part of spoken messages, or to the first few items in a set, but their performance deteriorates as the task continues. Complex materials usually increase the rate of noise buildup. Rest periods or time in tasks that are easy for the patient usually cause performance to recover. Relaxation training sometimes helps patients with noise buildup.

Patients with *retention deficits* have restricted short-term memory capacity, which prevents them from retaining longer strings of information. Most non-brain-damaged adults can retain from five to nine elements in short-term memory, but many brain-damaged patients cannot. Consequently, brain-damaged patients often have difficulty retaining sequences of numbers, sentences with several units of information, or other sequential verbal information. Many patients' deficient short-term memory is aggravated by general slowing of the rate at which they can analyze and make sense of incoming verbal information. The combination of decreased memory capacity and slowed information processing is particularly deleterious when incoming messages are mostly new information and the information comes in at a fast rate. Slowing the rate at which information is presented or pausing at appropriate places within messages may help these patients, sometimes dramatically.

Patients with *intermittent imperception* are the most difficult to characterize, because their performance fluctuates in apparently random fashion. Patients with intermittent imperception may perform errorlessly for intervals ranging from a few seconds to several minutes. Then, without observable changes in the task, the situation, or the patient, performance deteriorates. The poor performance may last for only a few seconds or several minutes, after which the patient's performance recovers. These periods of worsened performance usually are not predictable, but they may not be completely random, but related to subtle changes in the patient's attention, reactivity, or interest or to changes in the timing or content of stimuli. Some patients with intermittent imperception seem able to sense approaching periods of imperception. One such patient would stop the clinician when he sensed that he was going into an "imperceptive" state. When he recovered, he would signal the clinician to proceed.

Behaviors such as these led Wepman (1972) to propose a "shutter" effect to describe how some aphasic patients deal with verbal information. According to Wepman, many aphasic patients behave as if there were a "shutter" in the channels through which verbal materials are perceived. When the shutter is "open," the materials are perceived, and when it is closed, the materials are missed. According to Wepman, the shutter effect represents involuntary inhibition of the patient's ability to respond to language materials. This involuntary inhibition is automatic and takes place when the system is occupied with "processing" material that has just come in. Occasionally this automatic "closure" may be combined with a voluntary "shutting out" of competing stimuli by the patient as he or she attempts to process previously received materials.

Wepman believed that the shutter principle helps to account for the "unexplainable gaps" in receptivity of aphasic patients who, at other times, exhibit few receptive problems. Wepman's "shutter" phenomenon appears to be similar to Schuell's "intermittent imperception." Although both Schuell and Wepman were describing the behavior of aphasic adults, similar periods of intermittent imperception are often seen in the performance of brain-damaged adults with other communicative impairments.

Delayed Responses.—Brain-damaged persons' responses to stimuli often are characterized by delays between perception of the stimuli and their responses to them. The delays may range from a few seconds to several seconds. The delay interval may be unfilled, with the patient not doing anything observable, or it may be filled by attempts to facilitate a response—subvocal rehearsal, counting, saying letters of the alphabet, "writing" with a fingertip, and so forth. If delayed responses interfere with communication or if the patient's attempts to facilitate responses are counterproductive, the clinician may try to decrease or eliminate the delays and/or the counterproductive behaviors.

Sequential Ordering Deficits.—Some brain-damaged patients, have difficulty perceiving, retaining, reporting, and reproducing sequential information. This phenomenon was first described by Efron (1963) and subsequently elaborated on by Brookshire (1974, 1975). They found that brain-damaged persons (especially those with left anterior brain damage) frequently have difficulty perceiving and reporting the order of sequences of sounds or lights. Some of these patients also have problems with sequential organization in treatment activities; they cannot generate temporally ordered sequences of responses. Sometimes these patients are helped if the clinician provides cues to the proper sequence of responses by means of the spatial arrangement of stimuli (e.g., from left to right, in the order in which the responses to them are to be made).

SOME "PARALINGUISTIC" VARIABLES THAT MAY AFFECT RESPONSE ADEQUACY

The paralinguistic* characteristics of treatment stimuli and responses often affect the adequacy of patients' responses. Simple stimuli and short responses usually are easier than complex stimuli and long responses, and familiar stimuli and responses are easier than unfamiliar ones. However, brain-damaged patients may be idiosyncratic. Some tolerate noisy or distorted stimuli better than others. Some handle long or complex responses better than others. Consequently, the clinician is usually faced with some detective work at the beginning of treatment. The detective work is to deduce which stimulus characteristics and response requirements are likely to affect a particular patient, and in what way. Even though a patient may respond idiosyncratically to some stimulus manipulations, brain-damaged patients as a group tend to behave in predictable ways. In general, natural, familiar, short, simple, or interesting stimuli and responses are easier than unnatural, unfamiliar, long, complex, or uninteresting stimuli.

Stimulus Characteristics

Visual Stimuli.—During the 1970s several investigators set out to determine if the *form* of visual stimuli (whether they are objects, pictures, photographs, or line drawings, and whether they are representational or abstract) affects the performance of brain-damaged patients. Benton et al. (1972) asked aphasic subjects to name real objects and line drawings of real objects and found a small but statistically significant difference in favor of real objects. However, Corlew and Nation (1975) later found no meaningful difference between aphasic subjects' naming of objects and their naming of line drawings of those objects. Bisiach (1966) found small but significant differences between aphasic subjects' naming of realistic colored pictures and their naming of line drawings; the pictures were named better than the drawings. Kreindler et al. (1971) reported that aphasic subjects did better when they pointed to pictures of houses and flowers of different sizes and colors than they did when they were asked to point to colored circles and squares of different sizes and colors. Martino et al. (1976) reported a similar difference between common objects and tokens in a pointing task. LaPointe et al. (1985) reported that aphasic subjects' average scores were higher when they were asked to point to common objects than when they were asked to point to circles and squares of different colors and sizes.

These results suggest that the form of visual stimuli influences aphasic patients' responses to them, and it seems likely that similar effects would be seen with other brain-damaged patients. However, the magnitude of the effects usually was small, even when they were statistically significant, and when results for individual subjects

---

Paralinguistic refers to attributes of stimuli and responses that are not considered linguistic per se, but are related to linguistic processes. Vocal stress, speech rate, and the form of printed texts are examples of paralinguistic characteristics.

were reported, the performance of individual subjects frequently differed from that of the group. It probably makes little difference whether one uses objects, colored photographs, or line drawings in clinical activities, because most patients' responses to them are unlikely to differ in any important way. However, differences in the form of visual stimuli may be important for severely impaired patients or for patients with visual perceptual disabilities. In these cases, real objects and representations of real objects (pictures or drawings) are likely to be easier than nonrepresentational entities such as geometric forms or colored shapes.

Novelty and *context* seem to have somewhat more powerful effects on brain-damaged patients' performance. Many aphasic patients generate more speech, and more relevant speech, when they see pictures that are novel or heavily contextual, such as those "rich in context, relationships, action, and interdependencies, and which require some level of interpretation by the patient" (Myers, 1980). Norman Rockwell pictures, for example, are good for eliciting verbalization from aphasic persons, probably because they are interesting, novel, require interpretation of the inter-relationships depicted, and have a (usually humorous) "point."

Faber and Aten (1979) demonstrated that *novelty* can affect what aphasic patients say about stimulus pictures. They asked aphasic adults to describe pictures of intact objects and pictures of broken or altered objects. The pictures of broken and altered objects elicited more appropriate verbalization than the pictures of intact objects did, perhaps because there was something to talk about besides the names of the pictures.

Williams and Canter (1982) evaluated the effects of context on aphasic patients' picture naming. They asked aphasic subjects to name pictured objects that were shown either in isolation or in a pictorial context. Patients with Broca's aphasia were better at naming pictures of objects in isolation, and patients with Wernicke's aphasia were better at naming pictures of objects in contexts. Other groups of aphasic patients exhibited no group preference for contextual or acontextual pictures, but Williams and Canter reported that individual aphasic subjects in all groups showed marked differences in performance between the two conditions.

Patients with right-hemisphere brain damage and some traumatically brain-injured patients may have difficulty perceiving and communicating the complex relationships and interpretations represented by contextual pictures. They may tend to focus on tangential or irrelevant details rather than on the central theme of the pictures. For these patients, pictures with less contextual complexity may be easier.

The *size and nature of the array* in which visual stimuli are presented may affect brain-damaged patients' performance. As visual arrays become larger the difficulty of the task usually increases. Large arrays can lead to delays in responding by adding time for visual search to the time it takes the patient to comprehend the stimulus and execute a response. However, if the same array is used for a large number of trials, the effects of array size usually diminish as the patient learns where the elements of the array are located.

Helm-Estabrooks (1981) demonstrated that visual arrays can affect aphasic patients' performance in auditory comprehension tasks. She tested aphasic listeners in three conditions. In the *environment* condition, ten common objects were placed around the room, and the subjects were asked to point to them, either singly or in combination. In the *array* condition, the objects were shown as ten individual line drawings on 4 × 5 inch cards in two rows of five cards each. In the *composite* condition, the objects were shown as ten smaller line drawings on a single 7 × 7 inch card. The group's performance was significantly better when subjects pointed to pictures than when they pointed to objects located about the room. There was no difference between the two picture conditions for the group. However, many subjects showed differences among conditions that were not consistent with group performance. Some subjects were better in one of the picture conditions than the other, and some did better with real objects than they did with pictures. Helm-Estabrooks's results suggest that the form of visual stimuli and how they are arranged can affect brain-damaged persons' response accuracy, although the effects are not always predictable for individual patients.

Auditory Stimuli.— The *rate* at which auditory stimuli are presented may affect the ease with which they are comprehended by brain-damaged listeners. Sentences spoken at a fast speech rate often are comprehended less well than sentences spoken at a slow speech rate. The *fidelity* of auditory stimuli is also important. Distortion of spoken messages sometimes strongly affects brain-damaged listeners' comprehension of the messages. Fast speech rate and distortion most strongly affect patients with language comprehension impairments. Therefore, the effects of rate and fidelity on comprehension will be discussed in more detail when aphasic listeners' comprehension problems are addressed.

Response Requirements

Most treatment activities for persons with neurogenic communication disorders elicit large numbers of responses. The literature on learning suggests that speed of learning is directly related to the number of responses elicited. It seems reasonable that this relationship exists in treatment activities with brain-damaged adults, and few would disagree with Schuell et al.'s (1965) recommendation for intensive stimulation, with large numbers of stimulus presentations and a response by the patient to every stimulus.

Response requirements have strong effects on the difficulty of treatment activities. As response requirements escalate (in terms of length, effortfulness, complexity, or rate) the difficulty of the treatment activities increases. Increasing the rate at which responses must be made or decreasing the amount of delay that is permitted between stimulus and response usually makes the activity more difficult. (However, for some hyperresponsive patients, imposing a delay between stimulus and response may improve their performance.) Brookshire (1971) placed aphasic subjects in a picture-naming task in which the duration of stimulus exposure and the amount of time allocated for subjects' responses was manipulated. As stimulus exposure duration increased (from 3 to 30 seconds) the average number of correct naming responses also increased, with the greatest increment occurring from 3 to 5 seconds. However, allowing the subjects to control the rate of stimulus presentation proved most efficient in terms of number of correct responses per unit of treatment time. When the time allocated for subjects' responses (following 3-second stimulus exposure) increased from 0 to 30 seconds, there was a slight (but probably trivial) increase in the average number of correct naming responses. Brookshire reported that most correct naming responses occurred in the first 10 seconds after stimulus presentation, and suggested that providing more than 10 seconds is inefficient.

Providing more time for responses may also improve auditory comprehension. Yorkston et al. (1977) reported that imposing a time interval between delivery of *Token Test* commands and the opportunity for aphasic listeners to respond to the commands decreased anticipatory errors by some listeners. However, DeRenzi et al. (1978) and Toppin and Brookshire (1978) reported that imposing time intervals between stimulus presentation and pointing responses had no meaningful effects on aphasic listeners' comprehension.

The *meaningfulness* of responses usually has strong effects on a brain-damaged person's performance. More meaningful responses (in terms of their relationship to the person's experience) almost always are easier than less meaningful responses. The meaningfulness of responses appears to be related to two factors; (1) the number of times the person has performed the response, and (2) the relevance and naturalness of the response in the current situation.

The *context* in which responses are elicited also may have potent effects on response accuracy. One of the most striking characteristics of the behavior of brain-damaged adults is that responses that are difficult or impossible in one context can be easy in another context. Most adults with neurogenic communicative impairments say more and say it better when they talk in natural communicative interactions than they do when they are asked to respond in acontextual and unnatural situations. Similar effects of context on performance are seen in listening, reading, and writing. The major exceptions are some distractible or impulsive right-hemisphere-damaged patients and some traumatically brain-injured patients who cannot handle unstructured natural situations as well as they handle structured situations in which distractions are minimized and the focus of the interaction is carefully controlled.

CANDIDACY FOR TREATMENT

Assessment of a neurogenically compromised patient's communicative abilities permits clinicians to make decisions about whether to recommend treatment, and what the content of treatment should be. The processes involved in making these decisions have received little attention in the literature, perhaps because of the complexity and subjective nature of the decisions involved. Making decisions about whether to treat can be difficult, especially when treatment is not recommended. Few clinicians are comfortable with the recommendation that a patient not receive treatment for his or her communication disabilities.

Given unlimited professional and financial resources, every patient with a neurogenic communication disorder might get at least a trial period of treatment, and treatment might be provided to patients who are not improving much. Unfortunately, limitations on resources usually require that treatment be directed to those who are likely to receive the greatest benefit. Allocation of resources based on potential benefit generates another problem—that of how benefit is defined. Benefit may be defined in terms of the favorable effects of treatment on the patient and those around the patient—the "quality of life." Benefit also may be defined in terms of the degree to which treatment decreases the amount of resources that the community must allocate to the patient and family—the "cost-benefit ratio." The relative merits of the two kinds of benefits are, of course, arguable, and no standards for determining either exist. Clinicians tend to argue for quality of life, while funding agencies tend to think in terms of cost-benefit ratio. The issue of what constitutes a "benefit" is a complex one, and, as in the tale of the blind men and the elephant, one's attitude depends greatly on the direction from which one looks at the problem. The issue is one that every clinician must eventually face, although few clinicians believe they have satisfactorily resolved it.

Costs and benefits aside, one must consider whether a given patient's communicative abilities are likely to improve as the result of treatment. And, although we would sometimes like to believe otherwise, some patients' communicative impairments are irreversible, at least given our present level of sophistication. The primary determinant of whether a communicative impairment is reversible is the amount and location of brain damage. The greater the brain damage, and the more it involves areas of the brain involved in communication, the less likely recovery (with or without treatment) becomes. The size and location of a given patient's brain damage can be estimated directly from laboratory measures such as computed tomography (CT) or magnetic resonance imaging (MRI), or indirectly from behavioral measures, such as tests of speech, language, memory, and cognition. However, the relationship between lesion size and behavioral deficits may be weak immediately after strokes or traumatic brain injuries, when temporary bilateral reduction of cerebral blood flow, neurotransmitter release, cerebral edema, and diaschisis are present. For this reason, one would probably wait several weeks before deciding not to treat a patient because he or she is too severely impaired.

Complicating medical or physical conditions must also be considered when one predicts the outcome of treatment for a given patient. Illness, depression, or physical weakness diminish the probable effectiveness of treatment. Patients who cannot sit up and attend to a task for 30 minutes without undue fatigue may not be strong enough to tolerate intensive treatment. Such patients sometimes improve their performance on specific tasks in the clinic, but usually do not generalize the improvement to daily life outside the clinic. Sensory, perceptual, cognitive, attentional, or memory impairments also may compromise a patient's response to treatment. Patients who cannot attend to treatment tasks for at least a few minutes at a time are questionable candidates for treatment of their communicative impairments, although work on increasing their attention span may be appropriate. Patients who are extremely distractible likewise may be poor treatment candidates unless treatment can be structured to control the patient's distractibility. Depressed patients may not respond well to treatment until their depression has resolved.

Illness and weakness are frequent reasons for deferring treatment. For patients who are weak and ill, the issue may be survival rather than quality of life. However, if medical care and physiologic recovery lead to recovery of health and strength, these patients may be ready for treatment.

A patient's enthusiasm and motivation to recover often have powerful effects on the outcome of treatment. Some highly motivated and resourceful patients may benefit from treatment in spite of severe impairments. Some unmotivated or unconcerned patients may fail to benefit from treatment even though their impairments are not severe. A patient's life situation may also affect the outcome of treatment. A supportive, motivated, and caring family can enhance the effects of treatment programs, while a nonsupportive, unmotivated, and uncaring family may compromise them.

The patient's wishes must be considered when decisions about treatment are made. Patients have the right to refuse treatment, even though the clinician may think that treatment would be beneficial. If the patient understands the nature of his or her communication disabilities and the nature and potential benefits of treatment, then the patient's refusal must be accepted. If a patient is confused or has severe intellectual impairment, he or she may not be competent to make decisions about treatment, and family members or others with the right to represent the patient should make the decision.

THE TREATMENT TEAM

Speech-language pathologists who are responsible for patients with neurogenic communicative disorders usually work with other professionals as part of a treatment team. The composition of the team varies, depending on the treatment facility and the nature of a given patient's disabilities, but the speech-language pathologist usually works closely with other therapists, social workers, and psychologists. Each has primary responsibility for a given aspect of the patient's care, but responsibilities often intermix and overlap, so that planning, coordination, and communication among team members is necessary if the treatment program is to be both efficient and effective.

Physical Therapy.—Physical therapists evaluate patients' muscle strength and limb range of movement and carry out programs to help patients retain or regain muscle strength and limb movement. When a patient is confined to bed, physical therapy activities take place at bedside, and include teaching the patient how to turn over in bed, sit up, and transfer from the bed to a chair or wheelchair. Physical therapists also carry out passive range-of-movement exercises in which bedbound patients' limbs are moved and muscles are stretched to prevent *contractures* (permanent shortening of muscles resulting from spasticity), and to preserve muscle strength and tone. Other physical therapy activities take place in the physical therapy clinic, and include teaching patients how to transfer to and from a wheelchair, how to use braces, canes, and crutches, and how to get dressed, together with muscle strengthening and range-of-movement activities. If a patient is about to be discharged home or to a nursing home, the physical therapist may help the family or nursing home staff prepare the living environment for the special needs of the patient, and may provide the patient with exercise programs to be carried out at home.

Occupational Therapy.—Occupational therapists help patients regain abilities necessary for activities of daily living (ADLs). Activities of daily living include cooking, dressing, and grooming. Although both occupational and physical therapists work on muscle strengthening, occupational therapists usually work on movements within activities of daily living. A patient who needs to strengthen hands and arms might sand boards, saw wood, or weave on a loom. A patient with visual-spatial impairments might perform craft activities requiring eye-hand coordination. An important part of the occupational therapist's responsibilities is to help the patient resume daily life activities such as cooking, cleaning, and making beds. This is accomplished by teaching compensatory strategies, providing special tools and appliances, and modifying standard tools and appliances to compensate for the patient's disabilities. Occupational therapists also help patients develop skills and interests for leisure activities and hobbies. Occupational therapists sometimes test and treat patients for sensorimotor and visual-spatial disorders. Because occupational therapists often deal with visual perception, reading, and writing, speech-language pathologists often collaborate with them in working on daily life communicative skills.

In some facilities occupational therapists provide vocational testing and consultation. Patients may be given work aptitude tests and real or simulated on-the-job evaluations in order to (1) determine whether they may go back to work, (2) make appropriate job placements, and (3) modify a patient's work environment and responsibilities to enable the patient to perform the job successfully. In such cases occupational therapists may work closely with vocational counselors.

Corrective Therapy.—In some facilities corrective therapists may take responsibility for ambulation training. Corrective therapists usually work in collaboration with physical and occupational therapists, and help patients regain the strength, balance, and endurance needed for walking. They also may teach patients how to use crutches and canes, and how to climb and descend stairs.

Recreational Therapy.—Recreation therapists provide therapeutic recreational activities, and may introduce patients to leisure activities that they may continue after their discharge from treatment.

Physical, occupational, corrective, and recreational therapists work under the administrative supervision of *physiatrists,* who are specialists in *rehabilitation medicine,* the medical discipline responsible for helping physically disabled patients regain the use of impaired muscles.

Social Work.—Social workers play a major role in coordinating and managing interactions between the medical facility and patients and their families. The social worker often has primary responsibility for keeping the patient's family informed about the patient's status and about plans for treatment and eventual discharge. The social worker often serves as a referral source, suggesting, initiating, and coordinating referrals to medical, financial, and social service facilities and programs. Social workers may provide patients and families with information about nursing homes, county and state medical and family services, and other resources that may help the patient and family. The social worker may work with the patient's family to set up a home environment that is conducive to continued recovery and maximum self-sufficiency. The social worker has responsibility for making certain that physicians' orders for wheelchairs and other prosthetic appliances to be provided at discharge are carried out, and the social worker may make arrangements for programs such as "meals on wheels" or public health nurse visits to the patient in the home. The social worker may initiate and coordinate evaluations of legal competence for patients whose competence is questioned, and they make referrals to psychologic and mental health services, chemical dependency programs, social security or veterans administration counselors, financial advisors, vocational counselors, or family and marriage counselors. The social worker plays a major role in coordinating interactions among the medical facility, the patient, the patient's family, and community and state agencies. A competent and dedicated social worker can make a major contribution to the patient's and family's adjustment to changed life-styles, and can help to ensure that the patient's post-hospital placement represents the needs and the wishes of the patient and the family.

Neuropsychology.—Neuropsychologists often play an important part in assessment of brain-injured patients. They are usually concerned with measuring the patient's present level of mental functioning, and in comparing that level with the patient's assumed previous abilities. The results of testing help the neuropsychologist determine whether organic pathology accounts for the patient's symptoms, and, if so, test results may help to identify the nature of the pathology.

Neuropsychologists can choose from a large number of tests when they set out to evaluate a brain-injured patient. Which ones they will choose to administer depends, of course, on the nature and extent of the patient's problems, but when a patient has a brain injury, the neuropsychologist will almost always administer tests of verbal and nonverbal intelligence, memory, planning and foresight, and visual perception. Neuropsychologists and speech-language pathologists often collaborate on assessment of brain-injured patients, share the results of testing, and jointly make plans for the patient's management and rehabilitation.

Clinical and Counseling Psychology.—The services of clinical and counseling psychologists can be an important part of the care of many brain-injured patients. Psychologists administer and interpret tests of intelligence, cognition, and personality, and provide the patient-care team with information about the patient's intellectual, cognitive, and emotional state. The psychologist may help the patient and family deal with the emotional and psychologic effects of the patient's impairments on the family. When a patient is depressed, lonely, or anxious, the pyschologist may help the patient and family deal with the feelings. Some patients may exhibit behaviors resembling those seen in psychoses and neuroses. In these cases the psychologist or a psychiatrist may provide diagnostic, referral, and treatment services.

The Treatment Team.— The multidimensional nature of treatment usually requires that treatment be carried out by a professional team, rather than by one person or by independently operating professionals. The composition of the team may differ from patient to patient, depending on a particular patient's disabilities and needs, but it frequently includes a physician, a nurse, a speech-language pathologist, an occupational therapist, a physical therapist, and a social worker. Neuropsychologists, clinical psychologists, and vocational counselors may also participate, depending on a given patient's problems or needs. The speech-language pathologist is usually a central figure in treatment teams for aphasic patients. The speech-language pathologist is usually most skilled in communicating with aphasic people, and almost always has more experience in verbal interaction with any given aphasic patient than the other members of the team. The speech-language pathologist is likely to work with the aphasic patient more often and for longer than other members of the team. Because of this extended contact with the aphasic patient and his or her family, the speech-language pathologist often knows a great deal about the needs of the patient and family. The treatment team often depends on the speech-language pathologist to identify problems in management of the patient's case, to make appropriate referrals, and to suggest solutions to problems that may arise.

METHODS FOR DECIDING WHAT TO TREAT

How clinicians decide what to treat is more art than science, resulting from a combination of the clinician's conceptions of what the patient's communicative impairment represents, attitudes about what is important, opinions about the nature of therapy, and previous successes and failures with patients who resemble the current patient. There are no rules, and guiding principles are few. Yet there are some general approaches to making decisions about what to treat that characterize segments of the professional population.

Perhaps the most commonly used approach to planning treatment is the *relative level of impairment* approach, in which the patient's performance on various tests is analyzed to identify "peaks" and "valleys" in the patient's performance profile. These peaks and valleys are then given special attention in treatment. Clinicians sometimes choose to treat in the valleys (areas of relative impairment), but are more likely to treat at the peaks (areas in which impairments are less pronounced). The relative level of impairment approach has been clearly explicated with reference to aphasia, but the principles are relevant to treatment of patients with other neurogenic communication disorders as well.

Porch (1981b) suggested that differences in patients' performance across and within tests can be used in planning aphasia treatment. According to Porch, the test performance of most aphasic patients varies, so performance on some subtests is better than performance on others, and performance on some items within a subtest is better than the patient's average for the subtest. Porch has devised two measures of such variability—the *high-low gap* and *intrasubtest variability* (ISV). The high-low gap is calculated on the 18 subtests of the *Porch Index of Communicative Ability*

(PICA) (Porch, 1981a). The average for the 9 subtests with the highest scores and the average for the 9 subtests with the lowest scores are calculated. The difference is the high-low gap. The high-low gap, according to Porch, represents in part the amount of change that can be expected from treatment. Porch has suggested that when the high-low gap is closed (a difference at or near zero), the patient has achieved maximum treatment benefits and may be ready for discharge.

Porch also recommends consideration of ISV in treatment planning. Intrasubtest variability is the number of different scores within a subtest. A ten-item PICA subtest in which a patient receives eight scores of 13 (with the PICA 16-category scoring system) and two scores of 15 would have low ISV, while a subtest in which a patient's ten responses included scores of 7, 9, 10, 13, and 15 would have large ISV. According to Porch, ISV is related to a patient's potential for change in the task represented by the subtest, there being greater potential for change on subtests with high ISV than on subtests with low ISV. According to Porch, ISV decreases as the patient approaches the limits of his or her recovery potential.

Comparing test scores to identify areas of unusual impairment or unusual ability helps clinicians organize and consolidate the information gained during evaluation. Unfortunately, not all tests permit straightforward comparisons of performance across subtests. In order for such comparisons to be made, there must be a common reference value across subtests, so that differences across subtests can be interpreted. This common reference value usually is provided by statistics such as the mean and standard deviation or percentiles for scores on each subtest. By converting subtest scores into percentiles or Z-scores (based on the mean and standard deviation), clinicians can compare performance across subtests and identify subtests on which performance was unusually poor or unusually good.

In the *fundamental abilities approach* to treatment, clinicians attempt to identify impaired "processes" that underlie related linguistic or communicative abilities. Treatment is then focused on these processes, with the expectation that improving a process will improve the abilities that depend on the process. For example, Schuell et al. (1965) have claimed that impaired auditory comprehension is a central problem in aphasia, and that improving auditory comprehension is likely to lead to improvement in other language abilities. As a consequence, clinicians who agree with Schuell et al. are likely to test auditory comprehension in detail and to make auditory comprehension disabilities the focus of treatment, expecting that as auditory comprehension improves, so will general linguistic and communicative abilities. Gardner et al. (1983) and Myers (1990) have suggested that impaired capacity to make inferences is a central problem for many right-hemisphere-damaged persons. Those who subscribe to this view might focus treatment on inference-making, expecting that improvements there would generalize to other communicative abilities.

In the *functional abilities approach* to treatment, the clinician looks for competencies that are likely to be important in a patient's daily life communication, and focuses treatment on those competencies. For example, a clinician might teach a nonverbal patient to produce gestural yes-no responses, because the patient's acquisition of dependable yes-no responses would enhance communication with others in the patient's natural environment. Clinicians using the functional abilities approach often invite patients and family members to help decide what is to be worked on in treatment. Because the focus of treatment is on communication in daily life, families and caregivers often participate directly in treatment procedures.

Most clinicians combine the three approaches to test interpretation, data reduction, and treatment planning. Fundamental abilities that have little relationship to a patient's daily life probably would not be the focus of treatment, even by clinicians employing a "fundamental abilities" approach. Likewise, clinicians employing the "relative level of impairment" approach usually would consider how important a process or ability is in daily life when making decisions about what to treat.

GENERAL CHARACTERISTICS OF TREATMENT SESSIONS

Treatment sessions in which the patient and clinician work "one on one" usually have a relatively predictable form, regardless of the clinician's general approach to treatment, and regardless of the specific activities that take place in the session. The length and frequency of sessions is determined by the patient's tolerance and what the clinician wishes to get done. Most sessions begin and end with conversation, and the treatment "work" occupies the middle.

Length.—The length of treatment sessions depends on the patient's condition and the nature and duration of the treatment activities that are to be accomplished during the sessions. For patients who tire easily or who have a limited attention span, treatment sessions may be relatively short (15 to 30 minutes), whereas patients who are in good physical condition and are medically stable may work efficiently for an hour or more.

The content of treatment sessions also affects their length. As more treatment activities are included, treatment sessions must be longer to accommodate them. Three different activities might require 30-minute sessions, while five or six activities would probably require 1-hour sessions. Most patients (and perhaps clinicians too) cannot maintain maximum efficiency within a given treatment activity for more than about 8 to 10 minutes, so individual treatment tasks probably should not last much longer than this.

Frequency.—The frequency of treatment sessions is affected by the patient's tolerance, needs, and availability. Treatment sessions for patients who are seen a short time after onset tend to be shorter and more frequent than sessions for those who are seen a longer time after onset. Patients seen a short time after onset may be seen twice a day—once in the morning and once in the afternoon—or even four times a day. In this way, patients who cannot tolerate long treatment sessions may still receive adequate exposure to treatment. As these patients recover and can tolerate longer treatment sessions, the length of treatment sessions may be increased and their frequency may be decreased.

If a patient is close by and accessible, he or she is likely to be seen more often than if he or she were farther away or less accessible. Hospitalized patients, or those residing in or near the treatment facility, may be seen two or more times a day. Ambulatory hospitalized patients who can get themselves up, dressed, and to the clinic may be seen more frequently than patients for whom a journey to the clinic requires extensive time commitments from ward personnel. Patients who live at home and must travel to the clinic usually are not seen more frequently than once a day, two or three times a week. If an outpatient attends other clinics (such as physical therapy), the visits usually are scheduled so that both can be accomplished with one trip to the treatment facility.

Arrangement.— The arrangement of treatment sessions generally follows a consistent format. Most begin with a period of conversation, in which the clinician and the patient talk about what has happened since their last meeting, and the clinician deals with any problems that the patient might communicate (the *hello segment*). The clinician may use this time to evaluate the patient's overall level of communicative functioning relative to previous treatment sessions, to estimate the extent to which treated communicative behaviors are generalizing, and to ascertain the patient's mood and energy level. The hello segment gives the patient time to adjust to the clinician and the surroundings and to get problems or concerns out of the way before treatment begins. The hello segment may also help to create and maintain personal rapport between the patient and the clinician.

A short interval of work on activities that serve as "warm-ups" for the main treatment activities (the *accommodation segment*) usually follows the hello segment. The activities in the accommodation segment usually are activities from previous sessions with which the patient is comfortable and is successful. The accommodation segment permits the patient to adjust to the sequence and timing of treatment procedures before he or she is asked to deal with difficult tasks.

In the *work segment,* tasks become more difficult and challenging, and new or more difficult tasks are introduced (usually as extensions or modifications of previous tasks). Activities in the work segment usually are those with which the patient has some difficulty, but in which most responses are correct, delayed, or self-corrected. Three or four different activities at this level of difficulty may take place during the work segment. When the activities change, the clinician alerts the patient to the changes, explains the new requirements, and (if necessary) demonstrates the new task. (The exception is activities in which the objective is to teach the patient to adapt quickly to changing task requirements. They will be described subsequently.)

Following the work segment, a short interval of work with familiar activities in which most responses are successful may be provided (the *cool-down segment*). The cool-down segment helps the patient relax after working at challenging treatment tasks and may help the patient leave the treatment session feeling successful. At the very end of the session there may be a short period of conversation about the course of the day's session, about what the patient plans to do until the next session, and about what might happen in the next session (the *goodbye segment*).

TASK DIFFICULTY

Treatment activities usually are designed so that the patient's performance is slightly deficient, but not mostly or completely erroneous. This means that most responses are immediate and correct, while some are delayed but correct, or initially incorrect but corrected by the patient without clinician intervention. A few outright errors almost always occur in activities at this relatively low level of difficulty, but they should be few and scattered. If they are not, then the activity should be changed to decrease the frequency of errors. By placing patients in treatment activities in which most responses are immediate and correct, but in which some delayed or self-corrected responses occur, clinicians can ensure that patients are working at or near their limits, but not beyond them. Schuell et al. (1965) commented that the occurrence of a correct response is the primary way clinicians can tell whether a stimulus is adequate—that it "got into the brain." Treating neurogenic communicative impairments at this level of difficulty seems to be both effective and efficient.

Treatment activities should not be too easy. If a patient's responses are nearly all immediate and correct, the treatment is not likely to generate much improvement in communicative abilities. If a patient gives fewer than 10% delayed or self-corrected responses over a large number of trials, then the task is probably too easy. As a general rule, it is probably reasonable to keep patient performance at 60% to 80% immediate and correct responses during the beginning of a given activity, and to increase the difficulty of the task when immediate, correct responses exceed 90% to 95% over two or three sessions. Porch (1981b) advocates that one not change tasks or response criteria until 100% of a patient's responses are immediate and correct, and claims that responses trained to less-than-perfect levels will deteriorate in real-life situations or in more difficult treatment tasks. Extension of changes obtained in treatment activities from the clinic to daily life or to other treatment contexts seems more a problem of generalization than one of task difficulty within treatment tasks. Generalization is more likely if generalization procedures are incorporated into treatment than if one simply stays within treatment tasks until the patient's performance is essentially normal.

Another reason for structuring treatment activities so that few outright errors occur is that errors tend to create additional errors. Brookshire (1972) found that when aphasic patients misnamed pictures there was a strong tendency to misname subsequent items, even when those items ordinarily were easy to name. Brookshire (1976) later replicated this finding in a sentence comprehension task. Brookshire and Nicholas (1977) found a similar effect in videotaped aphasia treatment sessions. They reported that the probability that a patient would make an error increased dramatically following error responses. When uninterrupted strings of errors occurred, the probability of a correct response decreased with each error in the string, so that when three or four consecutive errors occurred, the probability of a correct response on the next attempt was near zero, unless the task or response requirements were changed by the clinician.

As a general rule, no more than 20% of a patient's responses in treatment activities should be errors. But, as with most rules, there are exceptions. If the adequacy of the patient's responses is gradually improving, even though they are mostly errors, then the clinician might be willing to allow higher error rates, because the patient appears to be learning something. Rosenbek et al. (1989) commented that a stimulus may be adequate even if it does not elicit a correct response as long as it leads to problem-solving, or if a series of incorrect responses moves in the direction of adequacy. However, if there is no improvement across sequences of off-target responses (especially if the patient gives the *same* response on every trial), the task should be made easier. If most of the patient's off-target responses consist of delayed responses and self-corrected errors, then a somewhat greater proportion of off-target responses may be permitted.

RESPONSE RECORDING AND CHARTING

Treatment procedures usually entail systematic scoring of patients' responses. Brookshire (1978) suggested that clinicians score every response made by patients in treatment sessions, but this may not always be reasonable. Sometimes responses occur so rapidly that one cannot keep up with the scoring, and if decisions about response acceptability take much time the clinician may not be able to score every response "on line" even when response rates are relatively low. When it is impossible or impractical to score every response, or if scoring every response would interrupt the "flow" of treatment, collecting a representative sample of the patient's responses is better than attempting to score every response.

If a sample of a treatment session is representative, the treatment stimuli and the patient's responses occur in the sample with the same relative frequency as they occur in the treatment session as a whole. How well a sample represents the entire session depends on the *frequency* with which the session is sampled, the *duration* of the sampled intervals, and the *distribution* of sampled intervals within the session. The more frequently the session is sampled, the longer the sampled intervals are, and the more evenly distributed the sampled intervals are across the session, the better the sample will resemble the session. Even if only one event in ten is sampled, the sample obtained usually will be representative of the entire session if samples are taken throughout the session (Brookshire et al., 1978).

When it is possible to score every patient response without disrupting the pace and cohesiveness of the treatment session, consistent procedures for tabulating and charting patients' responses may prove useful. LaPointe (1977) has described a system of treatment task specification and response recording called *Base-10 Programmed Stimulation*. Patients' responses are tabulated on a *Base-10 Response Form* (Fig 6–2), on which the clinician enters information about the nature of the treatment task, target performance criteria, the scoring system used, the stimuli presented, and the patient's responses. The response form also includes a graph on which a patient's performance can be charted over several treatment sessions. A different response form is used for each treatment task, so that several might be needed to record the activities within a treatment session.

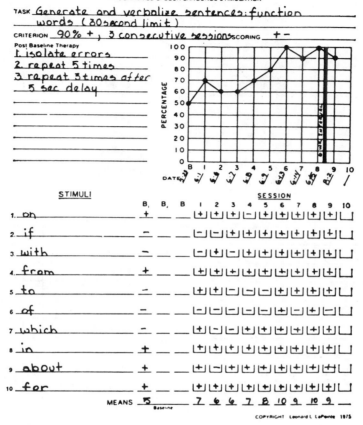

BASE 10 RESPONSE FORM
PROGRAMMED SPEECH-LANGUAGE STIMULATION

TASK _Generate and verbalize sentences: function words (30 second limit)_

CRITERION _90% + , 3 consecutive sessions_ SCORING _+ −_

Post Baseline Therapy
1. isolate errors
2. repeat 5 times
3. repeat 3 times after 5 sec delay

FIG 6–2.
The Base-10 task specification and response recording sheet. The task is described at the *top left* and the patient's responses to specific stimuli are recorded at the *bottom*. The patient's performance across time can be graphed at the *top right*.

When doing treatment in base-10 format, the clinician selects a task (or set of tasks) for a patient, and puts a description of each task on a response form. A target behavior and a target level of performance are established for each task and entered on the response form. Ten stimuli are selected (hence the label base-10) and listed on the response form. Each stimulus is presented and the patient's response to each stimulus is entered on the response form. The patient's session-by-session performance can be graphed on the response form to show changes in performance over time.

Whether or not one uses a formal system such as the base-10 system, patients' responses should be tabulated so that statistics such as averages for blocks of responses can easily be calculated. Commercially available data sheets can be used for

J. Doe   8-15-78

	Naming			Pointing by Name			Pointing by Function			Sentence Completion			Imitation			Pointing by Two's		
	1	2	3	5	6	7	9	10	11	13	14	15	17	18	19	21	22	23
Bedroom	15	13	15	13	15	15	13	15	15	15	15	15	15	15	13	13	13	15
Ball	15	15	15	15	15	13	13	13	15	15	15	15	15	15	15	13	15	13
Belt	13	15	13	13	13	10	13	9	10	15	13	15	13	15	15	15	15	15
Bicycle	15	15	15	13	13	12	15	15	15	13	15	13	15	14	14	13	10	15
Billfold	15	15	15	15	15	15	15	15	13	13	15	15	15	15	16	9	13	15
Birds	15	15	15	(5)	15	15	13	15	15	15	15	15	14	14	14	13	15	13
Black	13	13	15	10	15	15	10	15	15	15	15	15	15	15	15	13	13	15
Blue	15	15	15	15	15	15	15	13	15	15	15	15	15	15	15	15	15	9
Boat	10	15	15	13	15	16	15	15	15	15	15	13	15	15	15	10	15	15
Book	15	15	15	13	15	15	15	16	13	15	15	15	13	15	15	13	7	15
Mean Score	14.50			13.73			13.92			14.60			14.03			13.33		

A

FIG 6–3.
Examples of two forms for recording patients' performance in treatment. The form in **A** contains a record of a single session. The form in **B** permits the clinician to summarize the patient's performance on several tasks across several sessions.

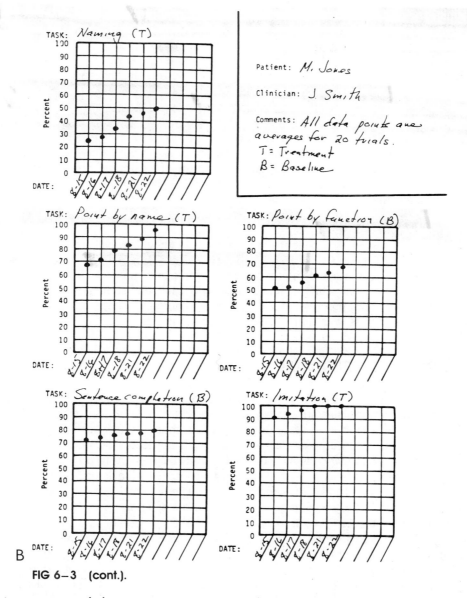

TASK: *Naming (T)*

Patient: *M. Jones*

Clinician: *J. Smith*

Comments: *All data points are averages for 20 trials.*
T = Treatment
B = Baseline

TASK: *Point by name (T)*

TASK: *Point by function (B)*

TASK: *Sentence completion (B)*

TASK: *Imitation (T)*

B

FIG 6–3   (cont.).

this purpose, and clinicians sometimes create their own personalized data sheets for this purpose. Figure 6–3 shows two examples of data sheets that we have found useful in clinical activities. The Data sheet A is a data form in which the clinician has entered treatment information for a patient. The Data sheet B provides a convenient way to summarize a large amount of information on a single page.

Keeping accurate records of patient performance in treatment activities is an important part of good treatment. Establishing stable baseline levels of performance permits one to document the effects of treatment procedures. Analysis of changes in patient performance over time or in response to certain treatment procedures may enable a clinician to modify existing treatment procedures or to introduce new procedures in order to maximize treatment effectiveness. In order to keep accurate records of treatment activities, the activities must be orderly and easily described. Consequently, the requirements of record-keeping may impose order and structure on treatment that otherwise might not be there. Finally, third-party payers (insurance companies, governmental units) and health-care accrediting agencies require that accurate records of patient performance and response to treatment be maintained.

However, when response-scoring and record-keeping procedures are cumbersome and intrusive, they may interrupt the rhythm of treatment, compromise the naturalness of the interaction between clinician and patient, and divert the attention of the patient and the clinician from the primary objectives of treatment. Consequently, response recording and record-keeping activities should be kept as simple and unobtrusive as possible.

Charts or graphs of a patient's responses in treatment activities can be useful when the clinician wishes to show the patient his or her progress. Showing the patient how much progress is being made can reinforce and motivate. Day-to-day improvement in treatment activities may be relatively small, and some patients may believe that they are not progressing and become discouraged. Graphic demonstration of a patient's progress in treatment may be helpful in such cases.

THE ROLE OF FEEDBACK

Brookshire (1973) identified two major categories of response-contingent feedback in treatment activities: *incentive feedback* and *information feedback. Incentive feedback* involves rewarding and punishing stimuli that can maintain (or eliminate) behaviors whose only purpose is to elicit (or avoid) the feedback. When the incentive feedback is no longer delivered, the behavior usually reverts to pretreatment levels. In most cases, increasing the magnitude of incentive feedback increases its effect, at least within certain ranges of magnitude. Incentive feedback is most useful when the objective is to change the frequency of behaviors when the person is capable of the behavior, but doesn't do it enough (e.g., make eye contact with listeners) or does it too much (e.g., shouts at doctors and nurses). Many stimuli may serve as incentive feedback, and what serves as an incentive for one person may not for another. The most generally effective stimuli are those with intrinsic rewarding or punishing properties (e.g., food, candy, money, electric shock, loud noise), although some stimuli that are not intrinsically rewarding or punishing may serve as incentive feedback because of the person's previous experience with them. Perhaps the best example of the latter kind of feedback is verbal approval and verbal reproof, which are not intrinsically rewarding or punishing but have acquired rewarding and punishing properties because of the individual's previous experience with them.

Incentive feedback usually is not required in treatment of neurogenic communicative impairments. Most patients are motivated to get better and are willing to work at it. They usually respond willingly without clinician-delivered incentives. Sometimes severely impaired, depressed, or confused patients may need response-contingent tangible incentives. Incentive feedback may help these patients get started, and when getting the targeted behavior out becomes less onerous, incentive feedback may be replaced by information feedback. Incentive feedback often is needed in treatment of traumatically brain-injured patients in the early stages of recovery. These patients are often minimally responsive to their environment, and may respond only to stimuli that are intrinsically rewarding. Incentive feedback also may be needed for patients in the late stages of dementia, when social rewards and penalties no longer function to maintain or change behavior.

Information feedback provides information about the degree to which responses approximate their targets. Information feedback comes in many forms, ranging from a tracing on an oscilloscope that tells the patient that his or her vocal intensity is on target, to the clinician's smile and spoken "good" that tells the patient that he or she has successfully communicated the intended message. Information feedback is most useful when the patient is motivated to respond, but does not know the "target" response, or does not know how closely his or her responses approximate the target. If the patient is motivated to respond, knows the target response, and knows how closely his or her attempts approximate the target, then *any* feedback may be trivial. Many patients with neurogenic communicative impairments meet these criteria. When they do, providing response-contingent feedback of any kind may have few important effects on the rate or quality of specific responses.

Even though it may technically be unnecessary, response-contingent feedback may affect the overall quality of the clinician-patient interaction. In addition to its role in providing information to the patient about the accuracy of his or her responses (which, though not *crucial,* may be *helpful),* response-contingent feedback serves several other functions. It provides a signal to the patient that the clinician has accepted the response, and that the patient can get ready for the next request. The clinician can manage the tempo of the treatment activity by manipulating the timing and frequency of feedback. The presence of feedback also contributes to the naturalness of treatment interactions by providing acknowledgment of the patient's responses, as participants in daily life interactions usually do.

Response-contingent feedback is always needed when the clinician wishes to use *shaping procedures,* in which abnormal responses are gradually changed into normal responses or simple responses are gradually changed into complex responses by means of *successive approximations* to the target responses. Shaping procedures depend on the systematic delivery of response-contingent feedback so that responses deviating in the direction of the target are reinforced and other responses are not. They permit the clinician to manipulate response requirements during treatment activities without interrupting the activities with instructions and explanations. Shaping procedures can be used when the patient does not know what the target response is or does not know how his or her responses differ from the target.

Regardless of the specific procedures used, almost all patients need *general encouragement.* General encouragement may consist of response-contingent positive feedback, or it may take the form of intermittent general positive statements that are not contingent on any given response— statements such as "you're doing fine," or "you're doing much better today."

Clinicians differ in their use of feedback. Brookshire et al. (1977), and Brookshire and Nicholas (1978) analyzed delivery of positive and negative feedback by clinicians in videotaped treatment sessions. They found that on average 55% of all patient responses received feedback. However, the percentage ranged from 9% to 98% across clinicians. Only 10% of unacceptable responses received negative feedback, and, surprisingly, 11% of *unacceptable* responses received *positive* feedback. Clinicians provided ambiguous feedback (feedback that was both positive and negative) for 20% of responses.

Brookshire and Nicholas (1978) reported that clinicians usually did more than just providing feedback following patients' responses. When a patient's spoken response was acceptable, they tended to repeat it, provide feedback, and then elaborate on the patient's response. (If the patient correctly named "table," the clinician might say "table—that's right—you sit at the *table*.") When a response was unacceptable, clinicians usually did not repeat it or provide feedback. When they did provide feedback, it could be either postive ("Nice try"), negative ("That's not it"), or a combination of the two. Following delivery of feedback, the clinician often provided the target response. (If a patient named "chair" as "table," the clinician might say, "no—*chair*.") Clinicians often provided explanation or instruction after unacceptable patient responses, even when the explanation or instruction was not needed by the patient. (If a patient named "chair" as "table," the clinician might say, "When I point to the picture, you tell me its name.") Offering instructions or explanations in such contexts usually led to additional unacceptable responses.

ENHANCING GENERALIZATION FROM THE CLINIC TO DAILY LIFE

Treatment of communication disorders should not be considered successful if the therapeutic changes achieved in the clinic do not transfer to the patient's daily life. Even though most clinicians recognize that transfer of treatment gains to daily life is important, until the 1970s most aphasia clinicians seemed to operate largely on the *train and hope* principle (Stokes and Baer, 1977), in which generalization of treatment effects from the clinic to outside contexts is hoped for, but neither actively pursued nor objectively measured. It is probably true that most aphasia clinicians (at least the better ones) either target communicative behaviors that are relevant to the patient's daily life environment, or target underlying processes that are assumed to enhance daily life communicative behavior, but most do not pursue generalization in a systematic way, nor measure it carefully. In the 1970s psychologists and behavior analysts began to address the problem of getting behavioral changes achieved in one setting to generalize to other settings. Literature on generalization accumulated, and procedures for enhancing generalization gradually made their way into clinical aphasiology. These procedures generally resemble those articulated by Stokes and

Baer (1977), the first of which (train and hope) is described above. The others include the following.

Take Advantage of Natural Maintaining Contingencies.—Stokes and Baer see this as "the most dependable of all generalization programming mechanisms." The easiest way to make use of natural contingencies is to target behaviors that will naturally elicit favorable consequences in the patient's daily life environment. For example, Thompson and Byrne (1984) trained patients with Broca's aphasia to produce various "social conventions" such as greetings, expecting that the patients' use of such social conventions would be naturally reinforced by those around them. Sometimes natural contingencies are not present in the patient's daily life environment, or are not consistent enough. Then one might redesign or restructure the environment so that the targeted behaviors receive enough payoff to maintain them. An example of such restructuring is provided by an aphasic patient who learned to produce one- and two-word requests in the clinic, but continued to communicate at home with grunts and gestures, by which he usually succeeded in getting family members to do what he wanted. The clinician taught family members to respond to spoken requests and to ignore or delay responses to grunts and gestures unaccompanied by speech. This soon brought the patient's clinic-learned spoken requests into his home environment, after which natural contingencies maintained them, both in the home and in other contexts with other listeners.

Train Sufficient Exemplars.—("Exemplar" is technical jargon with various meanings. As used here it means, roughly, "stimulus-response-reinforcement triads.") One way of *training sufficient exemplars* is to train a behavior in enough different settings that the behavior generalizes to all settings in which the behavior is desired. Once the behavior is dependably established in one context, the training is systematically extended to other contexts one or two at a time, with the expectation that at some point the behavior will generalize to all contexts of interest. Using social conventions as an example, this means that one might first train social conventions in the clinic, then extend the training to other rooms, other interactants, and, perhaps, to the patient's home or other community settings, expecting that at some point the patient's use of social conventions would generalize to all relevant communicative contexts. Another way of training sufficient exemplars is to train enough different representatives of a class of responses to ensure that a *class* of responses, rather than a *specific* response (or subset of responses), generalizes. Using social conventions as an example, one might successively train several social conventions of a given kind (e.g., greetings) with the expectation that increasing the frequency of greetings might naturally lead to increases in the frequency of other conventions, such as social questions ("How are you?") and self-disclosures ("I am fine").

Train Loosely.—To "train loosely" means to allow stimulus conditions, response requirements, and reinforcement contingencies to vary (within limits) to increase generalization across responses within a response class, and to increase generalization from the training environment to other environments. Loose training attempts to prevent a patient's responses from being tightly bound to specific contexts, which can often happen when treatment conditions are carefully controlled (as in clinic treatment activities). In loose training (1) a variety of stimuli are employed to elicit targeted responses, sometimes in different situational contexts; (2) a range of responses within a predefined response class is considered acceptable; and (3) response contingencies vary both in kind and schedule. Loose training is *not* unsystematic treatment. Specific response classes are targeted, eliciting stimuli and situational contexts are planned in advance, and response contingencies and their schedules are predefined. Prototypical loose training is as carefully thought out and as carefully controlled as more traditional structured intervention procedures. Thompson and Byrne (1984) used loose training procedures to train their aphasic patients to use social conventions. The social conventions were first established by asking the patients to imitate the clinician's production of them. Then the eliciting stimuli were systematically broadened to (1) requests by the clinician (e.g., "Tell me hello"); (2) naturalistic prompts given by the clinician (e.g., the clinician said "hello" and waited for a response from the patient); and (3) role-playing situations structured to resemble natural conversations. Verbal feedback (e.g., "Nice job") was provided contingent on responses, and the schedule of feedback was gradually "loosened," changing from feedback for every response in the early stages of training to a variable schedule (feedback for an average of one response in four) in the later stages. Thompson and Byrne reported that loose training increased their patients' production of social conventions, and that their increased use of social conventions generalized to novel social interactions. Although their procedures departed somewhat from prototypical "loose training" (they targeted specific responses for intervention), their study is a good example of how loose training can be incorporated into traditional treatment procedures.

Use Sequential Modification.—In sequential modification (Stokes and Baer, 1977), generalization across contexts is obtained by carrying out training in every context to which generalization is desired. For brain-injured persons, sequential modification may be practical (1) when a communicative behavior is appropriate (or important) in only a few contexts or when there are only a few contexts in which the person will be communicating; and (2) it is practical to carry out training in each context. It usually is difficult to identify all potential communicative contexts for a given brain-injured person, and it is almost always impractical in terms of time and resource allocation to carry out training in every context. Consequently, sequential modification is likely to have limited usefulness in treating neurogenic communicative disabilities (except, perhaps, for some patients with restricted communicative environments, such as those confined at home or in a nursing home, having contact with only a few others, and with communication limited to a small range of topics).

Use Indiscriminable Contingencies.—Stokes and Baer (1977) suggest that generalization to settings outside the treatment setting is enhanced if the response contingencies in treatment are gradually altered to make them more like those that can be expected in natural settings. These alterations may include (1) changing the schedule of contingencies from continuous (for every response) to intermittent (for every nth response) to intermittent and variable (for every nth response on the average, but varying around the average); (2) interposing delay between responses and their contingencies; and (3) choosing contingencies that resemble those expected in natural settings. Many clinicians routinely include alterations in contingencies in their treatment procedures to increase the likelihood of generalization to natural contexts. Making contingencies indiscriminable is an important part of other techniques such as loose training.

Program Common Stimuli.—Programming common stimuli means that the context in which behavior is trained is designed to resemble the context(s) to which the behavior is to generalize (the target context). Programming common stimuli manipulates *stimulus control* to enhance generalization across contexts. "Stimulus control" refers to how stimuli or stimulus complexes govern the occurrence of behavior. A laboratory rat that is reinforced with food pellets for pressing a bar when a green light is on but not when a red light is on soon presses the bar only when the green light is on. The rat has learned to *discriminate* the reinforcement condition from the nonreinforcment condition. To extend stimulus control to the patient's daily life environment, a clinician might incorporate stimuli from the environment into training, expecting that when the patient then encounters those stimuli in daily life, he or she will be more likely to exhibit the trained behavior. The greater the similarity between the training environment and daily life, the more likely it will be that the trained behavior(s) will generalize to daily life. The extent to which the training environment and the target environment (e.g., daily life) resemble each other usually is decided subjectively. In most cases certain key elements (e.g., eliciting stimuli, surroundings, and sometimes people) are selected to resemble those elements in the target environment. As is true for alterations in contingencies, programming common stimuli can be incorporated into any treatment approach to increase the likelihood of generalization to natural contexts.

Mediate Generalization.—*Mediation* refers to the elicitation of one response by another response. Mnemonic devices are one example of mediation. One attaches easily remembered verbal labels (the mnemonic devices) to difficult-to-remember material and uses the mnemonic devices to retrieve the difficult-to-remember material (as in the rhyme for remembering the names of the cranial nerves in Chapter 1). In *mediated generalization* easier responses are used to elicit more difficult responses. For example, an aphasic person might be taught to retrieve words by imagining their visual images. Most of the literature on mediated generalization has studied verbal mediation (Stokes and Baer, 1977), and verbal mediation may be inappropriate for many aphasic persons because of their language impairments. However, verbal mediation often is useful in treatment programs for persons with right-hemisphere syndrome or traumatic brain injuries.

Train Generalization.—Sometimes patients "spontaneously" generalize during treatment activities. For example, a patient who is working on improving syntax in written work may begin using better syntax in spoken utterances. These spontaneous generalizations might themselves be targeted for reinforcment, and reinforcement contingencies might be gradually modified so that such responses receive a greater proportion of reinforcement than "rote" responses to training stimuli.

Social Validation

Social validation is a procedure for evaluating the clinical significance of changes created by a treatment program. Social validation attempts to determine whether the patient is "better" in a real-world sense than he or she was before treatment. It can be accomplished in two ways (Kazdin, 1982). One way is to compare the (socially relevant) behavior of the person receiving treatment with the behavior of a "normal" group of peers. The greater the progression toward normalcy, the more "clinically significant" the change in behavior. The other way is to obtain subjective evaluations of the behaviors of interest from persons in the patient's natural environment. Although many clinicians have for years carried out informal social validation by soliciting family members' opinions about how the patient is communicating at home, structured procedures for socially validating the effects of treatment on neurogenically impaired patients' communication have only recently been described (Doyle et al., 1987; Thompson and Byrne, 1984). Doyle et al. trained four adults with Broca's aphasia to produce various syntactic forms in response to pictures. All improved on measures of accuracy, grammaticality, and utterance length. Doyle et al. then evaluated the social validity of the improvements by playing audiotape recordings of the aphasic persons describing pictures to five adults who did not know the aphasic people and who knew nothing about the study. Some of the recordings were made before treatment began and others were made after treatment had ended, and they were arranged so that pretreatment and post-treatment samples occurred in random order. The judges were asked to judge whether each sample was "adequate" or "inadequate." In spite of subjects' improvements on measures of accuracy, grammaticality, and utterance length during treatment, the social validation procedure revealed no general increase in judgments of adequacy by the judges, although there were significant increases in judgments of adequacy for some syntactic forms. Doyle et al. concluded that social validation measures are crucial for evaluating the effectiveness of treatment programs, and that they may be useful as pretreatment measures for selecting behaviors to treat.

Thompson and Byrne used a peer-group-comparison method to assess the social validity of changes in the use of social conventions by their aphasic subjects. They had each aphasic subject participate in a conversational interaction with a normal adult whom the subject had not met before. They then compared the aphasic subjects' use of social conventions with that of the normal adults. Before treatment the aphasic subjects' use of social conventions was well below the range of the normal subjects, but at the end of treatment aphasic subjects' performance approximated that of the normal ones.

Social validation in clinical management of adults with neurogenic communication disorders is in its infancy, but promises to become an increasingly important aspect of management as structured, reliable procedures for assessing and quantifying it are created, improved, and validated.

Treatment of Aphasia

In this chapter I will describe some of the assumptions that I believe underlie treatment, and how it seems to me that clinicians decide *who, what,* and *how* to treat. I will also discuss some of the principles that underlie treatment of aphasic adults' impairments in listening, reading, speaking, and writing. I will describe procedures that are commonly used in treating these impairments, and I will summarize some empirical findings that should affect what clinicians do in treatment.

CLINICIAN ASSUMPTIONS UNDERLYING TREATMENT FOR APHASIA

What clinicians do when they design and carry out treatment programs for aphasic adults is determined in large part by their assumptions about aphasia and about the nature of therapeutic processes. These assumptions govern *who* the clinician treats, *when* treatment begins, *how* treatment is carried out, and *when* treatment stops. Perhaps few clinicians ever verbalize their assumptions, and it is almost certain that few, if any, are universal. In the following section, I present some general assumptions that are, it seems to me, important not only in shaping one's attitudes about aphasia treatment, but in determining the general principles that govern if, when, and how one treats aphasic adults. Most of this chapter and the next reflect my own assumptions about treatment of aphasia, but I have chosen to state the following assumptions explicitly, because I believe that they are likely to have broad general effects on one's clinical behavior.

Assumption 1.—Treatment of aphasic adults' communicative disabilities provides significant benefits when treatment is delivered by appropriately trained personnel and when recipients are appropriately selected.

The question of whether treatment of aphasic persons' communication impairments is worthwhile has been a source of controversy for many years. Some have argued that no convincing scientific evidence exists for the efficacy of aphasia treatment, while others have argued that the efficacy of treatment is supported both by experimental evidence and by clinical experience. A number of investigators have concluded that treatment for aphasia provides no significant improvement in speech and language beyond that which would be generated by spontaneous recovery (Vignolo, 1964; Sarno et al., 1970; Lincoln et al., 1984). Others have reported positive effects of treatment (Butfield and Zangwill, 1946; West, 1973; Deal and Deal, 1978; Basso et al., 1979; Wertz et al., 1981; Wertz et al., 1984). In spite of numerous attempts to scientifically evaluate the effects of aphasia treatment, the evidence generated has not been conclusive, because most of the studies contain scientific, procedural, or logical flaws that compromise the interpretation of the results. In many cases, no control groups against which the effects of treatment programs can be measured have been included. When control groups have been included, assignment of subjects to groups often has been contaminated by sampling and assignment errors. Treatment procedures have been poorly designed, poorly documented, and poorly matched to the recipients of the treatment. The frequency of treatment sessions and the duration of treatment programs sometimes has been so limited that treatment had no chance to generate meaningful changes in patients' performance. In many cases, the measures used to document changes (or lack of changes) in response to treatment were nonstandardized, with undocumented reliability and dubious validity.

Wertz et al. (1981, 1984) reported two studies of the efficacy of aphasia treatment that satisfy most requirements for scientific quality, replicability, and dependability of results. Both were large, multicenter studies in which (1) patients were carefully selected and randomly assigned to groups; (2) patients' neurologic and speech and language status was measured periodically, using standardized and reliable tests; (3) the content of treatment was controlled and documented; and (4) the possibility of experimenter bias was eliminated. In both studies the results supported the conclusion that treatment of aphasic adults has significant positive effects beyond the changes that would be expected from spontaneous recovery.

Poeck et al. (1989) also concluded that aphasia treatment is efficacious, based on the results of a well-designed study in which they provided 6 to 8 weeks of intensive treatment to 68 aphasic adults divided into three groups. Those in the *early* group were from 1 to 4 months postonset of aphasia when they entered the study. Those in the *late* group were from 4 to 12 months postonset at entry, and those in the *chronic* group were more than 12 months postonset at entry. Ninety-two aphasic adults in a control group received no treatment, but were tested on the same schedule as the treated subjects. Poeck et al. reported that (1) both treated and untreated groups improved on measures of speech and language; and (2) subjects who received treatment improved more than those who did not receive treatment.

In addition to group studies of the effects of aphasia treatment, a number of single-case design studies (Kearns and Salmon, 1984; Thompson and Byrne, 1984) have demonstrated that carefully controlled treatment programs are effective in changing targeted aspects of aphasic patients' performance, and that generalization of the changes to other behaviors, as well as to patients' daily life environments, can be obtained. The weight of the evidence at this time clearly supports the efficacy of treatment for aphasia if the treatment is delivered by qualified persons, if patients with irreversible aphasia are excluded, and if the content, duration, and timing of treatment are appropriate for those receiving treatment.

Assumption 2.—Early treatment of aphasic patients' communication disabilities usually is better than later treatment.

Scientific studies of early versus late intervention have yielded equivocal results. Several investigators have reported that delaying treatment by 2 months or more after the onset of aphasia has significant negative effects on eventual recovery (Butfield and Zangwill, 1946; Wepman, 1951; Vignolo, 1964; Sands, 1969). For example, Vignolo studied the course of recovery of 69 aphasic patients. Some received treatment and some did not. Vignolo concluded that it is important that treatment begin during the time at which physiologic recovery is most rapid: "Only the period which extends from 2 to 6 months after the onset of aphasia seems to provide a ground where intrinsic capacity for recovery can be highly enhanced by the intervention of planned training."

Others have concluded that delaying treatment has no major effects on outcome. Wertz et al. (1986) randomly assigned aphasic patients to two groups. The patients in each group were from 2 to 24 weeks postonset of aphasia. One group received 12 weeks of treatment that began as soon as the patients qualified for the study. After waiting 12 weeks, the other group (matched with the first on numerous variables) received treatment equivalent to that given to the immediately treated group. At 12 weeks (when the immediate-treatment group had received 12 weeks of treatment and the delayed-treatment group had received none), the immediate-treatment group had improved significantly more (on Porch Index of Communicative Ability [PICA] overall scores) than the delayed-treatment group. However, when the delayed-treatment group then received 12 weeks of treatment while the immediate-treatment group received none, the delayed-treatment group made significant improvement and eventually caught up with the immediate-treatment group. Wertz et al. concluded that delaying treatment for 12 weeks had no irreversible effects on aphasic patients' eventual recovery.

Poeck et al. (1989) reported that neither age nor time after onset of aphasia significantly affected aphasic adults' recovery of language. However, time after onset appeared to affect the magnitude of patients' response to treatment. Of those who began treatment within the first 4 months postonset of aphasia, 78% improved significantly on a standardized aphasia test. In addition, 46% of those who began treatment from 4 to 12 months postonset improved significantly on the same test, even when subjects' test scores were corrected for the effects of "spontaneous" neurologic recovery.

Even if it were to be shown that delaying treatment has few or no significant effects on patient's scores on standardized tests of language and communication (the criterion used in the published studies), it may not be legitimate to conclude that delaying treatment has no negative effects on the patient or the patient's family. Clinicians do more than treat specific speech and language behaviors in the first weeks following the onset of a patient's aphasia. They provide reassurance, advice, and support to patients and families. They educate the patient and family about the causes of the patient's aphasia and how the patient and family can cope with it. They make referrals to members of other disciplines and help the patient and family make use of community resources. They keep the patient and family from responding in a maladaptive manner to the patient's communicative disabilities, and they teach the patient and family effective strategies for dealing with communication breakdown.

Education, counseling, support, and direction may not affect the patient's scores on standardized tests, yet they are important to patients and families immediately after onset of aphasia. Consequently, it seems inappropriate to suggest that clinicians have nothing to contribute to aphasic patients during the first 10 or 12 weeks postonset that cannot just as well be done later. It may be that delaying treatment of aphasic adults has no significant and irreversible effects on standardized test scores, but delaying or eliminating the counseling, education, support, and referrals provided during the first weeks after the patient becomes aphasic may have important and irreversible negative effects on the patient and the family.

Assumption 3.—A primary objective of treatment is to improve the aphasic person's communication in his or her daily life environment.

In 1965, Schuell et al. asserted that "The primary objective in treatment of aphasia is to increase communication. What the aphasic patient wants is to recover enough language to get on with his life." Holland (1977) observed that "traditional" didactic treatment approaches tend to focus on "activities such as matching, naming, and helping aphasics to comprehend utterances defined by their linguistic structure, instead of their likelihood of being heard in everyday communication. . . . Most therapy is disproportionately centered on the propositionality of an utterance, not on its communicative value." Holland went on to recommend that treatment focus on *communicative competence*—a person's *use* of language in naturalistic contexts. During the 1980s many clinicians moved away from the traditional linguistically oriented, didactic treatment that had predominated until that time, toward treatment that emphasized functional communication in naturalistic contexts. The new treatment programs typically relied on within-the-clinic analogues to naturalistic communicative interactions (e.g., conversations), with the expectation that communicative skills acquired in these situations would generalize to daily life. The best-known and most extensively documented program for teaching "functional" communication to aphasic adults is Promoting Aphasics' Communicative Effectiveness (PACE) therapy (Davis and Wilcox, 1985). It endeavors to place the aphasic person in communicative interactions that are governed by the same principles that govern daily life communicative interactions, e.g., patient and clinician participate as equals, there is exchange of new information, and adequacy is measured in terms of successful communication rather than linguistic integrity.

There is no convincing empirical evidence that "functional" approaches to treatment are more successful in creating improvement in daily life communication than "traditional" approaches, although it seems intuitively reasonable that this might be true. However, it also seems intuitively reasonable that "traditional" didactic approaches might also create comparable improvements in daily life communication *if* the behaviors targeted for treatment were important in daily life communicative interactions. That the *procedures* employed in treatment resemble natural communicative interactions may be less important than the fact that the *behaviors* (or processes) targeted for treatment are relevant to daily life communication. For example, it seems intuitively reasonable that placing an aphasic person in "unrealistic" activities in which he or she must quickly adjust to changes in stimuli or response requirements might enhance their comprehension in daily life interchanges in which topics and speakers change abruptly and without warning. Unfortunately, once again there is little empirical evidence that treatment directed toward "processes" that may underlie daily life communication actually improves daily life communication.

The really important issue here is that of *generalization*—the transfer of what is accomplished in the clinic to the aphasic person's daily life. Regardless of how one approaches treatment, unless one incorporates specific procedures for enhancing generalization into the treatment program, generalization to daily life often does not occur. Because improvements in communicative ability that do not extend outside the clinic are of little value, it behooves the clinician to plan for, work for, and test for generalization from the clinic to the patient's daily life.

Assumption 4.—Rehabilitation of aphasic persons requires attention to the linguistic, behavioral, emotional, social, and vocational consequences of aphasia and to associated medical and physical conditions.

Treatment of aphasic persons involves considerably more than direct treatment of speech and language abilities. It involves attention to the physical, emotional, and social consequences of the patient's physical and communicative disabilities. It involves making appropriate referrals, providing education, counseling, support, and reassurance for the patient, caregivers, and/or family members. The objectives of treatment always extend beyond communication to maximizing the patient's independence, competence, and happiness in daily life, and a comprehensive program of treatment must deal with the social, vocational, and familial consequences of aphasia, as well as their effects on communication.

Assumption 5.—Aphasia is not a loss of language, but is the result of impairments in processes that underlie speaking, listening, writing, and reading.

Most agree that aphasia is not a loss of language—either vocabulary or rules—but that it is the result of impairments in processes necessary for comprehending, formulating, and producing spoken and written language. For example, comprehension disability in aphasia may be caused by reduced speed and efficiency in attaching meaning to words, rather than loss of word meanings themselves, or it may be caused by reductions in speed, efficiency, or accuracy of retrieval from memory, rather than loss of vocabulary. Similarly, speech production problems may be caused by disruptions of word retrieval or phonologic selection and sequencing, rather than loss of words or syntactic rules.

If aphasia represents a reduction in the speed and efficiency of processes underlying language rather than loss of language, then treatment should focus on *reactivating* or *restimulating* language processes rather than on *teaching* specific responses (Schuell et al., 1965). For example, if an aphasic patient has a reading problem, the clinician might attempt to determine whether the problem is related to (1) eye movements and visual search; (2) word comprehension; (3) use of syntactic rules; (4) ability to deduce main ideas, make inferences, or draw conclusions; or (5) storage and recall of information gained from printed materials. After the determination is made, treatment is focused on the processes identified as deficient. One of the major advantages of a process-directed approach to treatment is that treating a general process may affect several specific communicative abilities that depend on the process.

CANDIDACY FOR TREATMENT

Not all aphasic patients are capable of recovering functional communication. There are several symptoms of severe aphasia (or bilateral brain damage) that suggest that a patient may not have the capacity to become a functional verbal communicator. The presence of one symptom in a patient who is neurologically stable is ominous, and the presence of more than one should make a clinician cautious about the functional outcome of speech and language treatment.

Verbal Stereotypes or Repetitive Utterances and Severely Impaired Comprehension.—The presence of repetitive, stereotypical, perseverative utterances ("me-me-me-me," "oh boy, oh boy, oh boy, oh boy," etc.) accompanied by severe disabilities in language comprehension in a neurologically recovered patient* suggests severe and irreversible aphasia. Few neurologically recovered patients who exhibit these symptoms become functional verbal communicators, even with treatment. A few may eventually learn to communicate a few basic needs using single words and gestures, and some may learn to communicate using alternative communication systems such as communication boards or communication books.

Inability to Match Identical Objects or Pictures and Objects.—If a neurologically recovered patient cannot match common objects (e.g., forks, pencils, keys) or cannot match common objects to pictures, they are unlikely to regain functional verbal communication, even with treatment. Inability to match objects to objects or ob-

---

*The adjective "neurologically recovered" will be used herein to denote patients for whom "spontaneous" physiologic recovery is mostly complete. For most patients with occlusive strokes, physiologic recovery is essentially complete within 4 to 6 weeks, although slow improvement beyond that time is common. For patients with hemorrhagic strokes and for those with traumatic brain injuries, physiologic recovery may last longer, but usually is essentially complete by 6 months or so.

jects to pictures is frequently (some would say always) associated with bilateral brain damage, and is unusual even in severely aphasic patients with unilateral brain damage.

Unreliable Yes-No Responses.—Neurologiclly recovered aphasic patients who cannot reliably indicate "yes" and "no" verbally, by gesture or head nod, or by pointing to cards showing words or symbols representing "yes" and "no," usually are not good candidates for treatment. A neurologically recovered patient's failure to develop dependable yes-no responses suggests severe aphasia. If such a patient cannot be taught reliable yes-no responses to simple *nonverbal* stimuli within an hour or two, the prospects for positive effects of treatment are poor.

Jargon and Empty Speech Without Self-Correction.—Some patients with severe comprehension disabilities emit either jargon (e.g., nonwords such as "kalimfropper") or empty speech (e.g., meaningless strings of words, such as "that's Sheila's aunt in a full subscription") without recognizing that there is anything wrong with what they say. Neurologically recovered patients who exhibit these behaviors usually are not good candidates for treatment directed toward speech and language disabilities.

These signs of irreversible aphasia include those that frequently influence decisions about aphasic patients' candidacy for treatment. Extended treatment to reinstate functional verbal communication for such patients is rarely appropriate. The speech-language pathologist's primary role with such patients usually is that of helping the family or other caregivers cope with the patient's communicative impairments, and helping family or other caregivers structure the patient's daily life environment to take advantage of the communicative abilities that the patient has retained. During the past few years several investigators have begun working on treatment programs for severely aphasic persons (Collins, 1986; Salvatore and Thompson, 1986). It may be that "irreversible" aphasia may become at least partially reversible, given specific treatment approaches.

TREATMENT OBJECTIVES

Most adults who remain aphasic for more than a month or so after onset do not completely regain their premorbid communicative ability. Some with very mild aphasia at a month or so after onset may eventually approximate their premorbid communicative abilities, but they are a small proportion of the aphasic population. Consequently, clinicians formulating treatment objectives usually expect that the patient will be left with residual communication impairments at the end of treatment. The objective of treatment usually is to enable the patient to communicate with maximum effectiveness in the face of these residual communicative impairments.

Unfortunately, many of the activities that traditionally have been incorporated into aphasia treatment appear not to be very relevant to daily life. Didactic treatment activities sometimes concentrate on specific and sometimes trivial skills that have little relationship to daily life communication activities. If the goal of treatment is to improve comprehension and retention of sequential information, a patient who has learned to touch squares and circles of various colors and sizes has accomplished less, in a real-world sense, than a patient who has learned to remember a telephone number from the directory long enough to dial it, even though the former may show greater "improvement" on a traditional aphasia examination than the latter.

As mentioned previously, Davis and Wilcox (1985) described a treatment approach that attempts to increase generalization of treatment from the clinic to daily life by making treatment activities resemble conversational interactions. This approach, PACE treatment, is based on four principles.

1. The patient and clinician alternate as senders and receivers of messages.
2. New information is exchanged between the clinician and the patient. The clinician does not know ahead of time what the patient will attempt to communicate on any given trial.
3. The patient has free choice of the communicative behaviors to be used in conveying a message. The clinician does not direct the patient to use a particular response modality, although the clinician may model communicative behaviors that would be useful to the patient.
4. Feedback is provided in response to the patient's success in conveying a message, and not according to the linguistic correctness of the message. Clinician feedback in PACE consists of (a) comprehension of the message, (b) misunderstanding the message, or (c) guesses about the content of the message.

Regardless of the techniques used in treatment, if treatment is to produce changes in a patient's daily life communication, it should target relevant communication, using relevant materials, in relevant contexts. If one teaches vocabulary, the vocabulary should be useful in the patient's daily life. If sentence comprehension is a treatment objective, sentences should be similar to those that the patient might encounter in daily life, and they should occur in contexts like those in daily life. The patient may be encouraged (or taught) to use nonverbal communication such as gestures and facial expression, and to make use of information provided by others' gestures and facial expressions and by situational contexts to enhance his or her comprehension. Aphasic persons need not be perfect speakers or perfect listeners to communicate adequately. Treatment objectives should respect this principle.

Usually there is an evolution of treatment as a patient progresses through a treatment program. Early in treatment the emphasis may be on measurement of residual abilities and treatment may be directed toward specific skills such as verbal retention, vocabulary, and grammar. As treatment progresses and the patient's eventual residual level of communicative ability becomes clearer, the emphasis may shift toward preparing the patient to deal with his or her daily life. By the end of treatment, activities may focus completely on communication in daily life.

THE FOCUS AND PROGRESSION OF TREATMENT

Aphasia is a communicative impairment. Consequently, most aphasia treatment attempts to remediate communicative deficiencies. How one partitions communication, or how one categorizes communicative deficits will determine, to some extent, how one approaches treatment of aphasia. The communicative deficits that characterize aphasia can be categorized in several ways (Table 7–1).

Most aphasia tests address the four primary language modalities—listening, speaking, reading, and writing—and permit evaluation at several levels in each modality (e.g., recognition, discrimination, comprehension, or selection, sequencing, and production).

Even though treatment programs may focus on a particular language modality, treatment usually is not confined to a single skill. Most aphasic patients have general impairments that cross modalities, and most clinicians treat several. Clinicians often treat both listening comprehension and speech production, and some simultaneously

TABLE 7–1.

Categories of Communicative Deficits That
Characterize Aphasia

By general processes
   Recognition
   Discrimination
   Comprehension
      or
   Selecting
   Sequencing
   Producing
By verbal processes
   Listening
   Speaking
   Reading
   Writing
By modalities
   Sensory (input)
      Auditory
      Visual
   Motor (output)
      Oral
      Graphic
By linguistic categories
   Phonologic
   Syntactic
   Semantic
   Pragmatic
By tasks
   Reading words
   Writing sentences
   Describing pictures, etc.

treat all four language skills—listening, reading, speaking, and writing. Some clinicians believe that comprehension should be treated before production, but they may treat both listening and reading comprehension, or they may treat comprehension at one level (usually higher) and production at another (usually lower) level. All treatment programs move the patient through a progression of tasks in which stimuli are gradually made more complex and response requirements gradually escalate.

When treatment is directed toward production, speech usually is treated before writing. There appear to be two reasons for this. First, speech usually is the patient's primary means of communication in daily life, and improving a patient's speech will have greater effects on daily life communication than improving his or her writing. Second, writing usually is more difficult than speaking for aphasic people, so it is most efficient to initially concentrate on speech and to follow with work on writing.

TREATMENT OF AUDITORY COMPREHENSION

Schuell et al. (1965) considered impairments in auditory comprehension and auditory retention span a central problem in aphasia. Since that time, treatment of auditory comprehension impairments has had a special status for many clinicians who believe that treatment of auditory comprehension impairments is the most efficient way of improving aphasic adults' general language competence. Even though this belief has not been directly supported by experimental evidence, treatment of auditory comprehension impairments continues to play a central role in many approaches to aphasia treatment.

For many years auditory comprehension was thought to proceed through a series of stages, from analyzing the acoustic characteristics of spoken messages to derivation of the meanings of utterances. Listeners were thought to identify the phonemes in the message, combine phonemes into representations of words, identify the words in the utterance, retrieve the meanings of the words, determine the relationships among words, and construct a mental representation for the meaning of the utterance, in that order. Such models of comprehension eventually became known as "bottom up" models, because listeners start with the physical characteristics of the message and work their way "up" through a series of levels to the "top," at which point the meaning of the utterance becomes apparent.

Other models of comprehension subsequently were proposed, in which listeners' general knowledge and expectations about what might be said play a role in comprehension. These models became known as "top down" models, because listeners start with expectations about what might be said, and confirm or change their expectations based on the information provided by the speaker. Research on normal listeners' comprehension suggests that how listeners go about making sense of what they hear often depends on the nature of the comprehension task, and that most listeners use combinations of top-down and bottom-up processes in daily life comprehension. It is clear that listeners are not bound to the literal content of spoken sentences; they use probablility, plausibility, and their general knowledge to arrive at the meaning of sentences, and resort to syntactic analysis of the relationships between words in the message primarily when the top-down approach fails or yields ambiguous meanings.

Auditory Memory and Auditory Comprehension

Listening comprehension and auditory memory cannot be separated. There seems to be at least general agreement about how the two interact, although terminology differs across models. Most models postulate three stages through which the information from a spoken sentence passes. The first stage is a *sensory register* in which acoustic characteristics of the utterance are briefly stored. The sensory register has limited capacity and information in that it decays quickly and cannot be maintained by rehearsal. The two most common labels for the second stage are *short-term memory* and *working memory*. The second stage also has limited capacity, and information quickly decays, but it can be maintained in consciousness by rehearsal. The exact syntactic structure of a sentence can be retained in working memory if it is rehearsed, and if no new information comes in to displace it. The two most common labels for the third stage are *long-term memory* and *secondary memory*. The third stage has very large (perhaps infinite) capacity and information at this stage decays slowly, if at all. The meanings of sentences are integrated into permanent memory at this stage.

Some contemporary models of memory (Craik and Lockhart, 1972) reject the "stages" conceptualization of memory in favor of a continuous "depth of processing" explanation. However, the general conceptualization of how comprehension proceeds in "depth of processing" models is similar to that for "stages" models.

The exact role of memory in aphasic patients' comprehension impairments is not well understood. Most aphasic patients have deficiencies in short-term verbal memory that interfere with recall of verbal messages. Most also have difficulty retrieving words and word meanings from long-term verbal memory. Treatment programs for aphasic patients' comprehension impairments often are directed toward improving short-term verbal memory by means of activities in which patients make immediate responses to spoken directions ("point-to" tasks). Many clinicians believe that if an aphasic patient's short-term verbal memory improves, his or her long-term verbal memory (and other language abilities) will also improve. At this time there is no empirical evidence to support this assumption, and evidence from studies of "normal" language comprehension suggest that the mental activity involved in comprehending language in natural situations depends on long-term memory more than short-term memory. Consequently, improving aphasic patients' short-term verbal memory may have weaker effects on daily life comprehension than many seem to believe.

Single-Word Comprehension

Disabilities in single-word comprehension need not necessarily affect daily life comprehension to any great degree. In most daily life listening activities, comprehension of speakers' utterances does not depend on comprehending every word in the utterances. The context (both verbal and situational) in which words occur often gives strong hints about their meanings, and the aphasic listener who can make use of context to deduce the meaning of uncomprehended words may do very well at comprehending utterances in daily life. However, sometimes disabilities in single-word comprehension are disruptive enough to warrant treatment.

Patients with severe comprehension impairments are the most likely candidates for treatment of single-word comprehension. However, treatment of single-word comprehension usually is not appropriate unless it is likely to contribute to development of higher-level communication skills. Training single-word comprehension by itself rarely creates meaningful changes in the communicative abilities of severely aphasic patients. Even if such patients acquire rudimentary single-word listening vocabularies, they are not likely to use them in a functional way outside the context in which they acquired the vocabularies. Exercises in single-word comprehension are most profitably used as stepping stones to more advanced comprehension skills. In these cases single-word comprehension exercises may lead to retention span and short-term memory exercises involving longer messages.

A small number of patients whose aphasia is not severe experience remarkable difficulties in attaching meanings to words that they hear (or read). They behave (usually intermittently) as if they do not know the meanings of spoken or printed words, even when the words are common in the language. Their performance is not word-specific—sometimes they comprehend a particular word and at other times they do not. Sometimes they behave as if they are hearing words from a foreign language. They may repeat an unrecognized word over and over, and they may even spell the word while attempting to associate it with a meaning. When such a patient is given a clue to the meaning of an unrecognized word (such as a synonym or antonym), comprehension of the word often occurs. Treatment for these patients usually involves exercises in which they match spoken words to pictures or give definitions, synonyms, or antonyms for spoken words. Unfortunately, such activities usually do not generate great improvements in single-word comprehension. However, one can sometimes improve such patients' single-word comprehension indirectly by improving their short-term auditory memory and sentence comprehension, and by teaching them to use context to arrive at the meaning of unrecognized words.

Variables Affecting Single-Word Comprehension

Several variables affect the accuracy of aphasic patients' responses in single-word comprehension tasks. A word's *frequency of occurrence* in the language often affects the ease with which it will be comprehended by aphasic listeners (Schuell et al., 1961). In general, as a word's frequency of occurrence decreases, the probability that it will be comprehended also decreases. However, for most aphasic patients, these effects usually are seen only with words that are infrequent in daily life, and the effects of word frequency can be overshadowed by other factors such as sentence context and semantic plausibility.

Semantic or acoustic similarity between target words and foils may affect aphasic patients' accuracy in single-word comprehension tasks. Semantic similarity appears to have a much stronger effect than acoustic similarity does. Schuell and Jenkins (1961) reported that semantic confusions are far more frequent than either acoustic confusions or random errors when aphasic patients match spoken words to pictures.

Part of speech may affect some aphasic listeners' single-word comprehension. Nouns usually are easier than adjectives, verbs, and adverbs. However, these differences may relate more to the ease with which nouns can be pictured relative to other parts of speech than to any inherent difference in comprehensibility between nouns and other parts of speech. Brookshire and Nicholas (1982) have shown that sentences containing picturable verbs (those that can be represented by objects, such as "hammering") are comprehended more quickly by aphasic listeners than nonpicturable verbs (such as "running") that cannot be represented by objects.

Referent ambiguity (ambiguity in pictured referents for spoken words) may affect aphasic patients' performance in matching spoken words to pictures. If pictorial referents are ambiguous or unclear, patients may respond inaccurately, not because they fail to comprehend the words, but because they are unable to deduce the intended meaning of the pictures.

Understanding Spoken Sentences

Comprehension of spoken sentences is an important part of communication in daily life, and impaired sentence comprehension is commonly targeted in treatment programs for aphasic adults, not only because it seems to be important in a daily life sense, but because of the central role played by auditory comprehension in some models of aphasia. Treatment activities for improving comprehension of spoken sentences usually rely on one or more of three tasks: *comprehension of spoken questions, following spoken directions,* and *sentence verification.*

Treatment involving *comprehension of spoken questions* can make use either of yes-no questions ("Is a horse larger than a kitten?") or open-ended questions ("What is your wife's name?"). Yes-no questions are less demanding in terms of patients' responses than open-ended questions. Even patients who have little or no functional speech may be able to respond to yes-no questions by pointing to the printed words "yes" and "no" or by head nods or head shakes. Yes-no questions can test recognition of information ("Is Mason City the capital of Iowa?"), verbal retention ("Are monkeys, horses, cows, and pigs animals?"), semantic discriminations ("Do you brush teeth with a comb?"), phonemic discriminations ("Do you wear a shirt and pie?"), syntactic analysis ("Do you wear feet on your shoes?"), or semantic relationships ("Is a banana a vegetable?").

Patients with retrieval, formulation, or production problems may perform poorly on open-ended questions because of their retrieval, formulation, or production problems, and not because they cannot comprehend the questions. However, open-ended questions are more versatile than yes-no questions; they permit one to sample a greater range and variety of information, and they permit greater flexibility in the structure of the questions. For patients whose output is sufficient for the task, treatment using open-ended questions has more flexibility than treatment using yes-no questions.

Treatment activities in which patients are asked to *follow spoken directions* typically require sequential pointing or manipulative responses in response to the spoken directions. Such activities are very common in treatment of comprehension impairments in aphasia, mainly because they eliminate the potential effects of verbal output problems on test performance. The *Token Test* (DeRenzi and Vignolo, 1962) is the prototypical example of such procedures. In the *Token Test*, the patient manipulates large and small colored circles and squares or rectangles in response to spoken directions that gradually increase in length and syntactic complexity. Most treatment procedures differ from the *Token Test* in that pictures or objects replace the geometric shapes, but the length and syntactic structure of spoken directions are manipulated in the same way as in the *Token Test*.

Kearns and Hubbard (1977) tested 10 aphasic listeners to evaluate the difficulty of 13 levels of spoken directions. The 13 levels, together with the average score for the 10 aphasic listeners (using the 16-category scoring system from the PICA) (Porch, 1967), were:

1. Point to one common object by name (14.30).
2. Point to one common object by function (14.02).
3. Point in sequence to two common objects by function (12.90).
4. Point in sequence to two common objects by name (12.67).
5. Point to one object spelled by the examiner (12.51).
6. Point to one object described by the examiner, using three descriptors (e.g., "Which one is white, plastic, and has bristles?") (12.23).
7. Follow one-verb instructions (e.g., "Pick up the pen") (12.05).
8. Point in sequence to three common objects by name (10.74).
9. Point in sequence to three common objects by function (10.72).
10. Carry out two-object location instructions (e.g., "Put the pen in front of the knife") (10.20).
11. Carry out, in sequence, two-verb instructions (e.g., "Point to the knife and turn over the fork") (9.77).
12. Carry out, in sequence, two-verb instructions with time constraint ("Before you pick up the knife, hand me the fork") (8.60).
13. Carry out three-verb instructions (e.g., "Point to the knife, turn over the fork, and hand me the pencil") (7.53).

Kearns and Hubbard identified the following four levels as representing significantly different levels of difficulty.

1. Point to one common object by function.
2. Point in sequence to two common objects by name.
3. Carry out, in sequence, two-verb instructions.
4. Carry out, in sequence, three-verb instructions.

Kearns and Hubbard suggested that these four tasks might be used as a screening test for comprehension impairments, and as measures of progress in treatment. Kearns and Hubbard's original list of 13 tasks also may be useful in setting up a hierarchy of task difficulty for a specific patient.

As a general rule, sentences that are difficult because of their length or the number of items of information they contain ("Point to the dog, the horse, and the farmer") depend primarily on short-term verbal memory. Sentences that impose time and response sequence constraints on the patient's responses ("Before touching the cup, give me the pen"), or include directional or locational information ("Put the pen behind the cup") require more complex linguistic analyses in addition to short-term verbal memory.

The sentences described above are *episodic,* that is, once the patient responds to the sentence, he or she can forget it without consequences. Many utterances in daily life are episodic (e.g., "Please pass the salt"). Comprehension of episodic sentences draws primarily on short-term memory. However, many daily-life sentences are not episodic. They must be remembered, integrated with existing knowledge, and retrieved and acted upon at a later time (e.g., "Call Mr. Jones as soon as you get home"). Such sentences make heavier demands on long-term memory and recall than episodic sentences do. Most sentence comprehension activities in aphasia treatment involve episodic sentences. Consequently, they may not require listeners to exercise long-term memory to any great extent, and they may not prepare listeners to deal with nonepisodic sentences in daily life. Comprehension activities in which instructions must be remembered and carried out later (e.g., "Put this pen in your pocket and give it back to me before you leave") may be more appropriate for this purpose.*

Sentence Verification

In sentence verification, sentences are spoken to the patient and the patient determines if each sentence is true or false. In one form of verification, a picture is presented along with each spoken sentence, and the listener decides whether the picture is a true representation of the meaning of the sentence. Usually a given sentence is presented several times, once with a picture that matches the sentence's meaning, as in Figure 7–1, **left** and at other times with a foil that assesses the patient's ability to discriminate the true meaning of the sentence from meanings that resemble the true meaning, as in Figure 7–1, **center** and **right.**

In another form of sentence verification, sentences are presented alone (e.g., "A sidewalk is wider than a highway") and the patient makes a decision about the truth of the sentences based on his or her general knowledge. This version of the verification procedure resembles yes-no questions. However, verification may be somewhat easier than yes-no questions for some aphasic listeners who may have difficulty comprehending interrogative structures.

---

*Such activities actually are exercises in delayed recall, rather than listening comprehension, because the difficulty lies more in *remembering* the instructions than in *comprehending* them.

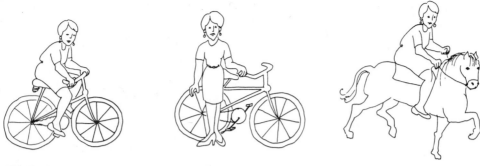

FIG 7–1.
A stimulus picture *(left)* and foils *(center, right)* for verification of the sentence, "The woman is riding the bicycle."

Sentence-to-Picture Match to Sample

The match-to-sample procedure resembles the picture-to-sentence verification procedure, except that target pictures (those that represent the true meaning of the sentences) and foils are presented together (as in Fig 7–2) and the patient points to the picture that best represents the meaning of a given sentence. The difficulty of match-to-sample tasks increases when sentences become longer or more complex, when correct choices and foils become more similar, or when the number of foils increases. Some standardized tests of sentence comprehension make use of the match-to-sample procedure. In these tests, foil pictures usually have systematic relationships to target pictures. Figure 7–2 shows a set of four pictures that might accompany the sentence "the man is hugging the woman." In order to respond correctly, listeners have to perceive subject, object, or verb mismatches between foil pictures and the stimulus sentence. Figure 7–3 shows a set of four pictures that might accompany the sentence "the boy is in the tree." In order to respond correctly, listeners have to comprehend the subject, the prepositional relationship, and the object of the preposition. (Remember that systematic relationships between pictured targets and foils sometimes may permit patients to choose the correct picture without comprehending the sentence, as was discussed earlier.)

Task Switching Activities

Many aphasic patients have difficulty comprehending spoken materials when task characteristics (stimulus materials, response requirements) change. Task switching exercises may teach such patients to deal with unexpected changes in communicative interactions. Task switching exercises require comprehension of sentences whose structure changes from trial to trial and execution of responses that change from trial to trial. A task switching exercise might include the following sequence of instructions.

1. Pick up the spoon.
2. Tell me the name of this (point) one.

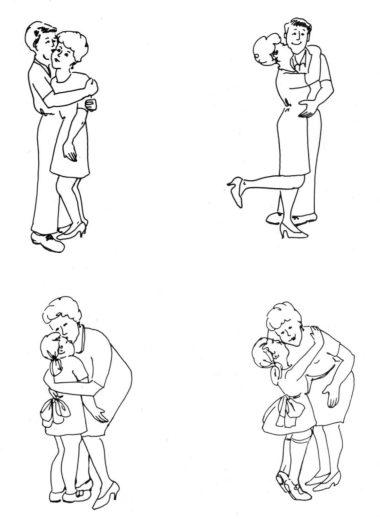

FIG 7–2.
A picture plate for verification of the sentence, "The man is hugging the woman."

3. Write the name of the one you drink from.
4. What day comes after Wednesday?
5. Spell "spoon."
6. Put the key in the cup.
7. Is your name Fred?

Variables Affecting Sentence Comprehension

Although several variables may affect aphasic listeners' comprehension of spoken sentences, two of the strongest are *length* and *syntactic complexity*. As spoken

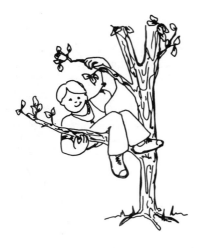
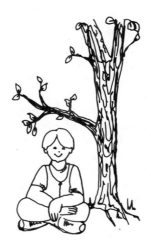
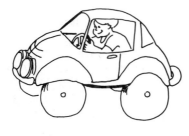
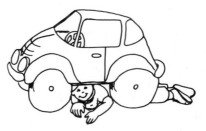

FIG 7–3.
A picture plate for verification of the sentence, "The boy is in the tree."

sentences become longer and syntactically more complex, they become more difficult for aphasic listeners to comprehend, provided that other characteristics of the sentences remain the same. Shewan and Canter (1971) found that syntactic complexity had stronger negative effects on aphasic listeners' comprehension of spoken sentences than either sentence length or vocabulary difficulty. Goodglass et al. (1979) and Nicholas and Brookshire (1983) also demonstrated that syntactic complexity has more detrimental effects on aphasic listeners' comprehension than sentence length. Goodglass et al. presented two sets of spoken sentences to aphasic listeners. One set was syntactically complex ("The man greeted by his wife was smoking a pipe") and the other contained syntactically simpler forms of the same sentences ("The man was greeted by his wife and he was smoking a pipe"). Goodglass et al. found that syntactically simpler sentences were comprehended better by aphasic listeners than syntactically complex ones, even though the simple sentences were longer than the complex versions.

In general, active sentences ("The dog bit the boy") are easier for aphasic listeners to comprehend than passive sentences ("The boy was bitten by the dog"). Conditional sentences ("If the cup is blue, give it to me"), sentences containing locational or directional prepositions ("Put the cup behind the box"), and comparative or relational sentences ("Is fire hotter than ice?") are difficult for many aphasic listeners. Embedded clause sentences ("The letter the girl wrote is on the table") are very difficult for almost all aphasic listeners (and for many nonaphasic ones).

Reversibility and plausibility affect aphasic listeners' comprehension of subject-verb-object sentences. Reversible sentences, in which subject and object can be transposed without creating an implausible sentence (e.g., "The man is hugging the woman" reverses to "The woman is hugging the man") are likely to be more difficult than sentences for which transposition generates an implausible sentence (e.g., "The man is carrying the book" reverses to "The book is carrying the man"). Sentences that become improbable (but not implausible) when subject and object are transposed (e.g., "The dog is chasing the cat" reverses to "The cat is chasing the dog") probably fall between the other two in difficulty. Caramazza and Zurif (1976) investigated the effects of reversibility on aphasic listeners' comprehension of embedded clause sentences ("The apple that the boy is eating is red"). They concluded that sentence comprehension of some aphasic patients was poorer when sentences were reversible than when they were not, although their major finding was that their aphasic subjects relied heavily on plausibility to comprehend syntactically complex sentences.

The *personal relevance* of questions strongly affects their difficulty for most aphasic listeners. Questions about personally relevant information usually are easier than questions about other information. Gray et al. (1977) and Busch and Brookshire (1982) evaluated aphasic subjects' responses to three categories of spoken yes-no questions: (1) questions that referred to nonpersonal factual information ("Do apples grow on trees?"); (2) questions that referred to information about the immediate environment ("Are we in a hospital?"); and (3) questions that referred to personal information about the patient ("Is your name _____?"). In both studies, aphasic subjects' responses to personal information questions were more accurate than their responses to questions about the immediate environment, and their responses to questions about the immediate environment were more accurate than their responses to questions about nonpersonal factual information. Although similar studies have not been carried out with open-ended questions, it seems reasonable to expect that their difficulty would be affected similarly by the personal relevance of the questions.

The difficulty of questions for aphasic listeners also appears to be affected by several other factors. Questions that test knowledge learned from teachers, books, or schooling ("Was Washington the first President of the United States?") usually are more difficult than questions that test knowledge gained from daily life experiences ("Is winter colder than summer?"). Questions that require reasoning or making inferences ("Why do farmers put hay in the barn?") usually are more difficult than questions that do not. The difficulty of these latter questions no doubt comes more from the fact that they require either memory search for the answers or logic, reasoning, and inference, rather than from the intrinsic difficulty of the questions. Questions such as "why do farmers put hay in the barn?" also require longer and more complex responses, so that verbal formulation and production problems may compromise performance on them.

The *rate* of auditory stimuli is likely to affect aphasic patients' responses in auditory comprehension tasks. Slowing the rate at which spoken materials are presented (either by speaking slowly or inserting pauses) improves many aphasic listeners' comprehension of the materials (Gordon, 1970; Parkhurst, 1970; Liles and Brookshire, 1975; Gardner et al., 1975; Lasky et al., 1976; Weidner and Lasky, 1976; Poeck and Pietron, 1981). Pashek and Brookshire (1982) found that a group of aphasic listeners comprehended spoken paragraphs better when they were spoken at 120 words per minute than when they were spoken at 150 words per minute. However, Brookshire and Nicholas (1984b) and Nicholas and Brookshire (1986) reported that not all aphasic listeners' comprehension improves when speech rate is slowed, and sometimes an aphasic listener will benefit from slowed speech rate at one time and not at another. They played recordings of sentences or short narrative stories to aphasic listeners at either 120 words per minute or 200 words per minute, and then tested their comprehension twice, not less than 2 weeks apart. The effects of speech rate on comprehension were not consistent across aphasic listeners, or within aphasic listeners across time. The facilitating group effects of slow speech rate found on the first test essentially disappeared by the second test. When a group of aphasic listeners exhibited a rate effect, it was always the case that some members of the group failed to exhibit the effect, exhibited it at one time and not another, or even exhibited effects opposite to that for the group. Consequently, clinicians should routinely assess the effects of rate manipulations (and the consistency of the effects) for patients with listening comprehension impairments.

Most aphasic listeners are sensitive to the *fidelity* of spoken messages. They have difficulty understanding speech in noisy conditions or when speech is distorted. Many aphasic listeners do poorly with tape-recorded auditory stimuli, especially if the recording introduces distortion. To avoid this problem, high quality recorders and audiotape should be used to record and play auditory materials used in aphasia testing or treatment. Because telephones introduce distortion, they often add to aphasic listeners' comprehension disability. Because some telephones have better fidelity than others, comparison shopping to find one with good fidelity is a good idea if there is an aphasic person in the family.

The *redundancy* of spoken directions sometimes affects their comprehensibility. West and Kaufman (1972) evaluated aphasic listeners' comprehension of *Token-Test*-like commands, in which some commands were redundant (certain elements were repeated, as in "Show me the big *blue circle* and the little *blue circle*"), and some were nonredundant (as in "Show me the big blue circle and the small red square"). They reported that redundant commands were easier than nonredundant commands, and suggested that clinicians consider redundancy of stimuli when constructing materials for treatment of auditory comprehension impairments. Gardner et al. (1975) concluded that aphasic listeners comprehended semantically redundant sentences ("You *see* a cat that is furry") better than semantically neutral sentences ("You *see* a cat that is nice"), although the statistical analyses did not strongly support the conclusion.

The *number of targets* available for pointing or manipulation and *similarity among targets* may affect the difficulty of tasks in which aphasic listeners point to or manipulate tokens, objects, or pictures in response to spoken directions. In general, increasing the number of targets for pointing or manipulation responses increases the difficulty of the task. For example, "point to the red circle" is less difficult if there are three choices (e.g., red circle, blue square, yellow triangle) than if there are six (e.g., red circle, blue circle, yellow circle, red square, blue square, yellow square). Increasing the similarity among targets also increases the difficulty of the task. For example, "point to the knife" is more difficult for aphasic listeners if the targets are semantically related (e.g., fork, knife, spoon) than when they are not (e.g., fork, umbrella, turtle).

The Relationship Between Sentence and Discourse Comprehension

The relationship between aphasic listeners' comprehension of single-sentence utterances and their comprehension of discourse (connected speech) seems not to be very strong. Stachowiak et al. (1977), Waller and Darley (1978), Pashek and Brookshire (1982), Brookshire and Nicholas (1984a), and Wegner et al. (1984) all compared aphasic listeners' comprehension of spoken discourse with their performance on tests of single-sentence comprehension. In every case, the relationship between performance on the two tests was weak, suggesting that one cannot predict an aphasic listener's comprehension of spoken discourse from his or her comprehension of spoken single sentences. Aphasic listeners' comprehension of discourse usually was better than their comprehension of single-sentence utterances would suggest that it should be. Since communication in daily life usually occurs more in the form of connected speech than as single-sentence utterances, it may be that a given aphasic listener's sentence comprehension performance gives a pessimistic estimate of daily life comprehension competence.

These results suggest that clinicians should be cautious in making inferences about aphasic listeners' daily life comprehension competence based on their performance on single-sentence comprehension tests, because aphasic listeners may perform better in daily life than their single-sentence comprehension test scores would predict. These results also suggest that treatment of comprehension disorders might incorporate spoken discourse to a greater extent than is presently the case. Treatment activities that include multiple-sentence spoken messages of the kinds that a patient would be likely to encounter in daily life might help to ensure that improvements created in the clinic would generalize to daily life communication.

Variables Affecting Comprehension of Discourse

Several variables appear to affect aphasic listeners' comprehension of information from spoken discourse. By far the strongest of these variables is *salience,* or the importance of a given piece of information in the discourse. Brookshire and Nicholas (1984a) and Wegner et al. (1984) tested aphasic listeners' comprehension and memory for information from narrative stories. They found that information that was central to the stories (*main ideas*) was comprehended and remembered better than information that was peripheral (*details*). *Directness,* or whether information was contained within the stories or had to be deduced or inferred by the listener, also affected aphasic listeners' comprehension, but not so strongly as salience. Information that was directly stated tended to be easier for aphasic listeners to comprehend and remember than information that had to be deduced or inferred (Brookshire and Nicholas, 1984).

Speech rate and *emphatic stress* also may affect aphasic listeners' comprehension of discourse in much the same way that it affects their comprehension of single sentences. Pashek and Brookshire (1982) presented spoken paragraphs at a slow speech rate (120 words/min) or a normal speech rate (150 words/min), with either normal stress or exaggerated stress (extra prosodic emphasis on important words). They found that (1) both slow rate and exaggerated stress facilitated aphasic listeners' comprehension of the paragraphs; (2) slow rate was slightly more effective in improving comprehension than exaggerated stress was; and (3) comprehension was best when slow rate and exaggerated stress were combined.

Kimelman and McNeil (1987) replicated the above study and reported similar results. However, Nicholas and Brookshire (1986) reported that the effects of slow rate on comprehension of discourse are not consistent from subject to subject or from test to test. They presented narrative stories to aphasic listeners at slow (120 words/min) and fast (200 words/min) speech rates and tested listeners' comprehension of stated and implied main ideas and details twice, with a week or more between tests. In the first session, slow speech rate improved comprehension of details for both high and low comprehension subjects, but it only improved comprehension of main ideas for subjects with poor comprehension. However, the effects of slow speech rate essentially disappeared by the second session, and there were many instances in which individual subjects failed to demonstrate rate effects exhibited by their group. Nicholas and Brookshire suggested that increasing the salience (or redundancy) of information in discourse and stating information directly are more dependable ways to improve aphasic listeners' comprehension of discourse than slowing the rate at which it is spoken. However, they recommend that clinicians still advise those who communicate with aphasic patients to speak slowly, because negative effects of slow speech rate were rare, and because some aphasic listeners did benefit from slow speech rate.

TREATMENT OF READING

Processes in Reading

Word Recognition.—Recognizing and attaching meanings to words is a prerequisite for comprehending printed texts. Word recognition quickly becomes automatic as readers develop skill in reading, and only unskilled readers appear to depend heavily on word-by-word reading. Skilled readers usually do not read sentences or texts word by word, unless they are complex or contain unfamiliar words. When readers must deduce the meaning of individual printed words, they may do so in four ways. In *whole word reading,* words are recognized as units. Analysis of letters or letter strings within words is not carried out. In *phonemic analysis,* the reader separates the word into letters or letter combinations, translates these letters or letter combinations into the sounds that they represent, blends the sound representations together, and identifies the word represented by the sequence of sounds. Definition by phonemic analysis requires that the unfamiliar word be in the reader's listening vocabulary. In *definition by context,* the reader uses the meaning of the context in which a word appears to guess that word's meaning. Definition by context does not require that the unfamiliar word be in the reader's listening vocabulary. Skilled readers read most words as whole words, and use phonemic analysis and definition by context only when they encounter unfamiliar words. In *dictionary definition,* the reader looks up unfamiliar words in a dictionary. Most readers resort to dictionary definition only when the other three methods fail.

Syntactic Analysis.—Syntactic analysis is the primary way in which readers deduce relationships among words. Syntactic analysis presupposes knowledge of syntactic rules and recognition of syntactic structures. Research in reading suggests that syntactic knowledge allows readers to combine word strings into units of meaning that can be stored in long-term memory. Failure to perform syntactic analysis overloads the reader's short-term memory, and errors in syntactic analysis lead to miscomprehension of sentence meanings. An important difference between failure to recognize a word and failure to recognize a syntactic structure is that readers usually know when they fail to recognize a word, but may be unaware when they miscomprehend a syntactic structure.

Semantic Mapping.—Semantic mapping is a process by which readers relate the writer's intended meanings to their own knowledge and experience. Semantic mapping is the stage at which a text can be said to "make sense" to the reader. Semantic mapping involves organizing the meanings conveyed by a text into a coherent and sensical whole, and integrating those meanings into memory. Failure to organize the information in a text leads to confusion about which elements of the text are important and which are unimportant. Failure to relate meanings from texts to knowledge leads to problems in appreciating the pragmatic dimensions of the texts, and to difficulties with metaphor and figurative language.

There was once general acceptance of the idea that if a reader could translate letters into their corresponding words, the problem of reading would be solved. This assumption is no longer considered valid, because it neglects the role of syntactic analysis in reading. Reading almost always depends on syntactic analysis more than listening does. In listening, syntactic information can be conveyed by pauses, intonation, word order, and syntactic markers. In reading, the reader depends completely on word order and syntactic markers to deduce syntactic structure. Furthermore, printed texts usually are grammatically more complex and more formal in style than spoken discourse, making most printed texts more difficult to comprehend than most spoken discourse.

Surface Dyslexia and Deep Dyslexia

Two patterns of reading impairment that may accompany aphasia have received considerable attention in recent years. They are *surface dyslexia* and *deep dyslexia* (Marshall and Newcombe, 1973). The two syndromes are based on a model of reading that postulates two routes to derivation of meaning. The *direct* (lexical) route provides access to the mental representations of words (and their associated meanings) directly, based on the visual forms of the words. The *indirect* (phonologic) route provides access to the mental representations of words and their meanings indirectly, by converting graphemes to phonologic mental representations and accessing meaning via these phonologic representations.

Patients with *surface dyslexia* have lost (or are impaired in) the direct (lexical) route, and depend on letter-by-letter decoding to deduce the meanings of the words they read. Such patients read regularly spelled words (e.g, "keep," "banana") accurately, but misread irregularly spelled words by regularizing their pronunciation (e.g., "neighbor" may be read as "negbor"). Patients with surface dyslexia can read aloud nonwords (such as "tobada") accurately. Because analysis is letter-by-letter, long words take longer to identify than short words.

Patients with *deep dyslexia* have lost (or are impaired in) the indirect (phonologic) route and must depend on whole-word recognition in reading. Such patients cannot read nonsense words, and their misreadings of real words tend to create semantic errors (e.g., reading "chair" as "table") rather than phonemic errors. Patients with deep dyslexia have more difficulty with "closed-class" words (articles, conjunctions, prepositions) than content words (nouns, verbs, adjectives, adverbs). Semantically supportive context often helps these patients recognize words that they otherwise would not recognize. Patients with deep dyslexia tend to make whole-word visual errors in oral reading, substituting a visually similar word for the target (e.g., substituting "cane" for "clean").

Treatment of Reading Impairments in Aphasia

Treatment of aphasic patients' reading impairments usually is most appropriate for mildly or moderately aphasic patients, whose reading comprehension is almost always more impaired than their listening comprehension. Severely aphasic patients usually need speech and listening comprehension more than they need reading comprehension, and few patients with severe aphasia ever regain functional reading.

Treatment of aphasic patients' reading impairments usually begins with measurement of reading vocabulary, sentence comprehension, and paragraph comprehension, using standardized timed reading tests. These tests assess both *capacity* (the level of vocabulary and complexity that the reader can comprehend) and *speed* (the rate at which the reader can progress through a text with acceptable comprehension). Reading test scores often are defined by *grade level.* Grade level quantifies the difficulty of the materials in terms of the school grade at which "average" students can comprehend them. Most newspapers, popular books, and magazines are at approximately grade 8 in reading difficulty. Consequently, those who are reading at 8th grade level or above are likely to comprehend most daily life reading materials (Chall, 1983).

The activities involved in treatment of aphasic patients' reading comprehension disabilities depend, of course, on the severity and nature of each patient's reading impairments. Patients with severe impairments are likely to start with single words. Patients with moderate or mild impairments are more likely to start with sentences or paragraphs.

Matching Printed Words to Pictures.—Aphasic patients who have difficulty deducing the meaning of printed words often work on development of reading vocabulary before working on longer units. Problems in comprehending printed words can arise from several sources. Most aphasic patients have difficulty in phonemic analysis of printed words. They have difficulty translating letters or letter strings into appropriate composite sound patterns, and they have difficulty blending individual sound representations into sound patterns for words (deep dyslexia). Some may have visual impairments that interfere with their perception of printed words. They confuse words that look alike, or they reverse or invert letters with similar configurations (e.g., b/d or m/w). Such patients may benefit from treatment directed toward single-word reading comprehension. Some aphasic patients can translate printed words into phonemic representations, but are unable to attach meaning to the representations (surface dyslexia). These patients may benefit from treatment directed toward the use of context to deduce word meanings and from treatment directed toward the underlying semantic impairment, using the auditory modality as well as the visual modality.

Treatment of single-word reading disabilities usually involves matching printed single words to pictures. The variables manipulated depend on the source of the patient's reading problems. If a patient has difficulty discriminating letters or words that look alike, treatment may focus on visual discrimination. If a patient has difficulty translating letter strings into sound patterns, treatment may focus on phonetic discrimination and combination. If a patient has difficulty attaching meaning to printed words, treatment may focus on word retrieval and definitions of words. (In the latter case, treatment might involve comprehension of spoken words and word retrieval for speech as well as reading because it would be unlikely that the semantic disability would be unique to reading.) In such cases it may be more efficient to treat the patient's word comprehension problems through the auditory modality and then treat whatever reading problems remain after auditory word comprehension has improved.

Understanding Printed Sentences.—Aphasic readers' comprehension of printed sentences is likely to be affected by the same variables that affect comprehension of spoken sentences. These variables have been discussed previously. However, most aphasic patients' reading comprehension is worse than their comprehension of equivalent spoken materials. There appear to be several reasons for this. Most aphasic patients have difficulty translating printed words into acoustic representations—a process that is vital in reading, but not needed in listening. Reading depends more on syntactic analysis than listening does, and most aphasic patients have problems with syntactic analysis. (Many aphasic readers overlook or misread the "small" words in sentences—function words such as "to," "but," and "by" that may be crucial to sentence meanings.) Finally, reading materials usually have less extra-linguistic support than discourse does. When one is listening, a speaker usually is present. When the listener fails to comprehend, the speaker may notice and repeat, paraphrase, or simplify in order to repair the failure. The speaker's pauses, intonation, stress, reiteration, paraphrasing, and gestures all help listeners to comprehend. The time of day, the location of the interaction, the speaker's identity, and other characteristics of spoken interactions also reduce the listener's dependence on the linguistic content of the speaker's utterances. Such contextual support is less common in reading. However, if an aphasic patient is given unlimited time to deduce the meaning of printed texts, their reading comprehension may approximate their listening comprehension. Printed texts are durable and remain available to the reader, while spoken messages are gone when the speaker stops talking. Some aphasic readers can read relatively complex texts if they are given enough time. However, their comprehension deteriorates if they are given only the amount of time that it would take a "normal" reader to read the material.

Understanding Printed Texts.—Aphasic readers are likely to be affected by the salience of information in printed texts in the same way that salience affects their comprehension of spoken discourse—main ideas are comprehended and remembered better than details, and stated information is comprehended better than implied information. The extra effort involved in translating printed materials into their acoustic representations may compromise aphasic readers' ability to remember information from a text and to integrate the information into their knowledge. However, in some cases, context provided by printed texts may compensate at least in part for these difficulties by diminishing the aphasic reader's dependence on the meanings of individual words and sentences within the text.

A number of remedial reading programs are commercially available. Most are designed for use with children, but some are designed for use with adults who have not learned to read. Neither is completely appropriate for use with aphasic adult readers, but those designed for adults usually are better because their content and subject matter are better suited to adult readers. The Barnell-Loft *Specific Skills Series* (Boning, 1976) was designed for use with children, but may be useful with aphasic adults because it divides text comprehension into several basic skills: *vocabulary skills, getting the main idea, using context, finding facts, following directions,* and *drawing conclusions*. Aphasic persons can be deficient in any or several of these skills. The *Specific Skills Series* can be useful for treatment of aphasic patients' reading disabilities because patients can be treated at appropriate levels of difficulty within each of the skills.

Treatment of aphasic patients' reading disabilities can make extensive use of homework. The patient can work on reading exercises at home or in his or her room, and can bring the completed exercises to the clinic, where the clinician goes over the patient's work, corrects and discusses errors, and provides instructions and practice for new materials. In many cases, work on auditory comprehension can be coordinated with work on reading so that skills learned in one generalize to the other. The use of homework in treating reading comprehension is an efficient and economical way to provide increased treatment time to the patient and to facilitate generalization of acquired skills from listening to reading and vice versa.

TREATMENT OF SPEECH PRODUCTION

Speech Movements

Most aphasic patients without coexisting apraxia of speech have little difficulty performing either isolated oral movements (stick out tongue, puff out cheeks, smile) or sequential oral movements (pucker and smile, pucker and puff out cheeks). Those with apraxia of speech (either in isolation or coexisting with aphasia) may have difficulty with oral movements. Impairments in oral movements are discussed in conjunction with apraxia of speech and will not be considered here.

Imitation

Imitation of words, phrases, or sentences spoken by the clinician is common in treatment procedures for dysarthric and apraxic patients, but is seen less frequently in treatment procedures for aphasic patients. When imitation is used with aphasic patients, the objective usually is to facilitate retention span rather than to improve the motoric aspects of speech production. The length of phrases or sentences to be imitated is manipulated so that the patient works at or near the limits of his or her retention span. A delay interval may be imposed between the clinician's model and the patient's response to increase the difficulty of the task. Sentence repetition to increase retention span may be appropriate for patients who have fluent speech and can repeat single words. If a patient has significant motor speech impairments, repetition drills for increasing retention span probably are not appropriate.

Naming

Confrontation naming, in which patients are asked to name pictures or objects designated by the clinician, is a frequent speech production activity in aphasia treatment programs. However, it is not clear that such activities provide much benefit. Brookshire (1975) evaluated confrontation naming with ten aphasic subjects who were asked to name pictures of common objects. He found that naming performance usually improved within training sessions but improvements did not carry over from day to day. Brookshire also found that improvements in naming pictures that the patient had been trained to name did not generalize to different pictures. He concluded that naming practice has little therapeutic value.

Confrontation naming exercises for aphasic patients also may be questioned on logical grounds. One is rarely called upon to name things in daily life unless one is a child or is learning the language. Furthermore, in confrontation naming, the referent for the name is present. Providing the name in this situation may be redundant, because a patient could communicate by pointing to the referent rather than by naming it.

In spite of the questionable value of confrontation naming as a therapeutic technique, it is still common in treatment programs (perhaps because it is easy to carry out and score) and a substantial literature on variables that affect aphasic patients' confrontation naming exists. *Word frequency* in the language may affect the probability that an aphasic patient will correctly name an object or a picture (Wiegel-Crump and Koenigsknecht, 1973; Rochford and Williams, 1965; Tweedy and Shulman, 1982). More frequent words usually are easier for aphasic patients than less frequent words. Unfortunately, in many studies of the effects of word frequency on naming, possible confounding variables such as length, abstractness, or phonologic complexity of words and ambiguity or uncertainty of pictures were not well controlled, making it difficult to reach definite conclusions about the effects of word frequency alone.

Stimulus uncertainty can also affect aphasic patients' naming. Mills et al. (1979) defined stimulus uncertainty in terms of the consistency with which a given referent (a picture, in this case) elicits a given name from a normal speaker. Pictures that elict many different names are said to be high in uncertainty and those that elicit few different names are said to be low in uncertainty. Mills et al. found that aphasic patients named pictures with low uncertainty faster and with fewer errors than they named pictures with high uncertainty. However, as Williams and Canter (1982) have observed, Mills et al. did not control for word frequency. Consequently we cannot be certain that stimulus uncertainty is the only explanation for their results.

Length and phonologic complexity also affect aphasic patients' naming. Goodglass et al. (1976) found that aphasic subjects' naming success decreased as the length (in number of syllables) of words increased. Articulatory complexity also may affect aphasic subjects' naming, probably because the number of syllables in a word is related to the ease with which it can be articulated. Word length and articulatory complexity affect the mechanical production of words, unlike variables such as word frequency or stimulus uncertainty, which are more likely to affect accessing words and retrieving them from memory.

Sentence Completion

In sentence completion, the clinician says a prompt sentence (a sentence that is missing the final word or the final few words) and the patient supplies the missing word or words. Sentence completion activities sometimes are appropriate for treating patients with moderate to severe speech production impairments. Many patients who cannot produce words in other contexts can do so when the words are elicited by a phrase or sentence. Sentence completion is almost always easier for aphasic speakers than confrontation naming (Barton et al., 1969; Wyke and Holgate, 1973; Podraza and Darley, 1977), and sentence completion usually is easier than providing words in response to definitions given by the clinician (Barton et al., 1969; Goodglass and Stuss, 1979).

The primary determinant of the effectiveness of prompt sentences is the amount of constraint they place on the word or words that can be used to complete them. The most effective prompt sentences are those containing word combinations that frequently occur in daily life (e.g., "A cup of _____" or "Some bacon and _____"). Other prompt sentences may depend on semantic relationships for their effectiveness (e.g., "Put a *stamp* on the _____" or "We wear *shoes* on our _____"). Prompt sentences in which the missing elements are not constrained (e.g., "Today Joe bought a _____") are not likely to be very effective in eliciting target words from aphasic speakers (or from nonaphasic speakers, for that matter). In general, the more "automatic" phrase completion is, the more effective the phrase will be in eliciting the target word(s) from aphasic speakers.

Behaviors Associated With Word-Retrieval Failure

Marshall (1976) has described five behaviors that accompany aphasic patients' word retrieval difficulties. They are *delay, semantic association, phonetic association, description,* and *generalization.* Marshall describes *delay* as a filled or unfilled pause or "some stalling tactic to let the listener know they did not want to be interrupted and needed more time to produce the word." In *semantic association* the patient produces one or more words that are semantically related to the target word, such as an antonym (front: *back*), class membership (fruit: *banana*), part and whole (foot: *toe*), or serial relationship (Sunday, Monday: *Tuesday*). In *phonetic association* the patient produces a word or words that are phonologically similar to the target word (hamper: *damper*). (Marshall excludes off-target phonemic productions generated by patients with apraxia of speech from this category.) In *description,* the patient produces descriptions of characteristics of the target ("It's round and red and it grows on trees." "It's an *apple")* rather than the target word. In *generalization,* the patient produces general words and phrases without specific meaning ("It's one of those *things."* "It's a *thing* that I know." "It's a *spider.").*

Marshall studied the incidence of these behaviors in the speech of 18 aphasic adults. He found that semantic association was the most frequent behavior, followed by description, generalization, delay, and phonetic association. He also evaluated the percentage of the time that each behavior was followed by the intended target word. Delay was most frequently followed by successful production of the target word (about 90% of the time). Semantic association and phonetic association were next most successful. They preceded correct production of the target about 55% of the time. Description and generalization were followed by their intended targets only 35% and 17% of the time, respectively. Marshall calls these behaviors strategies, implying that they are volitional and purposeful. It seems likely that at least some of the behaviors described by Marshall are unintentional *symptoms* of problems in word retrieval, rather than *strategies* used to access words. This is a crucial difference, because if the behaviors represent strategies, one might wish to encourage the patient to engage in those that have the greatest likelihood of success. If the behaviors represent symptoms, one would probably not wish to increase their frequency, and instead might search for ways to eliminate them because they may decrease communicative efficiency.

Sentence Production

In sentence production, the clinician provides a stimulus (a verb, a noun, a noun-verb combination, a picture, or some other prompt) and asks the patient to say a sentence related to the prompt. A number of variables may affect the difficulty of sentence production, including (1) the length and syntactic complexity of target sentences; (2) the amount of semantic or syntactic constraints on target sentences; (3) the amount of information about target sentences provided by prompts; (4) the characteristics of prompts (frequency of occurrence of words, modality in which prompts are given, and so forth); and (5) the overall relationships among prompts.

Semantic or syntactic constraints placed on target sentences affect task difficulty. The target sentence "the dog chased the rabbit" is semantically constrained because rabbits do not usually chase dogs. Consequently, such sentences usually will be easier than target sentences without such constraints (e.g., "The boy kissed the girl").

Prompts that contain frequently occurring words, common word combinations, or express commonly encountered relationships usually are easier than prompts that do not. For example, constructing a sentence with the prompts /coffee/man/drink/ would usually be easier than constructing a sentence with the prompts /vehicle/surveyed/mechanic. (Note, however, that semantic constraints may contribute to formulation of the latter target sentence.)

If prompts and target sentences are all related to a common theme, sentence formulation and production is easier than if there is no relationship among prompts and target sentences. The semantic context provided by a common topic for prompts and targets often facilitates aphasic patients' production of the target sentences.

Connected Speech

Several procedures are commonly used to elicit connected speech from aphasic patients. Those most frequently seen in treatment activities are *picture description, prompted story telling, procedural discourse,* and *conversation.*

In *picture description,* target sentences usually are not constrained. Instead, the patient has free choice of the kinds of sentences that he or she will produce as well as considerable latitude in word choice. However, the nature of the picture (or pictures) used to elicit descriptions may affect both the amount and the content of verbalizations elicited from the patient. The *familiarity* to the patient of occurrences or situations depicted in pictures is likely to affect the amount of verbalization produced. Familiar occurrences or situations are likely to elicit more verbalization than unfamiliar ones. The *thematic content* of pictures also may affect patients' verbalizations. Pictures that have a unifying theme and depict dynamic interactions usually elicit

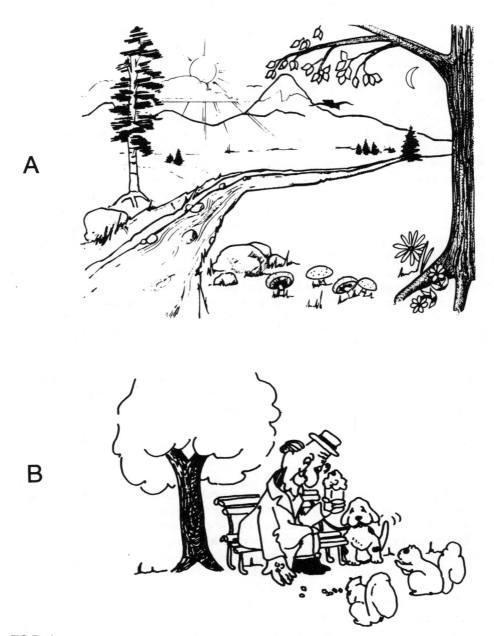

FIG 7–4.
Pictures that might be used to elicit connected speech. **A** is more likely to elicit enumeration than **B**.

more verbalization than those depicting static situations. Pictures depicting static situations tend to elicit enumeration (naming items in the picture), whereas those depicting dynamic interactions are more likely to elicit more elaborate descriptions. Figure 7–4 contains two pictures. The one on the the **top** depicts a static situation and would be more likely to elicit enumeration than the one on the **bottom,** which depicts a more dynamic situation.

The pictures most frequently used for eliciting connected speech from aphasic patients (Fig 7–5) are those from the *Boston Diagnostic Aphasia Examination* (Goodglass and Kaplan, 1983b), the *Western Aphasia Battery* (Kertesz, 1982), and the *Minnesota Test for Differential Diagnosis of Aphasia* (Schuell, 1972). Correia et al. (1990) reported that each elicits, on the average, about 100 words from aphasic speakers, but aphasic speakers have a greater tendency to name elements in the *Western Aphasia Battery* picture. However, aphasic speakers differed considerably in how much they said about the pictures. Their speech samples ranged from about 30 words per picture (for a nonfluent aphasic speaker) to 232 words per picture (for a fluent aphasic speaker).

Prompted story telling elicits stories by means of sequences of pictures that represent events in a story (Fig 7–6). The amount of speech that a picture sequence elicits often depends on the number of incidents pictured in the sequence, with more incidents generating longer speech samples. Brenneise-Sarshad et al. (1991) studied aphasic speakers' responses to 13-picture sequences taken from children's picture-story books. The sequences elicited, on the average, about 125 words from aphasic speakers. However, the number of words elicited varied greatly, ranging from 62 words (for a nonfluent aphasic speaker) to 219 words (for a fluent aphasic speaker). The picture sequence shown in Figure 7–6 elicited, on the average, slightly over 80 words from aphasic speakers, but again the range was substantial (from 23 words for a nonfluent patient to 164 words for a fluent patient).

Procedural discourse is connected speech elicited in response to requests such as "tell me how you make pumpkin pie." Procedures such as making scrambled eggs, writing and mailing a letter, and doing dishes by hand usually elicit speech samples ranging from 75 to 125 words, depending on the procedures (more complex procedures usually elicit longer samples). The range for aphasic speakers is great; some nonfluent aphasic speakers may generate only 25 to 30 words whereas some fluent aphasic speakers may generate nearly 300. Ulatowska et al. (1983) reported that the syntactic complexity of procedures generated by both nonaphasic and aphasic speakers was low. They commented that generating procedural discourse does not require very complex language, and that even patients with substantial aphasic impairments can produce adequate procedural discourse.

Conversation is sometimes used as a vehicle for eliciting speech from aphasic patients in treatment activities. However, many such conversations do not resemble natural conversations because the clinician does most of the talking and the patient's responses usually do not go beyond providing what the clinician specifically requests. The resulting interaction resembles an interview more than it resembles conversation; it becomes an extended series of requests for information from the clini-

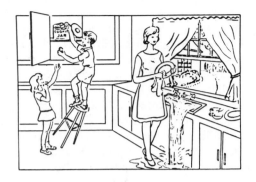

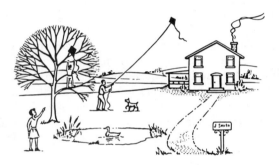

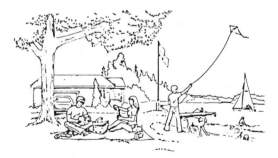

FIG 7–5.
Speech elicitation pictures from the *Boston Diagnostic Aphasia Examination,* the *Western Aphasia Battery,* and the *Minnesota Test for Differential Diagnosis of Aphasia.* (Used by permission.)

cian, with single-word, phrase, or short sentence responses by the patient, as in the following segment.

C: What kind of work did you do before your stroke?
P: Foreman.
C: A foreman. What company did you work for?

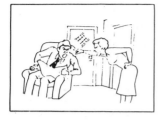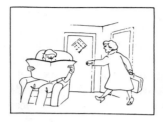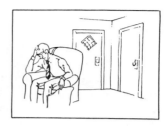

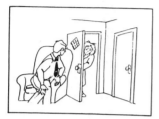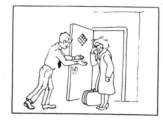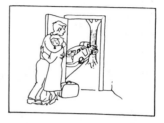

FIG 7–6.
A picture sequence that might be used to elicit connected speech. (Copyright 1991, Brookshire RH, Nicholas LE. Used by permission.)

> P: Amurcan.
> C: Amurcan? Do you mean American? American what?
> P: Amurican Freight.
> C: American Freight. Is that a trucking company?
> P: Yeah.
> C: And you were a foreman. Who did you supervise?
> P: Dock.
> C: People on the dock?
> P: Yeah.
> C: And what kind of jobs did they do?
> P: Oh—most ever'thing.

Unless carefully structured with pragmatic principles about formal conversational structures firmly in place, such clinician-patient interactions are not effective in eliciting connected speech from the patient. They are more appropriately employed when the objective is to improve the patient's conversational behaviors (e.g., turn-taking, eye contact, etc.).

Writing

Many of the same processes are used to generate spoken messages and written ones. It is only at the production stage that speaking and writing differ appreciably. Writers, unlike speakers, need a sense of how to spell. Writing requires visual-motor coordination and sufficient strength to produce written letters. Writers need better syntax than speakers, because speakers can compensate for deficient syntax by providing prosodic clues to meanings, while writers do not have this option. Written style is more formal and grammatically complex than spoken style. It should not be surprising that aphasic persons almost always write less well than they speak.

Aphasic patients' writing resembles their speech. Fluent speakers tend to be fluent writers. They write in cursive, produce well-shaped letters, and maintain horizontal and equally-spaced writing lines. Nonfluent speakers tend to be nonfluent writers (partly because they are using their nonpreferred hand). They produce distorted letters and their lines are uneven in contour and spacing. Nonfluent writers usually print, rather than writing in cursive. Agrammatic speakers are likely to be agrammatic writers, and aphasic speakers who generate "empty" speech (devoid of meaning) are likely to generate "empty" written materials. (See Figures 4–1 and 4–3 for examples.)

Treatment of Writing Impairments

Most aphasic patients have disabilities in spelling and syntax that make it difficult or impossible for them to communicate effectively by writing. Consequently, most writing treatment programs concentrate on spelling, syntax, and grammar. These programs tend to employ didactic procedures and to rely heavily on homework. Sometimes commercially available spelling and writing workbooks are used. Teaching written spelling and syntax to aphasic patients may be an exception to the general assumption that treatment involves "stimulation" or "reactivation" rather than "teaching." In most cases, procedures used in teaching aphasic persons to spell and write do not differ very much from those used to teach beginning writers.

It may be fortunate that most aphasic persons do not really need advanced writing skills in their daily lives. If a patient can write short notes, fill in forms, and write checks, he or she can probably get by in most daily life environments. Consequently, treatment programs that can get an aphasic writer to this level are likely to be sufficient in most cases. If this level cannot be achieved, then treatment focuses on writing skills that will make the greatest contribution to the patient's functional communication in daily life. Writing one's name is no doubt the most frequent single writing act that most of us do in daily life. Consequently, this may be the first treatment objective for patients who cannot write their name. (Writing one's name is one of our most highly automatized writing activities. Therefore, it is common to see aphasic patients who can write their name when they can write nothing else.)

Most of the linguistic variables (length, word frequency, syntactic complexity) that affect the difficulty of spoken sentences affect written sentences similarly. Context seems to affect aphasic persons' writing in the same way that it affects their speaking. If part of a sentence is provided and patients have only to complete the sentence, success rates are higher than if they have to produce the same words without contextual support. "Cloze" procedures, in which single words are deleted from printed passages, sometimes are appropriate for patients who cannot write phrases and sentences. (Many aphasic patients write single words better when they are given a sentence or paragraph context in which to write the words than they do when they are asked to write isolated single words.)

Haskins (1976) suggested a progression of tasks for treating aphasic patients' writing disabilities. The progression begins with auditory stimulation and progresses to graphic production. A modified version of Haskins's progression appears in Table 7–2.

Haskins recommends that clinicians expand or reduce the complexity of the treatment program to meet the needs of individual patients. Steps 1 and 2 may be difficult for many aphasic patients. In these cases, treatment could start with Step 3. Some patients will not need the training provided in early steps of the progression. They would begin at a point at which their performance begins to break down.

It would be unusual for treatment to concentrate exclusively on writing. In most cases, the emphasis is on listening, speaking, and (less frequently) reading. Treat-

---

TABLE 7–2.

Modified Version of Haskin's Progression

1. Point to letters after the clinician says the sound of the letter (not the letter name).
   1 letter
   2 letters
   3 letters, etc.
2. Point to printed words after the clinician says the sound sequence for the word (e.g., /k/–/a/–/t/).
3. Point to alphabet letters after the clinician names them.
   1 letter
   2 letters, etc.
4. Point to printed words after the clinician spells them.
5. Point to printed words after the clinician names them.
   1 word
   2 words, etc.
6. Trace letters of the alphabet.
7. Copy letters of the alphabet.
8. Write letters of the alphabet to dictation.
   Serial order
   Random order
9. Write words to dictation.
   Clinician spells word letter-by-letter as patient writes each letter.
   Clinician spells word, 1 second per letter and patient writes word.
   Clinician says word and patient writes it.
10. Copy structured sentences (e.g., "I eat pie," "I eat cake" etc.).
11. Write structured sentences to dictation.
    Word-by-word dictation
    Sentence dictation
12. Write sentences incorporating words provided by clinician.

---

ment of writing impairments usually is an adjunct to other treatment, with considerable reliance on homework. If the clinician plans carefully, treatment of writing disabilities can be coordinated with other treatment activities in order to create maximum generalization from one ability to another, and from the clinic to daily life.

GROUP ACTIVITIES FOR APHASIC ADULTS

Group activities for aphasic adults and family members sometimes are provided either as adjuncts to or as replacement for one-to-one clinician-patient treatment. Some groups include only aphasic patients, and some may include patients and family members. Group activities can be divided into four general categories, depending on their purpose: *treatment, transition, maintenance,* and *support.*

Treatment Groups.— The purpose of treatment groups is to provide structured experiences in communication among group members. For many patients, group treatment activities provide an environment where they can try out new behaviors or new ways of communicating in a situation that is more naturalistic than one-to-one treatment sessions with a clinician, but that is better controlled (and usually less threatening) than daily life social interactions. Activities for treatment groups tend to be clinician directed and controlled, relatively structured, and task-oriented. The clinician ensures that each group member receives stimulation appropriate to their abilities and consistent with the therapeutic objectives for the group member. Sometimes group activities are didactic and resemble the activities seen in individual clinician-patient treatment. Sometimes group activities resemble daily life conversational interactions, with emphasis on communication among group members. In the latter case, group treatment provides patients with experiences that are not possible in one-to-one treatment activities. Another advantage of group treatment is efficiency and cost effectiveness— more patients can be treated per unit of time and per clinician when patients are in group treatment than when they are in individualized one-to-one treatment.

Transition Groups.— Transition groups actually are a kind of treatment group, but in transition groups the emphasis is on preparing patients for the end of treatment. Activities for transition groups provide patients with experiences that prepare them for communication in daily life environments. Transition groups often teach strategies and problem-solving skills that are useful in daily life activities. Role-playing activities involving common experiences may be offered to give patients a chance to try out new strategies or problem-solving methods in a protected environment resembling real life. Transition groups also may provide patients with information and advice about how to find and make use of community services such as adult daycare centers, visiting nurse services, and senior citizens' centers. Transition group experiences are intended to provide a smooth and comfortable transition between treatment and discharge from treatment. Patients usually participate in transition groups for specified periods of time, usually from 4 to 6 weeks.

Maintenance Groups.—Maintenance groups usually are made up of aphasic patients who have been discharged from individual treatment. The activities that take place within maintenance groups are designed to keep participants' communicative abilities at optimum levels, and to prevent the deterioration that might occur when patients no longer receive regular treatment. Maintenance groups usually meet no more than once a week and sometimes as infrequently as once a month. Activities within maintenance groups tend to emphasize social interaction and communication in social contexts. Patients may stay in maintenance groups for several months or even years, depending on the needs of the patient and his or her family and the resources of the facility offering the group activities.

Support Groups.—Support groups for patients and family members serve several functions. They provide information to patients and families about the nature of aphasia. They help them understand the consequences of aphasia, and help them deal with the psychologic, social, and vocational effects of aphasia. Support groups may help patients and families cope with long-term changes in life-style that are caused by brain injuries and aphasia. They may provide emotional support and help patients and families find new friends and acquaintances. Support groups may offer activities such as:

1. Group discussions in which group members ask questions, exchange ideas and information, express attitudes, and discuss problems associated with aphasia and stroke.
2. Lectures or speeches by resource persons about problems related to stroke and aphasia.
3. Leisure and entertainment activities, either at the meeting site or at theaters, restaurants, or other such locations.

Support groups can help relieve feelings of confusion, loneliness, fear, anger, and hostility generated by the social and vocational disruptions caused by an aphasic patient's disabilities.

It is difficult to measure the value of group activities, and the value of group activities has not received much attention in the literature. According to Eisenson (1973) most of the literature on group treatment for aphasia consists of favorable testimonials with little empirical support. Schuell et al. (1965) suggest that group treatment may help patients feel less isolated and may provide patients with opportunities to observe others with aphasia. However, Schuell et al. believe that group treatment should be offered only as an adjunct to one-to-one individualized treatment, and group treatment should not be substituted for individual treatment:

> Treatment for aphasia must constantly be dovetailed to patient response. There are no mass methods, and none are possible. What reaches or helps one patient at one point in time loses another. For these reasons, we are unable to have confidence in group therapy as a basic method of treatment for aphasia.

Eisenson (1973) agrees that group treatment is not a substitute for individual treatment. Eisenson suggests that group activities may improve aphasic patients' adjustment, and it may help to reduce their anxiety. Eisenson believes that group activities should be designed to provide (1) psychologic support (according to Eisenson, the most important purpose of group activities); (2) practice in communicative interactions within a permissive and nonthreatening setting; and (3) some "teaching" regarding communication. According to Eisenson, group activities can provide patients with (1) an opportunity for socialization; (2) motivation from peers; (3) awareness of their own speech "habits"; (4) opportunities to observe the techniques with which other aphasic patients deal with communicative impairments; (5) practice in responding to speakers with different ways of using speech and language; and (6) an opportunity to ventilate feelings and air grievances.

Wertz et al. (1981) experimentally evaluated the effects of individual and group treatment on aphasia. Aphasic patients in *individual treatment* (Group A) received 4 hours of one-to-one direct stimulus-response type treatment with a speech-language pathologist and 4 hours of clinician-directed (but independently carried out) machine-assisted treatment and speech and language drill per week for 44 weeks. Patients in *group treatment* (Group B) received 4 hours of group treatment (three to seven patients in the group) designed to facilitate language use in a social setting. Group treatment sessions also were conducted by a speech-language pathologist. Patients in group B also participated in 4 hours of group recreational activities each week for 44 weeks. Patients' speech and language abilities were periodically assessed with several standardized measures. With minor exceptions, both groups made significant improvement on all speech and language measures between 4 weeks after onset (when they entered treatment) and tests at the end of 11, 22, 33, and 44 weeks of treatment. There were few significant differences between the two groups on any test occasion, although group A almost always performed somewhat better than group B. Both groups improved significantly between 26 and 48 weeks after onset (after 22 to 44 weeks of treatment, when, according to Wertz et al., spontaneous recovery should no longer be taking place). Wertz et al. concluded that both individual and group treatment of the kind provided in their study were efficacious. They suggested that individual treatment may be "slightly superior" to group treatment. However, they also suggested that the cost-effectiveness of group treatment "should prompt speech-language pathologists to consider it for at least part of an aphasic patient's care."

Kearns and Simmons (1985) surveyed 91 Veterans Administration Medical Centers to find out what kinds of group treatment activities they offered. Fifty-nine percent offered *treatment* groups and 54% sponsored *counseling* or *support* groups. Their report focused on treatment groups. The average treatment group size was 5.5 patients (89% of groups contained 8 or fewer patients). Eighty-nine percent of groups met either one or two times a week. Average session length was about 1 hour. Seventy-eight percent of patients in treatment groups were more than 1 year postonset, and 49% of group members received both individual treatment and group treatment. Most respondents (84%) reported that the primary goal of their treatment groups was language stimulation. However, many respondents reported other goals, which would be consistent with transition, maintenance, or support groups: emotional support (59%), carryover (47%), and socialization (45%). Treatment group activities fell into several categories: general discussion about a given topic (31%), individualized structured tasks (22%), nondirected social interactions (18%), multimodality stimulation (14%), and teaching communicative strategies (14%). Most respondents (73%) reported that the effects of group treatment were evaluated by periodic formal testing of group members, and 57% reported that periodic behavioral ratings were made. However, 20% reported that the effects of patients' participation in the treatment groups were not measured. Kearns and Simmons suggested that eclectic, multipurpose groups may not be the most effective form of patient management, and that treatment and maintenance groups have different goals and require different procedures. They also urged that the effects of group treatment on individual group members be documented, and that standard criteria be used in selecting patients for groups and in discharging them from the groups.

Chapter 8

Right Hemisphere Syndrome

That the two hemispheres of the human brain serve different functions has been suspected since the late 1800s. In 1861 Paul Broca reported that eight patients with language disturbance secondary to brain damage all had lesions in the left hemisphere. Within the next few years the dominance of the left hemisphere for language had become widely accepted.* During the next decade most believed that the left hemisphere was dominant for most cognitive functions, with the right hemisphere responsible only for perceptual and motor functions and perhaps some rudimentary mental processes. Then, in 1874 John Hughlings Jackson asserted that the two hemispheres serve different functions. He claimed that the left hemisphere is responsible for language and that the right hemisphere is responsible for visual recognition, discrimination, and recall. During the next 100 years the right hemisphere's contribution to cognition and intellect was largely neglected as investigators concentrated on exploring the allocation of responsibilities for language within the left hemisphere. It was not until the middle of the 20th century that investigators began to explore in any concerted fashion the organization and function of the right hemisphere. Our knowledge of what the right hemisphere does, and how it does it, remains imperfect, although we are slowly becoming more sophisticated. Unfortunately, the scientific and clinical literature on the right hemisphere is inconsistent and often contradictory. The number of cases on which claims about right hemisphere functions are usually made is small, subjects are not well described, and potentially important variables such as time after onset, handedness, etiology, location of lesion, and size of lesion often have not been controlled. Nevertheless, there seems to be at least general agreement about the major responsibilities of the right hemisphere in right-handed adults.

Early theories of hemispheric function speculated that the left hemisphere is specialized for language and reasoning whereas the right hemisphere is specialized for

*Statements about hemispheric specialization such as this one may be misleading unless the qualifier "in right-handed adults" is added. Few writers add the qualifier, and I will not belabor the reader with it. However, the reader should keep it in mind whenever reading descriptions of right-hemisphere-damaged adults.

music and visual processes. This concept of hemispheric specialization gradually changed as investigators found that the two hemispheres appeared to operate in fundamentally different ways. Writers began to describe the left hemisphere as "rational and analytic" and the right hemisphere as "intuitive and holistic." Contemporary models of hemispheric functions depict the left hemisphere as specialized for processing sequential, time-related material that requires linear (serial) processing, and the right hemisphere as specialized for processing nonlinear arrays that require holistic, gestalt-like (parallel) processing. Because auditory information often comes in time-ordered sequences (syllables in a word, words in a sentence), the left hemisphere may have greater responsibility for auditory events. Because visual information often comes in multidimensional arrays (pictures, scenes, faces), the right hemisphere may have greater responsibility for visual events. However, these hemispheric differences reflect the nature of the information that the brain must deal with, rather than the modality through which it enters the brain.

BEHAVIORAL AND COGNITIVE SYMPTOMS OF RIGHT HEMISPHERE BRAIN DAMAGE

The symptoms generated by right-hemisphere damage, like those generated by left-hemisphere damage, vary in their nature and severity depending on the site and extent of the brain injury causing them. Although the literature about the effects of right-hemisphere brain damage is often contradictory and the relationships between damage in given regions of the right hemisphere and behavioral symptoms have yet to be elucidated, there seems to be at least general agreement that right-hemisphere-damaged adults as a group are likely to exhibit distinctive perceptual and behavioral anomalies. Some of these anomalies are perceptual and attentional, some seem to be affective, and some affect communication in characteristic ways.

Perceptual and Attentional Anomalies

Neglect.—Right-hemisphere-damaged patients often exhibit *left hemispatial neglect*. These patients do not perceive left-sided tactile or visual stimuli. When asked to copy geometric designs they may copy only the right half (Fig 8–1). When orally reading printed materials they may read only the material on the right side of the page, even while they complain that the material does not make sense. When moving about they often bump into things on the left, and may become "trapped" against the left side of doorways or other obstructions because they fail to perceive the presence of the obstruction and remain unaware of its presence even after they encounter it. Patients with left neglect sometimes claim that their paralyzed left arm and leg do not exist, or that they belong to someone else. In its mildest form neglect may be detectable only with *simultaneous stimulation,* in which brief stimuli (flashes of light, light touch, pinpricks, etc.) are presented simultaneously on both sides. The patient with right-hemisphere damage and mild neglect (sometimes called *hemispatial inattention*) misses the stimulus on the left when both sides are stimulated, but

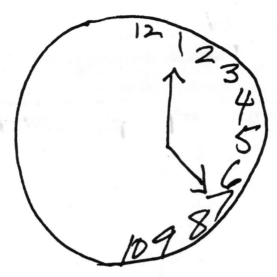

FIG 8–1.
A clock drawn from memory by a patient with right-hemisphere brain damage. The clock is flattened on the left and the numbers are displaced into the patient's (intact) right hemi-field.

perceives it when only the left side is stimulated. Patients with moderate neglect may attend to stimuli in their left hemispace if they are reminded to do so, but tend to bump into things on the left and may show other signs of inattention such as using only their right-side trousers pocket or the right-side drawers in dressers and bureaus (Lezak, 1983).

Neglect may follow damage in either hemisphere, but it is more severe and persistent following right-hemisphere damage (Cummings, 1983). It can occur after damage to any lobe, but it is most common and most severe after right parietal lobe damage (Mesulam, 1981; Heilman et al., 1985). It almost always affects visual, tactile, and auditory modalities. Same-sided visual field blindness often accompanies neglect, but visual neglect often is seen in patients with no visual field anomalies (Willanger et al., 1981). Neglect frequently resolves either partially or completely in the first few weeks or months after injury.

Facial Recognition Deficits (Prosopagnosia).—Many patients with right-hemisphere brain damage cannot recognize otherwise familiar persons by seeing their faces. These patients perform poorly on tasks that depend on perception and integration of facial features, such as identifying famous people from photographs and choosing pictures of people that they have just seen from a group of pictures. The recognition deficits usually affect perception of cartoons and line-drawn faces as well as actual faces and photographs, and may extend beyond facial recognition. For example, a birdwatcher who, after a right-hemisphere stroke, no longer recognized different species of birds, and a farmer who, after a right-hemisphere stroke, no longer recognized his cows (Albert et al., 1981). Patients with facial recognition deficits who fail to recognize friends and family members by their facial features recognize them when they speak. Facial recognition deficits are common after posterior right-hemisphere brain damage (Hecaen and Angelergues, 1962; Warrington and James, 1967; Whitely and Warrington, 1977), but persisting deficits may require bilateral damage (Albert et al., 1982; Cohn et al., 1977; Meadows, 1974). Facial recognition deficits seem to be independent of disordered visual-spatial perception (McKeever and Dixon, 1981) and of recognition of emotion (Cicone et al., 1980; Ley and Breyden, 1979).

Constructional Impairment.—Many brain-injured patients perform poorly on tests in which they must draw or copy geometric designs, create designs with colored blocks, reproduce two-dimensional stick figures, or reproduce three-dimensional constructions using wooden blocks. Deficient performance on such tasks, in the absence of visual perceptual or motor impairments that could account for the deficiencies, is called *constructional impairment* (sometimes erroneously called "constructional apraxia"). Constructional impairments may appear as a consequence of damage to either hemisphere, but they are more frequent and usually more severe after right-hemisphere brain damage. The frequency of errors on constructional tests does not differentiate between patients with left- or right-hemisphere damage, but the nature of the errors may (Gainotti and Tiacci, 1970). Patients with right-hemisphere damage often leave out details on the left side of figures or constructions or omit the left side entirely. When copying designs or figures they often draw over existing lines and add extraneous lines. They frequently rotate and fragment their drawings. Patients with left-hemisphere damage, in contrast, simplify figures or constructions and produce drawings in which the proportions are accurate, but angles and lines are distorted (Lezak, 1983). Figures copied by a left-hemisphere-damaged patient and a patient with right hemisphere damage are shown in Figure 8–2. Hecaen and Assal (1970) reported that patients with left-hemisphere lesions benefit from having a model to copy, while those with right-hemisphere lesions do not. Constructional impairments can follow damage anywhere in the right hemisphere, but they are most often seen following parietal or parieto-occipital damage.

Denial of Illness (Anosognosia).—Denial of illness is a frequent symptom of right-hemisphere brain damage, especially when the patient has parietal lobe damage. Denial can take several forms, ranging from (1) indifference to acknowledged disabilities, to (2) underestimating the severity of acknowledged disabilities, to (3) outright denial of major disabilities such as paralysis, sensory loss, or visual field blindness.

Affective Anomalies

Recognition and Expression of Emotion.—The experience of emotion is mediated by the limbic system, but the appreciation of others' emotions and the expression of emotion appear to be served by the right hemisphere in right-handed adults. Consequently, adults with right-hemisphere damage often seem to be deficient in

left hemisphere lesion

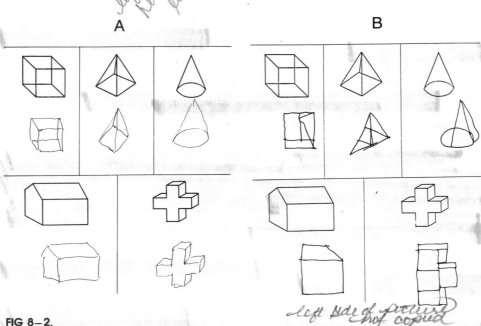

FIG 8–2.
Designs copied by a patient with left-hemisphere brain damage **(A)** and a patient with right-hemisphere damage **(B)**.

left side of picture not copied

recognizing and expressing emotion. They fail to relate others' facial expressions to their emotional state, and fail to make use of intonational cues to meaning and emotion. Their expression of emotion tends to be flattened, with a reduction in both facial expression of emotion and expression of emotion by intonation patterns of speech.

Communicative Impairments Associated With Right-Hemisphere Damage

Diminished Speech Prosody.—Right-hemisphere-damaged patients often lose the intonational characteristics of speech. As a consequence their speech sounds monotonous and devoid of emotion. Some right-hemisphere-damaged patients seem aware that their voice does not communicate their emotional state to listeners, and communicate their emotional state with propositional speech (e.g., "I am angry with you"). There is some evidence that right frontal lobe damage is most likely to cause diminished speech prosody, and that right parietal lobe damage is most likely to cause impaired appreciation of prosodic cues to meaning and emotion in the speech of others (Bryden and Ley, 1983).

Anomalous Content and Organization of Spontaneous Speech.—One of the most striking communicative impairments of right-hemisphere-damaged patients is their excessive, confabulatory, and sometimes inappropriate spontaneous speech. "The spontaneous speech of such patients is often excessive and rambling. Their comments may be off-color and their humor primitive and inappropriate; they tend to focus on insignificant details or make tangential remarks, and the usual range of intonation is frequently lacking" (Gardner et al., 1983). Right-hemisphere-damaged patients talk a lot, but they do not always make sense. They produce less information but use more words than either non-brain-damaged adults or left-hemisphere-damaged patients (Myers, 1979; Rivers and Love, 1980; Diggs and Basili, 1987). When asked to tell (or retell) a story, right-hemisphere-damaged patients tend to recall isolated details without organizing the material and establishing relationships among events. They often insert tangential and irrelevant comments and permit their personal experiences and opinions to intrude into their narratives.

Comprehension of Narratives and Conversations.—Patients with right hemisphere damage often exhibit striking impairments in comprehending implied meanings in narratives and conversations (Brownell et al., 1986). They seem unable to get beyond literal interpretations of what they hear or read. They tend to literally interpret idiomatic expressions, figures of speech, and metaphors. They often fail to identify incongruous, irrelevant, or absurd statements as such, and may offer confabulatory or bizarre reasons for accepting them as plausible. They are often unable to judge the appropriateness of facts, situations, or characterizations in stories or conversations, and they may be unable to extract morals from stories. If sentences in a story are separated and printed on cards, right-hemisphere-damaged patients usually have great difficulty organizing them into a coherent story (Delis et al., 1983). These deficiencies carry over into conversations. Right-hemisphere-damaged patients "often seem to lack a full understanding of the context of an utterance, the presuppositions entailed, the affective tone, or the point of a conversational exchange. They appear to have difficulties in processing abstract sentences, in reasoning logically, and in maintaining a coherent stream of thought . . ." (Gardner et al., 1983).

Pragmatic Impairments.—Pragmatic impairments are impairments in the social and interactional aspects of language, such as turn-taking, topic maintenance, social conventions, and eye contact. Impairments in the social and interactional aspects of language are a common consequence of right-hemisphere brain damage. Many right-hemisphere-damaged patients are poor at maintaining eye contact with conversational partners. They talk excessively, without regard for their listener. They have difficulty staying on topic and may interject irrelevant, tangential, and inappropriate comments. They tend to be insensitive to rules governing conversational turn-taking, especially those involved with "yielding the floor" to their conversational partners.

TESTS FOR ASSESSING PATIENTS WITH RIGHT-HEMISPHERE BRAIN INJURY

Objective assessment of right-hemisphere-damaged adults' linguistic, cognitive, and communicative abilities received little attention before the middle 1970s. Consequently, assessment of these patients is considerably less sophisticated than assessment of aphasic adults, which has been studied for over 50 years. At the time this is written, several nonstandardized procedures for evaluation of adults with right brain injury have been reported in the literature, and two standardized test batteries have been published.

Adamovich and Brooks (1981) described a procedure for evaluating communicative deficits of adults with right-hemisphere brain injury. Their procedure included auditory comprehension, oral expression, and reading subtests from the *Boston Diagnostic Aphasia Examination* (Goodglass and Kaplan, 1972); the *Revised Token Test* (McNeil and Prescott, 1978); the *Hooper Visual Organization Test* (Hooper, 1983); portions of the verbal absurdities, verbal opposites, and likenesses and differences subtests of the *Detroit Tests of Learning Aptitude* (Hammill, 1965); the *Boston Naming Test* (Kaplan et al., 1983); and the *Word Fluency Task* (Borkowski, Benton & Spreen, 1967).

Burns et al. (1985) described another procedure for evaluating deficits associated with right-hemisphere brain injury. The procedure includes (1) an interview with the patient; (2) observation of the patient in interactions with family members and hospital staff; (3) ratings of attention, eye contact, awareness of illness, orientation to place, time, and person, facial expression, speech intonation, and topic maintenance in conversations; (4) four tests of visual scanning and tracking; (5) ratings of written expression; (6) a scale for rating pragmatic communication skills; and (7) a metaphorical language test.

The procedures used by Adamovich and Brooks as well as those used by Burns et al. are unstandardized, do not have adequate norms, and do not have documented reliability or validity. However, they may prove useful as a source of materials and ideas for locally constructed protocols for evaluation of patients with right-hemisphere brain injury.

Gordon et al. (1984) also described a procedure for evaluation of adults with right-hemisphere damage. Their procedure assesses:

1. Visual scanning and visual inattention.
2. Activities of daily living skills.
3. Sensory-motor integration.
4. Perceptual (visual) integration.
5. Higher cognitive and perceptual functions (verbal and performance subtests from the *Wechsler Adult Intelligence Scale*).
6. Linguistic and cognitive flexibility.
7. Affective state.

They tested 385 right-hemisphere-damaged patients, but the number of patients tested differed across subtests. They provided raw scores, T scores, means, standard deviations, and percentiles for each subtest in their procedure. For many subtests the data are subdivided according to patient variables such as age, education, or presence of visual field deficit. Test-retest reliability coefficients are reported for each subtest. Although not a standardized test, the report by Gordon et al. describes materials and procedures for numerous tests of linguistic, cognitive, perceptual, and affective functions, and provides a large body of data about how adults with right-hemisphere damage perform on those tests.

The *Mini Inventory of Right Brain Injury* (MIRBI) (Pimental and Kingsbury, 1989) is a standardized test that, according to the authors, has six potential uses:

1. To identify adults who exhibit deficits in areas known to be compromised by right-hemisphere brain injury.
2. To determine relative severity of right brain injury.
3. To determine specific deficit areas of right-hemisphere dysfunction.
4. To earmark specific strengths and weaknesses of right-hemisphere dysfunction upon which treatment goals can be based.
5. To document patient progress as a consequence of right-hemisphere intervention programs.
6. To serve as a measurement device in research studies involving right brain injury.

The MIRBI contains 27 test items that test 10 categories of ability:

1. Visual scanning (2 items).
2. Integrity of gnosis (3 items).
3. Integrity of body image, schema (1 item).
4. Visual-verbal processing (reading and writing—5 items).
5. Visual-symbolic processing ("serial 7s"—subtracting 7 from 100, subtracting 7 from the remainder, and so on, for four subtractions—1 item).
6. Integrity of praxis associated with visual-motor skills (drawing a clock—1 item).
7. Affective language (speech intonation—2 items).
8. Higher level receptive and expressive language skills (humor, incongruities, absurdities, figurative language, similarities—8 items).
9. Affect (1 item).
10. General behavior (3 items).

A test booklet and score sheet is provided. The booklet contains instructions for administering each subtest, printed visual stimuli where appropriate, and a space in which to record the patient's score on each subtest. The front page includes a section in which the clinician can record biographic information about the patient, and spaces for listing the patient's score on each subtest in the MIRBI. A report form that could be placed in a patient's clinic or medical record is also included.

Sections on administration and scoring and test intepretation are provided in the test manual. Information about testing of 30 adults with right-hemisphere brain damage, 13 patients with left-hemisphere brain damage, and 30 non-brain-damaged adults is provided in the test manual. Correlations between MIRBI scores and age, education, and time postonset are reported. Comparisons of overall MIRBI scores and scores on each item are reported for the three groups. Sections on the reliability and validity of the MIRBI are also included in the manual.

The *Right Hemisphere Language Battery* (RHLB) (Bryan, 1989) was designed "to assess RHD [right-hemisphere-damaged] patients for the presence of language disorders. . . [and] in determining whether RH [right hemisphere] language skills are preserved in LHD [left-hemisphere-damaged] patients." It contains seven subtests:

1. Metaphor picture test (comprehension of spoken metaphors).
2. Written metaphor test (comprehension of printed metaphors).
3. Comprehension of inferred meaning (from printed paragraphs).
4. Appreciation of humor (from printed jokes).
5. Lexical semantic test (pointing to pictures by name).
6. Production of emphatic stress (in spoken sentences).
7. Discourse analysis (of spontaneous conversation).

Photocopy masters of the response forms for the subtests of the RHLB, a patient information form, and an individual profile form are provided. Users must make copies of the masters for recording the performance of individual patients.

The test manual contains (1) a general description of hemispheric specialization for language and a description of the major behavioral consequences of right-hemisphere brain damage; (2) a summary of the literature on language processing by the right hemisphere; (3) administration and scoring instructions for the subtests of the RHLB; (4) a summary of studies using the RHLB; (5) a section on test interpretation and applications; and (6) appendices containing a rating scale for discourse and a table for converting RHLB raw scores to T scores.

The manual provides a summary of results from testing 30 patients with vascular right-hemisphere damage, 10 patients with nonvascular right-hemisphere damage, 30 patients with vascular left-hemisphere damage, 10 patients with nonvascular left-hemisphere damage, and 30 neurologically normal adults. Means and standard deviations for right-hemisphere-damaged patients, left-hemisphere-damaged patients, and normal groups on each subtest are provided. Significant and nonsignificant differences among the three groups on each subtest (measured by analysis of variance) are reported. Test-retest reliability (evaluated by t-tests and correlation coefficients) are reported for each subtest, and correlations among the subtests of the RHLB are provided.

TESTS OF VISUAL PERCEPTION

Patients with nondominant-hemisphere brain damage often exhibit visual perceptual anomalies that affect both testing and treatment. These anomalies usually take the form of *visual inattention* and disruption of *visual organization*. Consequently, tests of visual attention and organization are an important part of the assessment protocol for patients who may have nondominant hemisphere damage.

Tests for *visual inattention* usually are paper-and-pencil tests in which the patient is asked to mark or cross out printed stimuli at various locations on a printed page. Albert's *Test of Visual Neglect* (1973) is typical. The patient is given a sheet of paper on which short lines have been drawn in random locations and is asked to cross out each line. Other tests present pages of circles, dots, crosses, etc., to be crossed out in similar fashion (Fig 8–3).

Line bisection tests sometimes are used to test for visual neglect. In these tests, the patient is given a page containing printed lines and asked to make a mark on each line to divide the line into two equal halves. Patients with inattention tend to mark the lines so that the segment in the neglected visual field is longer than the segment in the intact field (Fig 8–4).

Tests of visual organization, in which the patient is asked to identify incomplete or fragmented visual stimuli, and tests of figure-ground discrimination, in which the patient is asked to identify overlapping or partially occluded figures, are frequently administered to patients with right-hemisphere damage because they frequently ex-

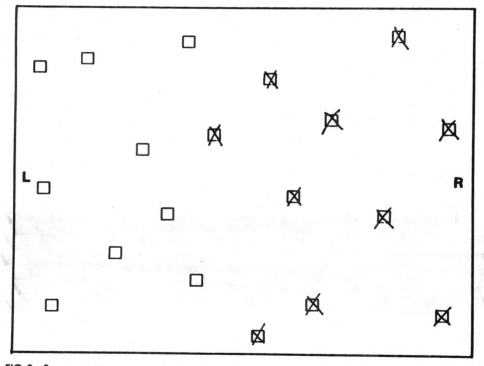

FIG 8–3.

An example of a visual neglect test. The examinee crosses out the squares. This patient exhibits left neglect.

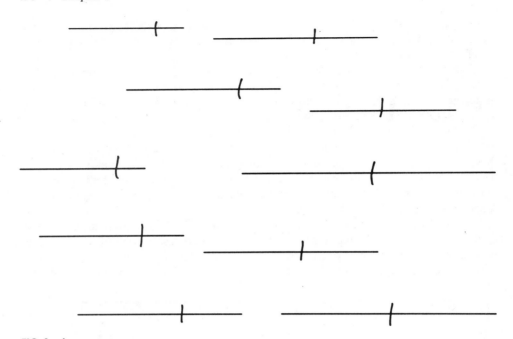

FIG 8–4.
Line bisection by a patient with right-hemisphere brain damage. The patient's bisection marks are displaced into the intact hemi-field.

hibit anomalies in visual discrimination and organization. Tests of visual discrimination and organization were described previously (see Chapter 5).

TREATMENT OF PATIENTS WITH RIGHT-HEMISPHERE BRAIN DAMAGE

We know less about treatment of right-hemisphere-damaged patients than we do about treatment of left-hemisphere-damaged (aphasic) patients, in part because the communicative impairments of right-hemisphere-damaged patients were largely unrecognized and untreated until about 10 years ago, and in part because focal right-hemisphere damage seems to produce more diffuse effects on behavior than left-hemisphere damage does. Consequently, identifiable (and treatable) right-hemisphere syndromes are not as well-described as left-hemisphere aphasic syndromes.

Within the last few years a treatment literature on right-hemisphere-damaged patients has begun to develop, but this literature is primarily anecdote and opinion, without much empirical support. We now know that right-hemisphere-damaged patients often (or usually) exhibit communicative impairments that can be objectively described, and that treatment can help at least some of these patients overcome or compensate for their impairments. However, there are several major differences between right-hemisphere-damaged patients and left-hemisphere-damaged (aphasic) patients that affect both the nature of treatment and its probable outcome. These differences are largely attributable to the fact that lesions in the left hemisphere tend to produce focal effects on specific linguistic and communicative abilities, whereas lesions in the right hemisphere tend to produce diffuse effects that are not readily reducible to specific communicative abilities.

Communicative impairments of patients with left-hemisphere damage are relatively discrete and can be identified, classified, and quantified with reasonable reliability. Their communicative failures are usually relatively easy to identify and most are characterized by countable "errors" (e.g., misnaming pictures, missing the last two parts of a three-part command). The relationships between diagnostic tests and the patient's underlying communicative impairments seem relatively straightforward—for example, the relationship between errors on tests of confrontation naming and impaired word retrieval. The communicative impairments of patients with right-hemisphere damage are less discrete and most are less amenable to simple counts of errors because their communicative impairments represent more diffuse failure, such as treating serious situations as humorous or failing to follow conversational rules. The relationships between diagnostic tests and the patient's underlying communicative impairments usually are less straightforward and require more assumptions than is the case with left-hemisphere-damaged patients—for example, the relationship between "inability to make inferences" and errors on tests requiring correct interpretations of idioms and metaphors.

Treatment of right-hemisphere-damaged patients' communicative impairments is most likely to focus on what Myers (1983) called "higher cognitive impairments":

1. Difficulty organizing and synthesizing information.
2. Impulsivity, tangentiality, and excessive detail in speech.
3. Difficulty separating what is important from what is not.
4. Inability to use contextual cues to ascertain meanings.
5. A tendency to interpret figurative language literally.
6. Overpersonalization.
7. Reduced sensitivity to pragmatic or extralinguistic aspects of communication.

Burns et al. (1985) suggest that treatment should also address:

1. Impairments in focusing, shifting, and maintaining attention.
2. Impaired orientation to place, time, and situation.
3. Impaired judgment and problem-solving.

Clinicians who provide treatment to right-hemisphere-damaged patients usually target these patients' cognitive and perceptual impairments, including impaired reasoning and problem-solving, pragmatic impairments, problems making inferences, and visual neglect. However, they must also deal with several behavioral anomalies that characteristically accompany right-hemisphere brain damage, including denial of illness, indifference and lack of apparent motivation, problems maintaining attention, distractibility, and impulsivity.

Lack of Awareness of Impairments.—Right-hemisphere-damaged patients often minimize or deny the existence of impairments, both physical and communicative. They tend to ignore errors when they occur, and may confabulate, argue, and justify the errors if they are called to the patient's attention. Right-hemisphere-damaged patients' indifference to or denial of errors often proves to be a major obstacle to successful treatment of their communicative impairments. Systematically treating these patients' indifference and denial may eventually get them to recognize their impairments and to become concerned with overcoming them. The process usually is long, and most patients retain some level of indifference and denial of impairment. Clinicians usually treat indifference and denial by (1) delivering immediate response-contingent feedback when errors occur during treatment activities; (2) gently confronting the patient when he or she denies errors or impairments; (3) teaching the patient self-monitoring skills in both structured and unstructured activities.

Lack of Apparent Motivation.—Right-hemisphere-damaged patients usually are compliant and willingly participate in treatment programs, but as passive participants rather than as active collaborators. They usually do not participate in making decisions about the content and focus of treatment. They often fail to carry out assigned activities unless closely supervised. Homework assignments are likely to be neglected unless someone in the patient's living environment provides supervision and direction.

For these reasons, treatment of patients with right-hemisphere damage tends to be highly prescriptive. Because right-hemisphere-damaged patients tend to be indifferent to or unaware of their impairments, they tend not to do more than is specifically required, and they may resist, either overtly or covertly, even doing what is specifically required. Consequently, it is important that the clinician define a clear set of treatment goals, and communicate them to the patient and his or her family, and that the patient and family understand the relationship between the treatment goals and what is done in treatment. Active participation by family members or other caregivers is important, both for ensuring that homework assignments are completed and for facilitating transfer of treatment gains from the clinic to the patient's daily life.

Impaired Attention, Distractibility.—Many patients with right-hemisphere damage (usually those with moderate to severe overall impairments) are unusually sensitive to background noise or movement and cannot maintain attention to treatment activities unless distracting background stimuli are controlled or eliminated. Burns et al. (1985) recommend that right-hemisphere-damaged patients' ability to deal with distractions be evaluated by testing them both in quiet, distraction-free conditions and in noisy conditions with background distractions. They also recommend that clinicians incorporate systematic manipulation of distractions and competing stimuli into treatment activities to enhance these patients' ability to deal with distractions in daily life.

Drills and exercises to increase sustained attention and resistance to distraction include (1) paper and pencil tasks calling for diligence and sustained attention, such as letter cancellation, solving mazes, and completing trail-making tasks; (2) com-

puter-based exercises that require monitoring of visual displays and making a keyboard response when the display changes; and (3) gradual introduction of distracting
or competing stimuli during treatment activities.

Impulsivity.—Right-hemisphere-damaged patients often are impulsive and respond to their first impressions of messages, events, or situations without taking time
to determine their actual meaning. In treatment activities they may respond to questions before the clinician has finished. They may ignore or get only part of instructions and directions, causing frequent mistakes. Impulsivity can be treated with behavior modification techniques, using various visual or auditory stimuli to control the
patient's impulsive behavior. The patient may be taught that a clinician-controlled
signal light or a tone means that he or she may not respond. The clinician incorporates the signal into treatment activities, using it to impose delays between task stimuli and the patient's responses. The light or tone is gradually faded out and replaced
by verbal cues, such as "wait" or "think before you act." When the clinician's verbal
cues control the patient's impulsivity, they are gradually replaced by self-cueing by
the patient.

COGNITIVE AND PERCEPTUAL IMPAIRMENTS

Impaired Reasoning and Problem-Solving.—Many right-hemisphere-damaged patients have difficulty with activities that require reasoning and problem-solving. They have difficulty organizing and planning activities such as shopping trips,
excursions, or parties. They tend to get lost in details and seem to lack an overall
concept of order and relative importance. They have difficulty anticipating consequences. They may suggest bizarre, unworkable, or dangerous schemes for accomplishing their wishes. Treatment of such impairments requires immersion in a variety
of activities that require reasoning, foresight, and problem-solving. The activities
might include role-playing situations in which problem-solving skills are needed (e.g.,
getting a refund for defective merchandise), proposing solutions to problems posed
by the clinician, and planning activities such as vacations, field trips, and picnics.

Pragmatic Impairments.—Many right-hemisphere-damaged patients exhibit
impairments in the pragmatics of language. These impairments range from diminished eye contact to disruptions of high-level processes such as the coherence and
relevance of spoken and written discourse. Three aspects of pragmatics—*eye contact, turn-taking,* and *topic maintenance*—are frequently treated, partly because they
are relatively easy to treat, and partly because improving them can have striking effects on the patient's conversational appropriateness. Both can be effectively treated
by means of behavior modification techniques. Increasing the patient's eye contact
usually requires only that the clinician say "look at me" at appropriate times in treatment interactions. This behavioral treatment usually is combined with discussions of
what constitutes appropriate eye contact and how it facilitates conversational interactions. When the patient responds consistently to the clinician's cues, they are gradu-

ally faded. Sometimes the clinician's cues are replaced by self-cueing by the patient. Giving the patient specific points at which to make eye contact may be necessary if the patient has difficulty making the transition from clinician cues to self-cues. Teaching the patient to make eye contact at the beginning and end of each of his or her utterances, then extending it to the beginning and end of each utterance by the conversational partner may be effective.

Teaching right-hemisphere-damaged patients to follow conversational turn-taking rules must be approached systematically and in stepwise fashion. Verbal instruction about turn-taking rules and how conversational participants know when to take or yield conversational turns precedes structured practice in turn-taking, but it is almost never sufficient by itself to improve right-hemisphere-damaged patients' turn-taking behaviors. The instruction usually is accompanied by structured practice in which the patient can concentrate on turn-taking without having to concentrate on other aspects of communication such as message formulation or inferential reasoning. The structured practice may include activities such as: (1) watching videotapes of conversational interactions (e.g., television talk shows) and discussing how the participants knew when to talk and when to let the other person talk; (2) preparing a script for a conversational interaction with appropriate conversational turns, videotaping it, then critiquing it; (3) videotaping a free conversation, viewing it, and identifying appropriate and inappropriate turn-taking behavior. When the patient begins to exhibit reasonably good appreciation of normal turn-taking, attention to turn-taking can be incorporated into other treatment activities and into free conversation with the clinician.

Teaching right-hemisphere-damaged patients to maintain conversational topics usually requires some instruction and much structured practice. The instruction usually involves pointing out to the patient that conversations usually have a central theme or topic that lasts through several conversational turns, and convincing the patient that he or she often inappropriately strays from the topic during conversations. The structured practice may involve activities such as (1) identifying topics in printed materials such as newspaper or magazine articles; (2) watching videotapes of conversational interactions and identifying topics, identifying when the topic changes, and discussing how the topic change was brought about by the participants; (3) engaging in structured conversations with the clinician while maintaining a specified topic for a given length of time or a given number of conversational turns.

Higher-level pragmatic disruptions, such as appreciating a speaker's implied intent and responding appropriately to figurative language, appear to represent problems in making inferences, rather than pragmatic impairments per se. These higher-level pragmatic disruptions probably can be more effectively and efficiently treated, at least in the initial stages of treatment, by treating the underlying deficiency in making inferences than by working on conversational interactions. In later stages of treatment, work on making inferences in conversational interactions may be appropriate.

Inference Failure.— Myers (1990) has recently argued that most (or all) of right-hemisphere-damaged patients' cognitive and communicative impairments may be explained by a central impairment in making inferences. She called this impairment "inference failure." According to Myers, inference "requires an interaction between two types of recognition—the recognition of key elements and the recognition of their relationship to one another and to other contextual cues." Myers considers right-hemisphere-damaged patients' tendency to interpret metaphor, humor, idioms, and indirect requests literally, their pragmatic deficits in conversations, their impaired expression of emotion, their impulsivity and denial of illness, their facial recognition deficits, their verbose, tangential, and inefficient speech, and their failure to produce integrated stories and descriptions to be the result of a general failure to go beyond the superficial meaning of events or situations to their deeper (implied) meanings. If Myers is right, treatment of right-hemisphere-damaged patients' communicative impairments would be most efficient and effective if it were focused on teaching them to make inferences. As their ability to make inferences improved, the surface impairments that depended on making inferences should improve. Myers's hypothesis has yet to be tested, but it suggests a promising alternative to current treatment-by-symptom approaches to remediation of right-hemisphere-damaged patients' communicative impairments.

If inference failure is the central problem of right-hemisphere-damaged patients, working on tasks that require making inferences should be the primary focus of treatment, and improved inference-making should generate improvements in many of the patient's specific disabilities. The following list of tasks provides examples of activities that would be appropriate for such a treatment focus.

1. *Appreciation of humor.*—The patient is given a printed joke, minus its punch line, and then chooses the humorous punch line from a set containing a humorous punch line and nonhumorous foils. The patient is given a cartoon minus its caption, and then chooses the humorous caption from a set containing a humorous caption and nonhumorous foils.

2. *Appreciation of the implied meanings of metaphors and idioms.*—The patient hears (or reads) a common metaphor or idiomatic expression, then chooses the correct interpretation from (a) a group of printed interpretations containing the correct interpretation and foils, including a literal interpretation of the metaphor or idiom; or (b) a set of pictures portraying the correct interpretation plus foils, as above.

3. *Identification of verbal and pictorial absurdities.*—The patient listens to a short spoken narrative in which there are absurd or inconsistent statements, identifies the absurd or inconsistent statements, and explains why they are absurd or inconsistent. The patient is shown pictures containing absurd or unlikely relationships (e.g., a rabbit chasing a dog) and identifies the absurd or unlikely relationships and explains why they are absurd or unlikely.

4. *Comprehension of indirectly stated information in stories and narratives.*—The patient listens to spoken stories or narratives, answers questions testing indirectly stated or implied information from the stories or narratives, and gives the main idea of the narrative or the moral of the story. The patient reads printed stories or narratives and does the same things.

5. *Retelling stories.*—The patient listens to a story, then retells it, paraphrasing and interpreting it, rather than repeating it verbatim.

6. *Perceiving relationships.*—The patient *categorizes* items according to similarities and differences or class membership, for example, telling why a scissors and a saw are alike, listing things that one might find at a picnic, naming ferocious animals, etc. The patient analyzes *familial relationships* (e.g., "How is your son's uncle related to you?"). The patient generates lists of *divergent functions* (Chapey et al, 1977), for example, "Tell me all the ways in which you could use a brick." (This task may exacerbate some patients' tendency toward tangentiality. If carefully controlled this task may provide a vehicle for working on tangentiality. If not carefully controlled, it may reinforce it.)

Neglect and Visual Perceptual Impairments.—Right-hemisphere-damaged patients' visual perceptual and visual-spatial impairments are also frequent targets for clinical intervention. Visual neglect is the most salient of these impairments and the one most frequently targeted, perhaps because it usually has direct effects on the patient's ability to read and comprehend printed materials. Visual perceptual and visual-spatial impairments frequently are treated by occupational therapists, whereas visual neglect may be treated by both occupational therapists and speech-language pathologists. Occupational therapists usually treat neglect in activities of daily living, and speech-language pathologists usually treat neglect in the context of reading printed materials.

Diller and Weinberg (1977) described a comprehensive treatment program for visual neglect in which patients received systematic practice in visual tasks such as (1) visual tracking of a moving target across visual fields; (2) detection of flashing lights in various locations in both visual fields; (3) letter cancellation; and (4) reading printed paragraphs projected on a wall so that they transcended both visual fields. The training program consisted of making the patient aware of his or her neglect, forcing the patient to view visual stimuli systematically, and massed repetition to make the systematic viewing automatic. Diller and Weinberg reported that 1 month of 1-hour-per day treatment sessions effectively reduced neglect in a group of right-hemisphere-damaged patients.

Stanton et al. (1981) described procedures for teaching reading to patients with left visual neglect. The procedures included (1) visual matching of printed stimuli arranged in columns—one column on the right and one on the left; (2) reading printed sentences, beginning with widely spaced sentences in large print and progressing to single-spaced small-print sentences; and (3) reading printed paragraphs, going from large print and double spacing to standard books, magazines, and newspapers, some in double-column format. Stanton et al. used verbal cues to help the patient attend to the left side of the materials. They began with the clinician instructing the patient to "tell yourself out loud, 'Look to the left'" at the end of each line, and progressed to self-initiated verbal cues by the patient. As the patient progressed, overt verbal cues were gradually eliminated. Stanton et al. recommend that clinicians take advantage of right-hemisphere-damaged patients' good verbal skills by having them ask themselves "does that make sense?" at the end of each sentence or periodically throughout their reading of texts.

Colored left-side margins, colored lines at the left margin, and rulers or other markers at the left margins of printed materials are frequently used to help patients attend to the left half of printed materials. The patient is instructed to find the red line (or other marker) each time he or she reaches the end of one line and begins a new line. Sometimes the patient is instructed to keep his finger on the margin and to track back to his finger when he begins a new line. These techniques for marking the left margin are eventually replaced by the patient's monitoring of whether the material makes sense (Stanton et al).

GENERALIZATION

Generalization Within Clinic Activities.— Many right-hemisphere-damaged patients do not make the inferences that allow them to generalize what they have learned from one level to another within treatment tasks, or from task to task within the treatment program. For this reason, treatment activities often have to be broken into small steps and generalization from one task to another must be carefully programmed, rather than assumed. Yorkston (1981) described a program to teach a right-hemisphere-damaged patient to transfer from his wheelchair to his bed. They began with a 7-step procedure, which proved ineffective. They then expanded it to 17 steps, then 27 steps, and eventually added the self-cue "have you finished this step?" at the end of each step before the patient eventually learned to transfer. Yorkston cautioned that clinicians should never assume that a right-hemisphere-damaged patient will make logical transitions from one step to another: "Rarely, if ever, does one err in the direction of breaking a task into too many steps."

Generalization From the Clinic to Daily Life.— Right-hemisphere-damaged patients, even those with relatively mild impairments, tend not to generalize what they learn in the clinic to outside situations. Treatment programs for right-hemisphere-damaged patients almost always must include careful, systematic attention to generalization, including extensive, carefully planned, and closely monitored participation of family members and caregivers. Even then, some right-hemisphere-damaged patients may fail to generalize what they learn in the clinic to their daily living environment.

Chapter 9

Traumatic Brain Injuries

NEUROPATHOLOGY

Traumatic brain injury (craniocerebral trauma) is caused by sudden deceleration or acceleration of the head, when (1) a rapidly moving object strikes the head or (2) the moving head strikes a stationary object. *Penetrating brain injuries* are injuries in which the skull is fractured or perforated and the meninges are torn or lacerated. Penetrating brain injuries are sometimes referred to as *open-head injuries. Nonpenetrating brain injuries* are injuries in which the meninges remain intact. Nonpenetrating injuries are often referred to as *closed-head injuries.*

PENETRATING BRAIN INJURIES

Penetrating brain injuries (open-head injuries) are most frequently caused by high velocity missiles (bullets or other projectiles). However, low velocity impacts (for example, blows to the head received in altercations or automobile accidents) may cause penetrating injuries if the force of the impact is concentrated in a small area. High velocity penetrating injuries perforate or fracture the skull and penetrate the brain substance. The projectile creates a pressure wave that has an explosive impact on the skull and brain, and causes destruction on both sides of the projectile's track. Hair, skin, and bone fragments are carried into the brain by the projectile, where they become potential sites for bacterial infections. In low velocity penetrating injuries, the skull usually is fractured, rather than perforated. If the fracture is severe, bone fragments may be carried into the brain, and there may be massive destruction of brain tissue at the impact site. Penetrating injuries to the brain often are survivable, but the patient is almost invariably left with physical, cognitive, or linguistic deficits. Penetrating injuries to the brain stem usually are fatal because of damage to structures that regulate respiratory, cardiac, and other vital functions. If the patient survives the first day after the injury, then infection, bleeding, and increased intracranial pressure, either from swelling of the brain or from hydrocephalus, become concerns.

NONPENETRATING BRAIN INJURIES

In nonpenetrating brain injuries (closed-head injuries) the meninges remain intact and foreign substances do not enter the brain. Nevertheless the brain and brain stem often sustain considerable indirect damage. The damage comes from *abrasions* (scrapes), *lacerations* (cuts), *contusions* (bruises), and *shearing* (tearing) of brain tissue. One source of damage is *impression trauma,* caused by deformation of the skull at the point of impact. It is not clear whether impression trauma is caused by the impact of the depressed skull on the brain, or if it is caused by negative pressure that develops when the skull snaps back into its orignal shape after being deformed inward by the impact.

Regardless of the mechanism of injury, trauma to the brain at the point of impact is a frequent consequence of closed-head injury. Trauma at the point of inpact is sometimes called *coup* (pronounced "coo") injury. Coup injuries can be caused either by compression of the skull into the brain or by rebound of the brain against the skull. Surprisingly, coup injuries contribute in a relatively minor way to the disabilities seen after closed-head injuries. Other mechanisms for brain injury are much more important. *Contrecoup injuries* are injuries to brain tissue on the opposite side of the brain from the impact. Contrecoup injuries result from the inertia of the brain, brain stem, and cerebellum, which causes these structures to lag behind the head as the head is propelled in the direction of the impact. When the head snaps back in the direction from which the blow came, the cranial contents continue moving in the opposite direction until they strike the skull, bruising and abrading brain tissue at the point of impact (*translational trauma*) (Teasdale and Mendelow, 1984). Blows to the front of the head frequently produce only coup injuries. Blows to the back of the head frequently produce only contrecoup injuries. Blows to the side of the head can produce coup injuries, contrecoup injuries, or both.

The movement of cranial contents within the skull also generates twisting and shearing forces within brain tissues (*rotational trauma*) (Teasdale and Mendelow, 1984). The forces are concentrated in the midbrain and brain stem, where the twisting movement of the brain mass is transferred to these structures. Shearing forces tend to be greatest at the boundaries between gray matter and white matter fiber tracts. For this reason one often sees bleeding and swelling from torn brain tissue around major white fiber tracts, especially the internal capsule, the corpus callosum, and brain stem fiber tracts.

Injuries to the cortex of the brain and cerebellum, in the form of abrasions and lacerations, are also common in closed-head injury. These injuries are caused by movement of the brain against sharp bony projections inside the skull. The bottom surface of the cranial vault is rough and uneven, with sharp projections, while the other surfaces are relatively smooth and featureless. Consequently, abrasions and contusions of the cortex tend to occur on the inferior surfaces of the frontal lobes, and on the bottom of the temporal lobes, where the brain rubs across the floor of the cranial vault. Abrasions and contusions of the parietal lobes, the occipital lobes, and the upper aspects of the frontal lobes are much less common in closed-head injury.

Some closed-head injuries are accompanied by skull fractures. Fractures at the base of the skull usually are more serious than those higher up, because basal skull fractures may damage cranial nerves or the carotid arteries. Regardless of its site, any skull fracture is dangerous if the meninges beneath the fracture are torn, because of bleeding from damaged meningeal blood vessels and because of the potential for infection by bacteria penetrating the damaged meninges. At one time the severity of closed head injuries was measured by whether the skull was fractured. However, it is now clear that the presence (or absence) of skull fracture does not predict the severity of central nervous system damage.

SECONDARY CONSEQUENCES OF TRAUMATIC BRAIN INJURY

Most traumatic brain injuries have a fairly predictable course. The patient usually loses consciousness immediately after the injury. The loss of consciousness can last from a few seconds to days, weeks, or months, and more severe injuries cause longer periods of unconsciousness. With the onset of unconsciousness comes transient interruption of respiration, slowing of heart rate, and a drop in blood pressure. These vital signs usually recover quickly, although the patient may remain unconscious. The patient's return to consciousness may be slow and spread over days, weeks, or months, or it may be rapid and abrupt, with only transitory impairments that quickly clear. Transient loss of consciousness without apparent permanent consequences is called *concussion* (or minor head injury). The patient loses consciousness immediately, opens his or her eyes within minutes, and regains apparently normal mentation within a few hours, although headache, dizziness, or other "minor" signs of nervous system instability may persist for days or even weeks. Contemporary studies of patients after concussion suggest that many do, in fact, have long-lasting and sometimes permanent subtle impairments of mental functions that are detectable by sensitive testing.

If the patient survives the first few hours after the accident, the secondary consequences of traumatic brain injury become important. Although no statistics are available, it is probably true that more patients with traumatic brain injuries die from the secondary consequences of the injury than from the immediate injuries sustained in the accident. Death rates from traumatic brain injuries are highest in the first 3 days, with 50% to 75% of deaths occurring within 72 hours. The major secondary consequences of traumatic injury are *traumatic hematoma, cerebral edema,* and *increased intracranial pressure.*

Traumatic Hematoma

Hematomas are accumulations of blood caused by hemorrhages. There are three major categories of traumatic hematoma, depending on where the blood accumulates. They are *epidural hematoma, subdural hematoma,* and *intracerebral hematoma.*

Epidural Hematoma.—Epidural hematomas, as the label suggests, are accumulations of blood between the dura mater and the skull. They are caused by lacerations of the middle meningeal artery, middle meningeal vein, or the dural venous sinus. Automobile accidents are their most common cause, but minor falls and sports injuries are frequent causes of epidural hematoma. Ninety percent of epidural hematomas are consequences of skull fracture (Teasdale and Mendelow, 1984). About 20% to 30% of patients with epidural hematoma die as a consequence of their head injuries. Mortality from epidural hematoma is strongly related to whether the bleeding is from an artery (about 85% of cases die) or a vein (about 15% of cases die). Arterial bleeding usually is marked by massive hemorrhage, with symptoms progressing rapidly, often culminating in death within a few hours. Venous bleeding usually follows a less dramatic course, with slow progression of symptoms. Small venous hemorrhages may ooze blood so slowly that they produce no overt symptoms, and the bleeding may be detected only with computed tomography (CT) scans of the head during evaluation of the patient. The magnitude of the symptoms caused by epidural hemorrhages depends to some extent on the location of the hematoma. Bleeding into the posterior inferior epidural space often causes compression of the brain stem, with respiratory depression, decreased heart rate, and increased blood pressure. Bleeding into the frontal and superior epidural space is likely to be less serious, because centers for vital functions are far away, and because there is more epidural space for the hematoma before it begins to displace brain structures. The most common treatment for epidural hematomas is surgical evacuation, which can usually be done relatively easily because of the hematoma's accessibility, just beneath the skull.

Subdural Hematoma.—Subdural hematomas, as the name suggests, are accumulations of blood between the dura and the arachnoid. Subdural hematomas are twice as common as epidural hematomas, and are twice as deadly, with 60% (or greater) mortality. Motor vehicle accidents are their most common cause, and about half are associated with skull fractures. The source of most subdural hematomas is laceration of cortical blood vessels caused by abrasions and contusions on the brain surface. *Acute subdural hematomas* usually develop within a few hours, and almost always within a week of the injury. The combination of increasing pressure and displacement of brain tissue by the expanding hematoma, if not controlled, usually leads to coma and death within several hours. Surgical excavation of the hematoma is the most common treatment for acute subdural hematomas. In some cases surgical removal of swollen brain tissue caused by contusions is also necessary to control increased intracranial pressure, if medications (steroids, mannitol) are unsuccessful.

Chronic subdural hematomas are most common in older patients and in patients with long-term alchoholism, who usually have some brain atrophy with a consequent enlargement of the size of the subdural space. In many, if not most cases, the injury that precipitates the hematoma is relatively trivial (usually a fall, with a bump on the head). The hemorrhage gradually fills the subdural space, and within a few weeks a membrane forms around it. Eventually the hematoma may increase in size until it produces symptoms, which often wax and wane. Headache and tenderness in the affected area are the most common symptoms, although progressive dementia and decreasing levels of consciousness may develop. Surgical evacuation of the hematoma was for many years the treatment of choice, but mortality rates were distressingly high. In the last decade or so, a more conservative procedure has been successful. In this procedure, a catheter is inserted into the hematoma through a burr hole in the skull. The fluid is then continuously drained into a container below the level of the head. However, some cases require opening the cranial vault and removing the membranes.

Increased Intracranial Pressure

Perhaps the most dramatic (and deadly) consequence of brain injury is increased pressure within the cranial vault. The pressure is a consequence of increases in the volume of the cranial contents, caused by accumulating fluid (blood, cerebrospinal fluid, or water) within the skull. Accumulation of fluid is the brain's generic response to a wide variety of insults, such as trauma, anoxia, infection, and inflammation. The fluid may accumulate between the brain and skull (hematoma), within the ventricles (hydrocephalus), or within brain tissues (cerebral edema). The resulting pressure buildup compresses and displaces brain tissues, causing increasing neurologic impairment as the pressure increases. Increased intracranial pressure is the most frequent cause of death from traumatic brain injury, and one of the primary concerns in medical management of traumatically brain injured patients is monitoring and controlling intracranial pressure.

Generalized pressure on brain tissue can by itself cause neurologic impairments, but only if the pressure becomes very high, because the brain seems reasonably tolerant of modest increases in pressure if they are distributed equally throughout the cranial vault. The most dangerous consequences of elevated intracranial pressure come from distortion and displacement of tissues within the cranial vault caused by localized increases in intracranial pressure. Most traumatic injuries produce pressure gradients in which pressure is greatest at and around the site of injury, with decreasing pressure with increasing distance from the site of injury. These differences in pressure displace brain tissues away from areas of high pressure into areas of low pressure. Brain tissues are compressed, distorted, stretched, forced against the skull, and forced against and across protruberances within the skull, usually with ominous consequences, for the brain is as intolerant of displacement and distortion as it is tolerant of moderate increments in general intracranial pressure. Damaged cell walls leak fluid into extracellular space. Damaged blood vessels leak into brain tissue or into convenient spaces. The already swelled brain swells further, increasing the forces that displace and distort it. Uncontrolled, this sequence of events may lead quickly to coma and brain death.

The most dangerous consequence of regional increases in intracranial pressure is *herniation,* in which cerebral structures are pushed around rigid partitions in the cranial vault or extruded through cranial orifices. Pang (1989) describes four major types of herniation.

Subfalcine herniation is, according to Pang, most common and least ominous. It occurs when one cingulate gyrus is pushed across the falx cerebri, a rigid sheet of dura that projects downward into the superior longitudinal fissure. Most cases of subfalcine herniation do not generate observable neurologic symptoms unless the anterior cerebral artery is compressed, in which case numbness and weakness of the contralateral leg may be observed.

Lateral transtentorial herniation usually occurs as a consequence of injury to the temporal lobe. The mesial surface of the temporal lobe is squeezed against the tentorium, a rigid sheet of dura that separates the space occupied by the brain from that occupied by the cerebellum. The herniation creates pressure on cranial nerve III, causing ipsilateral pupillary dilation. The pressure also forces the brain substance downward into the foramen magnum, stretching tissues and blood vessels at the base of the brain and in the brain stem. The resulting brain stem ischemia may lead to coma, and if brain stem hemorrhages occur, to irreversible coma or death.

Central transtentorial herniation is caused by swelling near the apex of the brain or in the frontal lobes. The brain mass is pushed downward into the foramen magnum. As in lateral transtentorial hernia, structures and blood vessels at the base of the brain and in the midbrain are stretched and distorted, with consequent impairment of vital functions. Irreversible coma or death are common consequences of central transtentorial herniation.

Tonsillar herniation is caused by swelling in the cerebellum, pons, or medulla. The cerebellar tonsils (hence the name *tonsillar*) are extruded through the foramen magnum, where they exert pressure on the medulla. The brain stem is displaced downward, with consequent shearing and distortion. Respiration is compromised, heart rate decreases, blood pressure rapidly increases, and coma soon follows.

Prolonged high levels of intracranial pressure inevitably cause irreversible brain damage, with coma and death the frequent outcome. Fortunately, intracranial pressure is controllable in many cases. The patient may be hyperventilated. Increased blood oxygen causes constriction of cerebral arteries, decreases cerebral blood volume, and provides at least temporary reductions in intracranial pressure. Steroids (anti-inflammatory medications) may be administered to reduce cerebral edema. Diuretics (medications that increase the body's excretion of fluids) may be administered. If these treatments are unsuccessful, the patient may be put into a barbiturate coma to decrease cerebral metabolism and constrict cerebral blood vessels.

ISCHEMIC BRAIN DAMAGE

In addition to the impairments caused by the effects of tissue destruction, swelling, and tissue displacement, most traumatically brain-injured patients will suffer from some degree of ischemic brain damage. Graham et al. (1978) reported ischemic damage in 91% of patients who had died of head injuries. Ischemic brain damage can occur for numerous reasons. Reduced respiratory and cardiac output may contribute to decrements in blood oxygenation and reduced blood supply to the brain. Elevated intracranial pressure and pressure on blood vessels may prevent adequate amounts of blood from reaching the brain. Cerebral vasospasm (see below) may decrease the carrying capacity of the cerebral vessels, especially in cases in which cardiac output is below normal. The distribution of damage from these ischemic processes varies, but damage commonly occurs in the basal ganglia, hippocampus, and in the "watershed" areas separating the distributions of the three major cerebral arteries.

CEREBRAL VASOSPASM

Cerebral vasospasm (contraction of the muscular layer surrounding blood vessels) occurs in 15% to 20% of head injuries. The most frequent are spasms of cortical arteries that are irritated by blood from a subarachnoid hemorrage. Other causes include stimulation of cerebral blood vessels by chemicals such as serotonin, which are released by the injury, or injury to control centers that regulate dilation and constriction of cerebral arteries. Cerebral vasospasm by itself is rarely responsible for major neurologic complications. However, when it is inflicted on a system already compromised by the other consequences of brain injury, it may be responsible for significant worsening of the patient's condition.

ASSESSMENT OF TRAUMATICALLY BRAIN-INJURED PATIENTS

Behavioral and Cognitive Recovery After Traumatic Brain Injury

The general course of recovery after traumatic brain injury is one of improvement, but the pattern of improvement usually differs from that seen after vascular accidents. Recovery from vascular accidents usually progresses predictably and regularly, with relatively rapid recovery in the early postonset period and gradually slowing recovery thereafter. Recovery from traumatic brain injuries usually progresses in stepwise fashion, with periods of little or no change interspersed with periods of sometimes rapid improvement. The relationship between the severity of the patient's impairments in the first few weeks postonset and the eventual chronic level of impairment is much stronger for vascular accidents than it is for traumatic brain injury. Consequently, it is more difficult to predict a traumatically brain-injured patient's permanent level of impairment than it is to predict it for vascular patients.

Traumatically brain-injured patients typically progress through a fairly predictable sequence of stages during recovery. The patient almost always loses consciousness immediately after the accident, with the duration of unconsciousness lasting from a few seconds to weeks or, rarely, months. Return to consciousness begins a period of undifferentiated activity, in which the patient is awake, but his or her responses to the environment are inconsistent, nonpurposeful, and disorganized. During this period the patient is likely to be agitated and irritable. Gradually the patient becomes more lucid and behavior becomes more purposeful, although he or she may continue to be restless, agitated, and irritable. Orientation to time and place develops during this stage, and the patient begins to respond appropriately to simple requests, although attention span is short and distractibility is high. With the passage of time the patient begins to manage his or her daily routine with careful supervision and directions, but judgment, memory, and abstract reasoning continue to be impaired. Eventually the patient may reach a level at which he or she can function independently in familiar situations, but almost all continue to have problems with memory and abstract reasoning. A few patients eventually resume premorbid activities, but almost always with subtle (but important) deficiencies in memory, abstract reasoning, and tolerance for noise and distractions.

The *Rancho Los Amigos Scale of Cognitive Levels* (Hagen and Malkamus, 1979) summarizes the typical course of cognitive and behavioral recovery after traumatic brain injury (Table 9–1). Rancho Los Amigos levels are commonly used by clinicians to identify a traumatically brain-injured patient's level of cognitive and behavioral recovery. There is some evidence that length of time spent at the lower levels is related to eventual outcome. The longer the patient remains at levels I through IV, the poorer the prognosis for recovery, but the relationship is far from perfect, and sizeable errors in prediction can occur.

Assessment of Severely Impaired Patients

Most severely impaired traumatically brain-injured patients are first seen at bedside. The clinician's purpose at this time usually is to determine the patient's general

TABLE 9–1.

The Rancho Los Amigos Scale of Cognitive Levels

Level I: No response
  No response to pain, touch, sound, or sight.
Level II: Generalized response
  Inconsistent, nonpurposeful, nonspecific responses to intense stimuli. Responds to pain, but response may be delayed.
Level III: Localized response
  Blinks to strong light, turns toward/away from sound, responds to physical discomfort. Inconsistent responses to some commands.
Level IV: Confused-agitated
  Alert, very active, with aggressive and/or bizarre behaviors. Attention span is short. Behavior is nonpurposeful, and patient is disoriented and unaware of present events.
Level V: Confused-nonagitated
  Exhibits gross attention to environment. Is highly distractible, requires continual redirection to keep on task. Is alert and responds to simple commands. Performs previously learned tasks but has great difficulty learning new ones. Becomes agitated by too much stimulation. May engage in social conversation, but with inappropriate verbalizations.
Level VI: Confused-appropriate
  Behavior is goal-directed, with assistance. Inconsistent orientation to time and place. Retention span and recent memory are impaired. Consistently follows simple directions.
Level VII: Automatic-appropriate
  Performs daily routine in highly familiar environments without confusion, but in an automatic robot-like manner. Is oriented to setting, but insight, judgment, and problem-solving are poor.
Level VIII: Purposeful-appropriate
  Responds appropriately in most situations. Can generalize new learning across situations. Does not require daily supervision. May have poor tolerance for stress and may exhibit some abstract reasoning disabilities.

level of consciousness and overall level of mentation. The *Glasgow Coma Scale* (GCS) (Teasdale and Jennett, 1976) is frequently used to summarize such patients' overall level of consciousness and orientation (Table 9–2). The patient's highest level of eye-opening, motor, and verbal responses is determined, and the scores for the three levels are summed. Total scores on the GCS can range from 3 to 15; *coma* frequently is operationally defined as a GCS total score of 8 or less (Eisenberg and Weiner, 1987). Initial GCS scores have been shown to be strong predictors of patients' eventual recovery, if the patient is assessed during the early stages of recovery but long enough after injury for noncranial contributors to the patient's impairment to dissipate (e.g., alcohol intoxication). Most studies of the relationship between GCS scores and outcome have used the GCS score at 6 hours after the accident as the reference value for predicting outcome.

The GCS has been shown to be highly reliable (Teasdale and Jennett, 1976), but it is relatively insensitive because wide ranges of behavior are reduced to a limited number of possible scores. Because no exceptions are made for untestable categories of behavior, the GCS may overestimate the severity of impairment for some patients (e.g., intubated patients who are verbally competent but who cannot talk because of the intubation).

If the patient is conscious, attends to his or her environment, and follows simple instructions, the clinician may wish to get a general idea of the patient's memory and orientation at bedside. The *Galveston Orientation and Amnesia Test* (GOAT) (Levin et al., 1979) is useful for such screening purposes. As the title implies, the GOAT tests patients' *memory, orientation,* and *amnesia.*

The *amnesia* section of the GOAT contains four questions: "What is your name?," "When were you born?," "How old are you?," and "Where do you live?"

TABLE 9–2.

The Glasgow Coma Scale

Category of Behavior	Behavior	Value
Eye opening	Opens eyes spontaneously	4
	Opens eyes to verbal command	3
	Opens eyes in response to pain	2
	No response	1
Motor responses	Obeys verbal commands	6
	Attempts to pull examiner's hand away during painful stimulation	5
	Moves limb away from painful stimulus	4
	Flexes body in response to pain	3
	Extends limbs, becomes rigid in response to pain	2
	No response	1
Verbal responses	Converses and is oriented	5
	Converses but is disoriented	4
	Utters intelligible words, but does not make sense	3
	Produces unintelligible sounds	2
	No response	1

The *orientation* section tests the patient's orientation to *location* (where the patient is) and *time* (year, month, day, hour).

The *memory* section contains tests of short-term memory for words, the alphabet, and backward counting. The highest possible GOAT score is 100. Scores from 80 to 100 are considered average, scores from 66 to 79 are considered borderline, and scores from 0 to 65 are considered impaired. The GOAT is a useful screening test for getting a general idea of a patient's level of cognitive functioning. Orientation is weighted more heavily than amnesia and memory. Because it requires spoken responses, it may overestimate the severity of impairment for patients with focal language-dominant-hemisphere pathology in addition to the diffuse damage typical of traumatic brain injury.

Assessment of Moderately and Mildly Impaired Patients

Because cerebral damage in most cases of traumatic brain injury is diffuse, traumatically brain-injured patients usually exhibit diffuse cognitive and behavioral impairments, although their impairments sometimes may have focal components. The most pervasive and consistent mental consequence of traumatic brain injury is a general slowing of information processing and responding. Most traumatically brain-injured patients perform poorly on tasks involving memory, and for most, "nonverbal" skills (visual perception and organization, drawing, constructions) are more impaired than "verbal" skills (naming, repetition, following directions). Recall and use of information acquired before the accident is almost always better than recall and use of information acquired after the accident. Although the choice of which tests to administer depends on the nature and severity of the patient's impairments, general assessment of traumatically brain-injured patients usually involves assessment of verbal and nonverbal "intelligence," speed of information processing, memory, alertness and vigilance, selective attention, concentration and mental tracking, and language.

Verbal and Nonverbal Intelligence.— A general intelligence test such as the *Wechsler Adult Intelligence Scale—Revised* (WAIS-R) (Wechsler, 1981) can provide an overall estimate of a traumatically brain-injured patient's abilities and disabilities in a variety of test tasks. Traumatically brain-injured patients usually do best on untimed subtests that assess abilities that were well-established prior to the patient's brain injury (Lezak, 1983). They usually do poorly on subtests that require sustained attention, visual-spatial organization, and mental flexibility. Of the verbal subtests, traumatically brain-injured patients usually have the most difficulty with the *similarities* subtest and the *digit span* subtest, especially *digits backward*. Of the performance subtests, traumatically brain-injured patients usually have the most difficulty with the *digit symbol, block design,* and *object assembly* subtests. Some patients who have difficulty learning new response sets may consistently make errors on the first trials of "unusual" subtests such as block design, followed by improved performance on later (and more difficult) trials in that subtest (Lezak, 1983).

Speed of Information Processing.— General slowing of mental processes is a universal consequence of traumatic brain injury. The slowing is unselective and nonspecific; it affects all mental processes, regardless of stimulus input or response output modality. The slowing is easily seen when the patient's performance on timed and untimed versions of the same test are compared. When the patient is tested under time constraints, performance is markedly poorer than it is when the patient is given unlimited time to complete the test. Most timed tests are sensitive to this slowing, but timed versions of attention, vigilance, and tracking tasks are among the most sensitive.

Memory.—Memory disturbances are one of the most salient early consequences of traumatic brain injury, and one of the traumatically brain-injured patient's most serious long-term impairments. Memory disturbances in traumatic brain injury usually are divided into two general categories—*pretraumatic amnesia* (sometimes called "retrograde amnesia") and *posttraumatic amnesia* (sometimes called "anterograde amnesia").

Pretraumatic amnesia is loss of memory for events occurring before the accident. It appears to be a problem of retrieval, in which the patient cannot retrieve previously stored information from memory. The patient often cannot remember the minutes (sometimes hours, rarely days) before the accident. Pretraumatic amnesia is almost always shorter in duration than posttraumatic amnesia. It usually lasts for a few minutes to a few hours. Russell and Nathan (1946) reported the duration of pretraumatic amnesia in 973 patients with traumatic brain injury. Fourteen percent had no detectable pretraumatic amnesia, 73% had amnesia lasting less than 30 minutes, and 14% had pretraumatic amnesia lasting longer than 30 minutes. Pretraumatic amnesia tends to shrink, primarily during the first year postonset.

Posttraumatic amnesia is loss of memory for current events. It appears to be a problem of getting information into memory. The patient may not remember meetings, conversations, or people from hour to hour or from morning to afternoon. The duration of posttraumatic amnesia is moderately related to the duration of coma, and it may be a better predictor of eventual recovery than duration of coma (Levin et al., 1982), with longer posttraumatic amnesia suggesting greater residual deficits. Patients with posttraumatic amnesia of 1 month or more are likely to have permanent cognitive deficits, and patients with posttraumatic amnesia of 3 months or more are likely to have permanent and substantial impairments of cognition, learning, and memory (Brooks, 1989). Russell (1971) measured the duration of posttraumatic amnesia in 1,324 closed-head injury patients and reported that 11% had no measurable posttraumatic amnesia, 21% had posttraumatic amnesia lasting less than 1 hour, 25% had posttraumatic amnesia lasting from 1 to 24 hours, 24% had posttraumatic amnesia lasting from 1 to 7 days, and 19% had posttraumatic amnesia lasting more than 7 days. Jennett (1976) reported a greater incidence of longer intervals of posttraumatic amnesia in a study of 139 patients. He reported that only 8% of his patients had posttraumatic amnesia lasting less than 7 days, 19% had posttraumatic amnesia lasting from 7 to 14 days, 27% had posttraumatic amnesia lasting from 14 to 28 days, and 45% had posttraumatic amnesia lasting longer than 28 days. Posttraumatic amnesia is far more serious than pretraumatic amnesia and causes the greatest disruption in the patient's daily life. According to Lezak (1983) traumatically brain-injured patients are most troubled by posttraumatic amnesia, whereas their lawyers are most troubled by pretraumatic amnesia.

Residual memory deficits often persist after the full-blown amnesia resolves. These memory deficits seem to reflect a combination of impaired retrieval from memory and abnormal decay of memory traces. Immediate memory usually is relatively unaffected, but long-term memory is reduced. Traumatically brain-injured patients with residual memory impairment are likely to perform in the normal range on tests of short-term retention and immediate recall, such as forward digit span, but will perform poorly on tests requiring both recall and mental manipulations, such as backward digit span. Traumatically brain-injured patients also usually do poorly on tests of short-term visual memory, such as the Memory for Designs Test (Graham and Kendall, 1960). Patients with damage in the left temporal lobe may be aphasic and are likely to exhibit significant impairment of both short-term and long-term verbal memory.

Alertness and Vigilance.—Van Zomeren et al. (1984) divide alertness into *tonic alertness* and *phasic alertness*. *Tonic alertness* refers to an individual's ongoing, continuing receptivity to stimulation. Tonic alertness changes slowly and reflects the individual's overall state of arousal. Diurnal rhythms, increasing drowsiness in monotonous tasks, and the "midafternoon slump" are examples of changes in tonic alertness. *Phasic alertness* refers to momentary, rapidly occurring changes in receptivity to stimulation. Changes in phasic alertness occur within milliseconds. Phasic alertness is strongly affected by the individual's intentions and interests. Increased alertness in response to warning signals or important events are examples of changes in phasic alertness.

Most traumatically brain-injured patients appear to have lower-than-normal "resting" levels of tonic alertness, but the magnitude of their "cycles" of tonic alertness does not seem greater than normal. Traumatically brain-injured patients who "drift off" or fall asleep during testing or treatment are examples of lowered tonic alertness.

Lowered tonic alertness is an inconvenience for the patient and those around him or her, and may slow the patient's progress in treatment, but diminished phasic alertness usually is more disruptive, both in treatment activities and in daily life. In treatment tasks patients with diminished phasic alertness tend to make errors on initial stimulus items, with consequent disruption of performance when treatment tasks change. They may fail to perceive short-duration stimuli, unless given a warning signal, and they may fail to perceive subtle changes in instructions or treatment stimuli. In daily life they may miss key elements in others' spoken messages, and they may respond slowly or erroneously to rapidly occurring events or stimuli, such as traffic signals. Impaired phasic alertness may be related to "mental slowness" (see above).

Selective Attention.—Most traumatically brain-injured patients are distractible and have difficulty maintaining attention in the face of competing stimuli. In figure-ground tasks (both visual and auditory) these patients may have difficulty discriminating figures from backgrounds, or they may be distracted by the background and be unable to maintain attention to the figure. They may be distracted by irrelevant aspects of stimuli, such as the border around a picture or irrelevant details in stories or events. Patients with impaired selective attention perform poorly on visual figure-ground tests (embedded figures, overlapping figures, masked or occluded figures), picture description, and storytelling or story-retelling tasks.

Sustained Attention.—Impairments in sustained attention are not clearly separable from impairments in alertness, vigilance, and selective attention. Clearly, diminished alertness and impaired selective attention will disrupt performance on tasks that require sustained attention. However, there are patients who perform well on tasks requiring momentary alertness and who have few problems discriminating figure from background who then perform poorly on tests requiring sustained attention. These patients' performance deteriorates as the interval during which attention must be sustained increases, and as the complexity of the task increases. They do poorly on tests such as digits backward, backward spelling, oral arithmetic, and challenging vigilance tasks.

Language.—Traumatically brain-injured patients with brain stem or cerebellar damage often are dysarthric. Assessment of these patients follows the same course as assessment of patients with dysarthria from other causes (see Chapter 11). Except for dysarthria, speech and language impairments usually are a minor consequence of traumatic brain injury. Traumatically brain-injured patients usually produce syntactically well-formed and meaningful spoken and written sentences, but their written sentences are likely to contain spelling errors. Word retrieval in spontaneous speech usually is not significantly impaired. Traumatically brain-injured patients often make errors on tests of confrontation naming, but the errors usually reflect visual misperceptions or the patient's inability to inhibit competing responses, rather than word-retrieval impairments per se. Comprehension of commonplace spoken and printed verbal material usually is normal, but some traumatically brain-injured patients may have difficulty appreciating the meaning of implied and nonliteral information. Responses to open-ended questions may be irrelevant and confabulatory, but generally are linguistically acceptable. Bernstein-Ellis et al. (1985) compared the *Porch Index of Communicative Ability* (Porch, 1981a) performance of 15 left-hemisphere-damaged aphasic adults with that of 15 traumatically brain-injured adults. They found significant differences between the groups on one visual subtest and three writing subtests (of 18 subtests). Aphasic subjects performed better on the visual subtest, and traumatically brain-injured patients performed better on the writing subtests. Aphasia test batteries are usually of limited value in assessing patients with traumatic brain injury because they focus on linguistic disabilities that are unlikely to be impaired in traumatic brain injury. Selective testing of reading, writing, speaking, and listening abilities of traumatically brain-injured patients with tests that focus on perceptual and processing impairments likely to be affected by traumatic brain injury is preferable to testing with standard aphasia tests.

REHABILITATION OF TRAUMATICALLY BRAIN-INJURED PATIENTS

Rehabilitation of traumatically brain-injured patients requires participation and collaboration of physicians, nurses, speech-language pathologists, occupational therapists, physical therapists, neuropsychologists, clinical psychologists, social workers, and vocational counselors. Interdisciplinary collaboration is especially important in the early stages of the patient's recovery, when medical, physical, and behavioral impairments are most severe. The physical, cognitive, and behavioral impairments exhibited by traumatically brain-injured patients cross professional boundaries, and require a unified, integrated program of treatment that extends from the clinic to the patient's daily environment. According to Kay and Silver (1989), "rehabilitation [of traumatically brain-injured patients] must be interdisciplinary in the truest sense of the word. There must be ongoing communication among team members (not just with a central leader), care planning that cuts across disciplines, and coordination by a professional who is an expert in the cognitive and behavioral problems of head injured persons."

Treatment During the Early Stages of Recovery

Medical stabilization of the patient is the primary concern immediately after traumatic brain injury. During this period treatment is primarily medical, and focuses on ensuring the patient's survival and preventing cerebral damage caused by the delayed effects of brain injury. If the patient cannot talk, establishing a reliable means of communication may be an important aspect of care at this time. Establishing communication may include teaching the patient how to indicate "yes" and "no" and how to make simple requests by gestures, nods, eye-blinks, or other alternatives to speech. Treatment directed toward the patient's behavioral and mental condition also begins at this time. Treatment at this stage of recovery often focuses on *sensorimotor stimulation* and *management of agitated, confused behavior.*

Sensorimotor Stimulation.—Comatose patients often receive several periods of repetitive auditory, tactile, olfactory, and visual stimulation every day, together with passive range-of-motion activities to prevent muscle deterioration. Many practitioners believe that sensorimotor stimulation hastens the patient's emergence from coma, but there is no empirical evidence supporting this belief. Nevertheless, the idea makes intuitive sense, and as Kay and Silver (1989) point out, "It would seem to make sense on rational grounds that it is better to provide regular, gentle sensory input to comatose patients than to let them lie unattended and unstimulated (physically and sensorially) for long periods of time."

The nature of sensorimotor stimulation depends on the patient's general level of arousal. Stuporous and lethargic patients may be bombarded with dramatic and intense stimuli to increase their level of arousal. Excitable and restless patients may receive gentle, rhythmic stimulation to calm them. Family members often participate in sensorimotor stimulation programs. It may be that familiar voices, touches, and activity are intrinsically more effective than unfamiliar ones, but there is no evidence confirming this.

Management of Confused, Agitated Behavior.—Most traumatically brain-injured patients go through a period of agitation, disorientation, and confusion as they emerge from coma. Management during this period is concerned with reducing agitation and confusion and increasing the patient's constructive interaction with the environment. *Environmental control* and *response contingencies* are the primary vehicles for achieving these objectives.

Environmental control provides a stable and predictable "prosthetic environment" within which the patient's confusion and agitation can be minimized, while his or her successful interactions with the environment are maximized. The key element in environmental control is creation of a predictable and familiar environment wherein (1) the significant events (therapy appointments, meals, etc.) are arranged into a consistent routine, so that they happen at the same time and in the same place each day; (2) significant locations (the patient's room, lounges, etc.) are vividly identified with signs, posters, and pictures; (3) staff and others who interact with the patient (including family members) do so in a coordinated, consistent way.

The patient's room may be identified by signs ("This is David Smith's room"), posters, and pictures of home and family members. Therapy sessions are scheduled at the same time, in the same room, with the same clinician every day. Visual prompts such as signs, notes, appointment calendars, and appointment books help the patient anticipate upcoming events and gain active control of the environment. Environmental control changes as the patient acquires increasing self-sufficiency. The frequency and salience of prompts and visual cues decrease, and the predictability of the environment diminishes. Treatment during this period emphasizes:

1. *Increasing the patient's orientation* to *place* (where he or she is), *person* (who he or she is and who others are), *time* (what time of the day or year it is and when things happen during the day), and *the therapeutic mileau* (why the patient is hospitalized, the purposes of testing and treatment activities).
2. *Increasing the patient's attention* to his surroundings, the people around him or her, and to activities of daily life.
3. *Stimulating the patient's mentation* by providing challenging but manageable activities and daily life experiences.

Environmental control relies on manipulation of *antecedent stimuli* to regulate the patient's behavior and maximize therapeutic environmental stimulation. *Response contingencies* modify, control, or eliminate behaviors by manipulating the consequences of the behaviors. Traumatically brain-injured patients who are in the early stages of recovery usually are not affected by intangible consequences such as verbal praise or reproof.* Tangible, primary consequences (incentive feedback) are needed. Tangible consequences include both positive consequences, such as sweets, music, touching, massaging, or other pleasurable stimuli, and negative consequences, such as noise, bright light, or painful stimuli.

Response contingencies can be manipulated in four ways: (1) *positive reinforcement*, in which positive consequences are delivered contingent on desired responses; (2) *negative reinforcement*, in which negative consequences are removed contingent on desired responses; (3) *punishment*, in which negative consequences are delivered contingent on undesired responses, and (4) *extinction*, in which positive consequences are removed from undesired responses. Positive reinforcement is socially the most acceptable procedure, although its effects on behavior at this stage of the patient's recovery may be limited. It is often difficult to find consequences that have positive reinforcement value, because traumatically brain-injured patients at this level may find few externally delivered stimuli rewarding. Punishment is socially the least desirable procedure, and is used only when there are no alternatives, such as physical restraint. Physical punishment (slapping, pinching, etc.) is in almost all cases legally impermissible. Milder forms of punishment, such as the sound of a buzzer or loud verbal reproof may sometimes reduce a patient's inappropriate behavior. However, punishment often causes only temporary suppression of behavior. More lasting behavior change usually is obtainable by other forms of reinforcement and by controlling the patient's environment to minimize undesirable behavior.

Negative reinforcement is sometimes effective in modifying patients' behavior at this stage of recovery. These patients often find almost any kind of stimulation aversive, and are often intolerant of demands made upon them by treatment personnel. Caregivers can sometimes negatively reinforce desirable patient behaviors by making termination of stimulation and/or departure of the clinician contingent upon certain desired behaviors (the "if you do this one thing for me, I'll go away and leave you alone" approach). Negative reinforcement is initially made contingent on one or two simple responses, then the number, complexity, and/or difficulty of the responses required to terminate the (aversive) stimulation is gradually increased. As positive reinforcers become available, control of behavior can be gradually shifted from negative reinforcers to positive ones.

Sometimes caregivers unintentionally provide positive reinforcement for undesirable behaviors by giving the patient attention when he or she "misbehaves" and ignoring the patient at other times. Extinction (removing positive consequences for certain behaviors) may eliminate such misbehavior, especially if extinction is combined with positive reinforcement of alternative behaviors.

The response contingencies employed and the schedule on which they are delivered change as the patient recovers. In the very early stages of recovery, when the patient has just emerged from coma, only a few important behaviors are treated, re-

---

*These patients do not meet the conditions set forth earlier (see pages 138–140) under which intangible consequences (information feedback) is effective. They are not internally motivated to "get better." Much of their behavior is primitive and unmodulated by cortical control mechanisms. Consequences requiring interpretation by the cerebral cortex are unlikely to affect these patients' behavior.

sponse-contingent stimuli must have primary reinforcing value, and consequences follow almost every occurrence of the targeted behavior. Negative reinforcement and punishment often are salient at this time. As the patient continues to recover, the number and complexity of behaviors that are targeted for treatment increase, the emphasis shifts from negative reinforcement and punishment to positive reinforcement, and partial reinforcement schedules, in which not every occurrence of the target behavior receives consequences, become prevalent. During this time the emphasis shifts from *controlling* the patient's behavior to *teaching* new behaviors, and to *generalizing* new behaviors from the clinic to the patient's daily life environment.

Treatment During the Middle Stages of Recovery

During the middle stages of recovery the patient becomes a more active participant in the rehabilitation process. The environmental control begun in the previous stage continues, but with gradually increasing flexibility. Treatment of specific cognitive disabilities is now superimposed on the program of environmental control. The primary objectives at this stage of recovery are to increase the patient's independence and control of the environment, to increase the adequacy and appropriateness of the patient's interactions with the environment, to stimulate organized, purposeful thinking and use of knowledge, and to help the patient compensate for physical or intellectual impairments.

During this stage of recovery the frequency and intensity of environmental prompts and cues gradually diminish. Posters, signs, and labels are replaced by personal appointment sheets, calendars, and daily logs. The patient is given greater responsibility for daily self-care and for remembering and keeping appointments. The rigid, unchanging daily schedule becomes less predictable, and the patient is given responsibility for dealing with changes in the schedule constructively. Treatment activities now focus on specific cognitive impairments, including *attention, perception, memory, organization and planning, abstract thinking,* and *judgment.* Intensive stimulation (within the limits of the patient's capacity) and massed practice are important during this period, and careful design of activities to enhance carry-over of learning from the clinic to the patient's daily life environment is crucial.

Treatment During the Late Stages of Recovery

During the late stages of recovery the patient becomes an active partner and collaborator in setting goals and planning and carrying out treatment activities. The overall objective of treatment at this stage is to enable the patient to function independently in as many situations as are practical, given the patient's residual impairments. Control of the patient's environment is further diminished, or, when practical, eliminated, and real-life inconsistencies and stresses are introduced (changes in schedules, time limits for getting things done, etc.). Treatment of specific cognitive impairments may continue during these stages, but the emphasis of treatment changes to helping the patient prepare for independent functioning in daily life. The focus of treatment at this stage is on helping the patient discover and learn *compen-*

satory strategies to minimize the effects of residual impairments, teaching the patient how to use *environmental control* to keep daily life events and situations within his or her capabilities, and helping the patient devise and implement a system of *prompts and cues* to organize and carry out daily life activities.

Compensatory strategies for patients at this stage of recovery might include:

1. Breaking complex and demanding tasks into smaller segments to minimize the effects of fatigue and attentional impairments.
2. Requesting time, date, and other orienting information from others when necessary.
3. Writing down main ideas and periodically summarizing when reading printed materials.
4. Rehearsing spoken or written material, either covertly or overtly, to help remember it.
5. Relating new information to what the patient already knows to improve retention.
6. Mentally rehearsing potentially difficult situations. Using visual imagery and written plans to organize responses to such situations.
7. Developing standard routines for organizing thinking, e.g., from first to last, most important to least important, from best known to least known, etc.
8. Asking for clarification or repetition when confused about others' wishes or intents.
9. Asking others to write down complex instructions and schedules.

Environmental controls for patients at this stage of recovery might include:

1. Establishing consistent routines and regular schedules for daily life activities.
2. Instructing family members, friends, and associates in how best to facilitate the patient's success in daily life activities.
3. Limiting or eliminating distractions by keeping radios and televisions turned down, and closing doors and windows to reduce noise from outside or from other rooms.
4. Keeping possessions in designated places, and putting them away when they are not being used.
5. Organizing the workspace and setting aside specific times for work at difficult tasks—times at which the patient is rested and alert.
6. Setting time limits (using alarms, timers) for working at difficult tasks to avoid fatigue and minimize mistakes.

Prompts and cues might include:

1. A written daily schedule of events and appointments, with a place to check off events and appointments when they are completed. The schedule may be placed on a clipboard to which an inexpensive stick-on digital clock is attached, or in a noteboook.

2. An alarm watch or timer that can be set to signal appointments or remind the patient of scheduled duties or events.
3. A daily log or journal in which the day's events can be recorded, by the patient and/or those around him or her.
4. Signs or notes placed in strategic locations to remind the patient to carry out certain activities (e.g., "Have you made the bed?," "Do you have your keys?").

Working With the Family

Providing support, reassurance, information, and direction to family members is an important part of the clinical management of patients with traumatic brain injuries. The family's need for support, reassurance, and information is greatest in the acute postinjury interval, and their need for direction is greatest in the middle and later stages of recovery. Polinko (1985) has divided the time following traumatic brain injury into three stages: *injury to stabilization, return to consciousness,* and *rehabilitation.* For the family, the first stage (injury to stabilization), when the patient remains unconscious, is a period of apprehensive waiting. The patient is in the care of strangers, and is surrounded by an alarming array of monitors and support systems. The family may have been told that the patient may not regain consciousness. They anxiously watch for the first signs of return to consciousness, and may be compelled to interpret the patient's purposeless activity as a sign that the patient is waking up. According to Polinko, this is a time of shock and denial, with occasional breakthroughs of panic, and family members need extensive support and reassurance. During this time, family members also need objective information about what has happened and what the outcome is likely to be, but because of their emotional state they are likely to have difficulty assimilating it. Consequently, information may have to be reiterated a number of times in order for it to "get through." As time goes on, denial may be replaced by "bargaining," in which family members attempt to strike a deal with a deity or with fate by promising acceptance of the patient's condition, acts of contrition, changes in attitudes, or changes in behavior, if only the patient survives.

The second stage (return to consciousness) usually brings feelings of relief that the patient will live, together with apprehension about the extent to which he or she will recover. Family members continue to watch anxiously for hopeful signs, and may continue to interpret incidental patient behaviors as signs of recovery. Because the patient's emergence from coma often occurs rapidly, family members may respond with overly optimistic predictions about the patient's eventual recovery. Educating family members about the usual course of recovery from traumatic brain injury and helping them to separate true prognostic indicators from fallacious ones is an important part of the clinician's responsibility during this stage. When it becomes apparent that the patient will not fully recover, the family will need help in planning how they will cope with a future that includes an impaired family member.

By the time the third stage (rehabilitation) is reached, most families will have accommodated to the accident and its aftermath, and will have moved past the stage of denial to relatively realistic expectations about the future. The beginning of structured treatment activities usually is a time of increased hope and optimism for family members, often leading to rosy expectations of what will be accomplished in treatment. This time of hope and optimism often gives way to anxiety, confusion, and eventually anger with the patient and with professional staff, as the patient's recovery fails to meet their optimistic expectations. The unpredictable nature of recovery from traumatic brain injury adds to the family's confusion and sometimes to their anger. When periods of rapid recovery alternate with periods of little change, family members may accuse the patient of slacking off, or clinicians of not doing their job. As time goes on, families usually return to a semblance of normal functioning. Family members who once stayed with the patient during long parts of the day return to work, and the patient no longer is the central focus of family life. Responsibility for the patient may be divided among family members. One family member may assume primary responsibility for visiting the patient and interacting with caregivers, and another may take responsibility for dealing with financial and logistical adjustments. During this time the family may need the help of psychologists, social workers, rehabilitation therapists, speech-language pathologists, and community service agencies in setting up a long-term plan for incorporating the brain-injured patient into family life in a way that is maximally beneficial for the patient and the family. Throughout the course of the patient's recovery the family will need continuing and conscientious assistance from all members of the patient-care team in order to survive the mental, emotional, and physical consequences of the patient's injury.

Chapter 10 _____

Dementia

Dementia is "an acquired persistent impairment of intellectual function with compromise in at least three of the following spheres of mental activity: language, memory, visuospatial skills, emotion or personality, and cognition (abstraction, calculation, judgment, etc.)" (Cummings and Benson, 1983). The definition requires that the condition is acquired, distinguishing it from congenital conditions such as mental retardation; that it is persistent, distinguishing it from transitory states such as acute confusional states; and that the deficits cross several areas of mental function, distinguishing it from more focal impairments such as aphasia or psychiatric disturbances.

Dementia almost always begins late in life, and its incidence increases rapidly with age. Dementia is the most common single diagnosis in nursing-home occupants. Estimates of its prevalence vary greatly, because of differences in where samples were obtained, definitions of dementia, and the age of the patients in the sample. Estimates of the prevalence of dementia in the over-65 population range from 6% to about 20%, with the highest rates in the oldest age groups. Because of declining birth rates and longer life expectancy, the proportion of elderly persons in the world population is increasing, and with it the incidence of age-related illnesses, including dementia.

CAUSES OF DEMENTIA

Dementia often occurs as the primary (or only) symptom of neurologic impairment, as in Alzheimer's disease and Pick's disease. It often occurs as a consequence of vascular disease, and may appear in the late stages of extrapyramidal diseases such as Huntington's or Parkinson's disease. Metabolic disorders, nutritional deficiencies, infections (encephalitis, meningitis), and poisoning with toxic substances (mercury, lead, arsenic) also may contribute to dementia. Some dementias (primarily those caused by metabolic and nutritional disorders) are reversible, but most are irreversible and progressive. The two most frequent causes of dementia are *Alzheimer's disease* and *vascular disease*. Alzheimer's disease accounts for approximately

224

half the reported cases of dementia, and vascular disease accounts for 15% to 20% (Bayles et al., 1987).

Alzheimer's Disease

Those with Alzheimer's disease constitute the fastest growing and most expensive clinical population in the United States (Bayles et al., 1987). Alzheimer's disease is two to three times more common in women than in men (Cummings and Benson, 1983). Its cause is not known, and a massive research effort is currently underway to determine its causes, and to develop preventive and palliative medical treatments.

Alzheimer's disease is characterized by microscopic changes within the neurons of the brain, particularly the cerebral cortex. These changes are detectable only by direct examination of brain tissue; they are not visible on computed tomography (CT) scans or magnetic resonance imaging (MRI) scans until the late stages of the disease, when the brain becomes atrophic, with increased ventricular volume, widened sulci, and decreased mass. These changes are readily seen on CT and MRI scans, but definitive diagnosis of Alzheimer's disease depends on the presence of three microscopic changes in neuronal tissue: *neurofibrillary tangles, senile plaques,* and *granulovacuolar degeneration.*

Neurofibrillary Tangles.—Neurofibrils are "filamentous structures seen with the light microscope in the nerve cell's body, dendrites, axon, and sometimes synaptic endings" (*Stedman's Medical Dictionary,* 1990). In Alzheimer's disease, the neurofibrils become twisted, tangled, and contorted. These changes are easily seen using standard microscopic techniques. Neurofibrillary tangles are not unique to Alzheimer's disease. They sometimes are present in the brains of patients with Parkinson's disease, patients with hereditary cerebellar ataxia, and occasionally elderly patients with no obvious neurologic disease. Neurofibrillary tangles may be the neuron's nonspecific reaction to central nervous system damage (Cummings and Benson, 1983; Bayles et al., 1987).

Senile Plaques.—Senile plaques are "minute areas of tissue degeneration consisting of granular deposits and remnants of neuronal processes" (Cummings and Benson, 1983). Senile plaques tend to concentrate in the cortex and subcortical regions of the brain. Neuronal synapses are markedly reduced by senile plaques; consequently, synaptic transmission is adversely affected. In addition to Alzheimer's disease, senile plaques are seen in Down's syndrome, Creutzfeldt-Jakob disease (a rare disease characterized by progressive degeneration of corticospinal nerve fibers), and in the brains of some "normal" elderly persons.

Granulovacuolar Degeneration.—Granulovacuolar degeneration refers to a condition in which small fluid-filled cavities containing granular debris appear within nerve cells. The pyramidal neurons in the hippocampus (a deep brain structure that seems to be important in memory) are most frequently affected. Granulovacuolar degeneration also is seen in other diseases, and occasionally in the brains of "normal" elderly persons. However, Tomlinson and Henderson (1976) report that if 10% or more of hippocampal neurons are affected, dementia is always present.

Neuropathologic changes in Alzheimer's disease are not diffuse and equally distributed throughout the brain. Neurofibrillary tangles and senile plaques are most frequent in the temporoparietal-occipital junctions and the inferior temporal lobes. The frontal lobes, the motor and sensory cortex, and the occipital lobes are usually spared (Fig 10–1).

The cause of Alzheimer's disease is unknown, although several causes have been proposed, including aluminum intoxication, disturbed immune functions, infections with a "slow virus," and genetically transmitted disturbances of neuronal functions. There is no cure for Alzheimer's disease, and there is no specific medical treatment other than management of the patient's symptoms. Tranquilizers may be administered to control combativeness and aggression. If the patient is depressed, antidepressants may be administered. The patient's diet and fluid intake can be monitored and managed to avoid dehydration and maintain adequate nutrition. The patient's environment can be managed to stimulate the patient, maintain orientation and cognitive abilities, and to prevent social isolation. Counseling and other support services can be provided to the patient's family.

The general course of Alzheimer's disease is one of gradual deterioration. The first symptoms are subtle, and include lapses of memory (usually the first symptoms

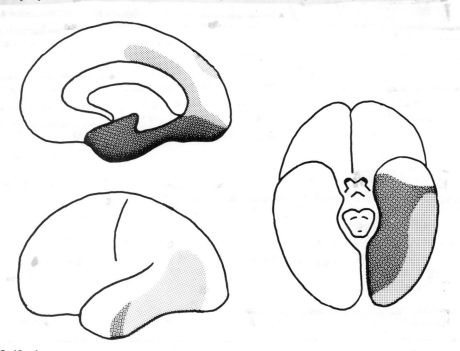

FIG 10–1.
The most frequent sites of neuropathology in Alzheimer's dementia. (Adapted from Cumming's JL, Benson DF: *Dementia: A Clinical Approach.* Boston, Butterworths, 1983.)

reported), impairments in reasoning, periods of poor judgment, disorientation (except in highly familiar environments), and alterations of mood (usually depression and apathy). Personality and social behavior remain "remarkably intact" during the early stages of the disease (Cummings and Benson, 1983). As the disease progresses the patient's mental impairments become more obvious and general. Intellect and cognition become increasingly impaired, and disturbances of language and communication appear. The patient may become restless and agitated, and may wander off when not supervised. Depression may resolve as the patient's sensitivity to self declines. Periodic incontinence may be seen. These symptoms gradually worsen, and in the final stages leave the patient with profound motor problems (rigidity or spasticity), complete incontinence, and loss of almost all intellectual and cognitive abilities. The patient usually dies of aspiration pneumonia or infection.

Language is usually less affected than cognition and intellect in the early stages, although some aspects of language are affected relatively early. Mild anomia and subtle problems in comprehension of ambiguous, nonliteral, and abstract language often appear early. Phonology and syntax usually are well-preserved until the late stages. Articulation and voice quality usually are unaffected until the terminal stages, when the patient often becomes mute. As a general rule, automatic responses are spared (e.g., counting, saying the alphabet, saying days of the week) whereas responses calling for sustained attention (e.g., describing pictures, explaining proverbs) are compromised early. Confrontation naming rarely is impaired until later stages, but word-retrieval errors and verbal paraphasias in conversation are common in the early stages of Alzheimer's disease. Perseverative responses often appear in the middle stages.* As the dementia progresses, literal paraphasias appear, and by the late stages the patient's speech is circumlocutory, semantically "empty," and riddled with jargon.† In the late stages, the patient with Alzheimer's disease may become hyperfluent, speaking rapidly and incoherently ("flight of ideas").

Auditory and reading comprehension become progressively impaired as the disease progresses, but repetition and oral reading usually remain intact until the very late stages. Reiterative speech disturbances (echolalia, palilalia)‡ often become prominent in the late stages.

Language pragmatics usually are affected early and progressively deteriorate as the disease progresses. In the early stages the patient observes conversational turn-taking rules, but talks too long, strays from the topic, and repeats himself or herself without awareness. The patient has difficulty grasping implicit meanings such as

---

*The perseverative responses of patients with Alzheimer's disease differ from those of aphasic patients, representing intrusion of unrelated repetitive thoughts rather than persistence of response sets. An aphasic patient might say "that's a comb" to *comb,* and "that's a comb" to *fork* on the next trial, while the patient with Alzheimer's disease might say "a comb—I lost my comb when I was four" to *comb,* and "it was a pretty red comb" to *fork* on the next trial.

†The circumlocution seen in Alzheimer's disease differs from that in aphasia. The patient with Alzheimer's disease circumlocutes because he or she has forgotten the topic or lost his or her "train of thought" whereas the aphasic patient circumlocutes because of word-retrieval failure. The aphasic patient's circumlocution is goal-directed, but the Alzheimer's patient's is not.

‡*Echolalia*: uncontrollable repetition of what others say. *Palilalia*: uncontrollable repetition of what the patient says.

those involved in humor, sarcasm, or nonliteral statements. As the disease progresses the patient stops initiating conversations and ignores social conventions such as greetings and farewells. In the terminal stages the patient loses all orientation to self and surroundings, and does not use language in any meaningful way.

Pick's Disease

Pick's disease, like Alzheimer's disease, is a degenerative disease affecting neurons in the cerebral cortex. Its etiology is unknown. It is characterized by two neuronal abnormalities—the presence of *Pick bodies* within neurons and a proliferation of *enlarged neurons.* Pick bodies are dense globular formations within the neuron cytoplasm. They are about the same size as the cell nucleus and contain numerous neurofibrils. The progression of Pick's disease is marked by gradual reduction in brain mass (particularly in the temporal and frontal lobes) and neuron loss throughout the cortex. Treatment of Pick's disease, like that of Alzheimer's disease, is symptomatic, consisting of medications to control changes in mood and temperament, and behavioral treatment to maintain orientation and manage the patient's daily life behavior.

The progression of symptoms in Pick's disease differs from that of Alzheimer's disease. Whereas intellect is compromised early in Alzheimer's disease while personality is spared, in Pick's disease personality disturbances usually are the first symptoms reported. The initial stages of Pick's disease are dominated by alterations in personality and emotion. Social behavior usually deteriorates early, with general disinhibition of behavior—inappropriate jocularity, inappropriate comments and behavior (often sexual), and "loss of personal propriety" (Cummings and Benson, 1983). Judgment and insight are soon compromised, and stereotypical repetitive sequences of behavior often develop (e.g., folding napkins and putting them away, taking them out, refolding them, and putting them away again and again). Increased eating and weight gain are common in the early stages of Pick's disease.

As the disease progresses the patient's intellectual functions begin to deteriorate. The pattern of deterioration differs from that in Alzheimer's disease. In Pick's disease, unlike in Alzheimer's disease, memory and orientation to place usually are spared, but linguistic breakdowns appear. The patient's spontaneous speech becomes anomic and circumlocutory. Echolalia and verbal stereotypies may be present. The patient may repeat the same story over and over (the "gramophone syndrome") (Cummings and Benson, 1983). Confrontation naming is impaired. Comprehension impairments for both spoken and printed materials appear. In the final stages patients with Pick's disease become completely mute and profoundly demented, with severely impaired memory, orientation, and cognition. Like patients with Alzheimer's disease, those with Pick's disease usually succumb to aspiration pneumonia or infection.

Cerebrovascular Dementia

Vascular disease is second to Alzheimer's disease as a cause of dementia. Its clinical characteristics include a history of hypertension and strokes, stepwise progression, and focal neurologic signs. Personality and general intellectual abilities tend to be better preserved than in other varieties of dementia, and focal deficits (visual and somatosensory anomalies, aphasia, apraxia, etc.) often appear after individual cerebrovascular incidents. Three etiologic subgroups of cerebrovascular dementia frequently are described. *Multiple bilateral cortical infarcts* cause focal neurologic symptoms that progress in stepwise fashion to dementia. The symptoms depend on the cortical areas involved in each incident, and include those commonly associated with cortical damage (aphasia, apraxia, neglect, etc.). *Lacunar state* results from multiple small infarcts in the basal ganglia, thalamus, midbrain, and brain stem. The symptoms usually include dysarthria, swallowing disturbances, pseudobulbar palsy, weakness, and sometimes tremor. The progression of symptoms is stepwise and involvement of intellect and language occur late in the course of the disease. *Binswanger's disease* is a rare disease, caused by multiple infarcts in subcortical white matter, usually in patients with severe hypertension. The first symptoms of Binswanger's disease usually are focal and the disease progresses in stepwise fashion, culminating in dementia. Motor abnormalities often develop, but later than in lacunar state.

Subcortical Disease and Dementia

Alzheimer's and Pick's disease and bilateral cortical infarcts primarily involve cortical neurons. Consequently, impairments of cortical functions (memory, intellect, language) are seen early, and motor impairments are seen late in the course of the disease. In lacunar state and Binswanger's disease, subcortical neurons are most affected. Patients with degenerative diseases affecting subcortical structures also may become demented in the late stages of their disease. Whether the dementia is caused by the degenerative disease itself or arises from an extraneous cause is not now known. Dementia is often seen in the late stages of more than a dozen subcortical degenerative diseases. Although there are differences in symptoms and in the manner in which they appear, all dementias associated with subcortical pathology are characterized by early motor impairments and preservation of mental abilities until late in the course of the disease.

Parkinsons's Disease

The first symptom of Parkinson's disease reported usually is tremor, but in many cases immobility and "poverty of movement" (Adams and Victor, 1981) are noted by family members before tremor appears. As the disease progresses, the patient's mental functions often become increasingly impaired. Memory, problem-solving, abstract reasoning, and other mental functions requiring sustained mental effort become increasingly compromised. Affect usually becomes progressively flattened, and many patients become depressed. Treatment with L-dopa or similar medications suppresses dyskinesia and slows mental deterioration for about two thirds of patients with Parkinson's disease, although depression, if present, often is unaffected. Many patients eventually reach the point at which their disease progresses in spite of medications, at which time their mental functions also deteriorate.

Huntington's Disease

Huntington's disease is a hereditary degenerative neurologic disorder characterized by increasingly severe chorea and dementia. The first symptoms usually are personality changes. "Patients begin to find fault and complain about everything and to nag other members of the family; they may be suspicious, irritable, impulsive, eccentric, or excessively religious, or may exhibit a false sense of superiority" (Adams and Victor, 1981). Irritability is common, and emotional outbursts frequently occur. Chorea and mental impairment develop slowly and insidiously and usually together. However, mental deterioration may begin later, sometimes several years after the first signs of chorea. Memory usually is affected first, followed by general mental slowing and attentional impairments. Language usually remains relatively intact until the late stages of the disease, except for tests requiring sustained attention, memory, and judgment. Dysarthria frequently accompanies the development of the patient's movement disorder. In the final stages of the disease patients with Huntington's disease are mute, incontinent, and profoundly demented. Death usually occurs within 10 to 20 years of onset of symptoms.

Progressive Supranuclear Palsy

Progressive supranuclear palsy is a rare progressive disorder that usually begins during the sixth or seventh decade of life, with death in 5 to 7 years after onset of symptoms. The first symptoms are motor abnormalities: paresis of gaze (downward gaze first, then upward gaze), rigidity of the neck and trunk (axial rigidity) that gradually extends to the limbs, and pseudobulbar palsy (exaggerated palatal and laryngeal reflexes, drooling, swallowing disturbances, and heightened emotionality). Slowly progressive dementia may eventually appear but usually remains mild. Language usually remains well-preserved, but the patient's speech may be slow and deficient in loudness, sometimes with stuttering-like repetitions (Albert et al., 1974).

Human Immunodeficiency Virus Encephalopathy

Active human immunodeficiency infections often lead to pathologic changes in the subcortical white matter and basal ganglia. These changes lead to characteristic extrapyramidal motor signs (weakness, slowness, rigidity, dyskinesia), and eventually to general intellectual impairment. Spontaneous speech usually is slow, labored, sparse, and dysarthric, but language usually is well-preserved until the late stages of the disease. The patient eventually becomes mute and immobile and death usually occurs within 6 months after onset of central nervous system pathology.

CLINICAL MANAGEMENT OF DEMENTIA

Assessment

The speech-language pathologist's role in assessing patients with dementia is not well defined. Bayles (1986) asserts that speech-language pathologists have an important role in diagnosis of dementia and in monitoring its progression, because performance on language tests correlates strongly with the severity of dementia. Bayles also asserts that measuring patients' communicative abilities can provide information about the effectiveness of therapies, and can provide information useful in advising families about the effects of dementia on communication. Because dementia causes a multitude of intellectual, cognitive, behavioral, communicative, and social problems, diagnosis and evaluation of dementia is carried out by a team of professionals, and the speech-language pathologist usually collaborates with neuropsychologists, clinical psychologists, neurologists, and other health-care professionals.

Diagnosis of Dementia.—Assessing communication is an important part of the diagnosis of dementia (Bayles, 1986; Rosenbek et al., 1989), although Bayles sees assessment of communication as most important in diagnosing mild dementia, because "it is not difficult to identify moderate or severe dementia." According to Bayles language tests most sensitive to dementia are those that require active, creative thought and the use of reason. Bayles suggests that *verbal description* (describing common objects), immediate and delayed *story retelling,* and *verbal fluency* ("Tell me all the words you can think of that start with the letter S") tasks are sensitive to mild dementia, whereas simpler and more automatic tasks, such as pointing to objects by name or reciting the alphabet or the days of the week, are not.

Rarely is the diagnosis of dementia made only from a patient's performance on tests of language and communication. Other tests of memory, attention, perception, and intellect are important in confirming that the patient has general impairment of intellect, rather than a more focal impairment such as aphasia. The patient's medical history also plays an important part in the diagnosis. Dementias usually develop slowly, with gradual progression of symptoms from subtle impairments of memory, reasoning, and problem-solving to gross impairments of intellect, personality, and behavior. Other less generalized impairments such as aphasia usually develop rapidly, and in most cases their course is one of improvement, rather than deterioration.* Tests of communicative abilities by themselves are of limited value in determining that a patient has dementia, rather than some other condition. Together with information from the patient's medical history and the results of other tests of memory, perception, and intellect, the patient's pattern of performance on tests of communicative ability may contribute to the diagnosis.

Measuring the Patient's Impairments and Plotting Their Course.—Speech-language pathologists also contribute to management of dementia by administering standardized, reliable tests that permit the treatment team to identify the patient's communicative strengths and weaknesses, to provide dependable baseline measures against which the effects of interventions can be assessed, and to help structure a comfortable, safe, and stimulating environment for the patient. Tests of language and communication supplement tests of verbal and nonverbal intelligence, tests of

*Several cases of slowly progressive aphasia have been reported in the literature (Heath et al., 1983; Holland et al., 1985; Mesulam, 1982). Such cases are rare, but their existence lessens our confidence in rate of onset to discriminate demented from aphasic persons.

immediate and remote memory, and tests of attention and perception to provide a comprehensive description of the patient's impairments. Evaluation of the patient's speech, language, and communicative abilities may include a comprehensive aphasia test such as the *Boston Diagnostic Aphasia Examination* (Goodglass and Kaplan, 1983b), the *Western Aphasia Battery* (Kertesz, 1982), or a test of functional communication such as *Communicative Abilities in Daily Living*) (Holland, 1980).* Tests of auditory and reading comprehension, spelling, arithmetic, vocabulary, and confrontation naming may also be appropriate. As the patient's dementia progresses, tests of more basic abilities (e.g., orientation) may replace some of the more difficult tests in the battery.

The *Arizona Battery for Communication Disorders of Dementia (Research Edition)* (ABCD) (Bayles and Tomoeda, 1991) is a clinical assessment instrument for identifying and quantifying the communicative deficits of persons with dementia (specifically that caused by Alzheimer's disease). The ABCD contains 4 screening subtests (speech discrimination, visual perception and literacy, visual fields, and visual agnosia) and 14 subtests to evaluate *mental status, linguistic expression, linguistic comprehension,* and *visual-spatial construction.* The subtests in the ABCD are based on the authors' research on the language performance of 175 "normal" older adults and 300 adults with dementia-producing illnesses. The ABCD is standardized on 50 adults with Alzheimer's disease and 50 age-matched normal adults. Reliability and validity information and cutoff scores for normal performance are provided in the test manual. The ABCD appears to be an efficient and informative instrument for assessing communicative disabilities of persons with either suspected or confirmed dementia.

Management

When dementia is progressive (as most are), the objectives of treatment are to slow the progression of the dementia, facilitate constructive interactions between the patient and his or her environment, ensure the patient's safety, keep the patient healthy, and provide support and direction for caregivers. Achieving these objectives requires the coordinated efforts of several disciplines—medicine, nursing, speech-language pathology, neuropsychology and clinical psychology, occupational, recreational, and physical therapy, social work, dietetics, and others.

Maintaining and Enhancing the Patient's Communicative Ability.—Speech-language pathologists play an important part in facilitating communication between the demented patient and his or her caregivers, and in helping the patient maintain communicative competence. This requires attention to both the patient and his or her caregivers. During the early stages, when the patient's dementia is mild, the patient can be an active participant in efforts to maintain and enhance communication. As the patient becomes less able to comprehend instructions, remember communi-

*The *Western Aphasia Battery* and *Communicative Abilities in Daily Living* have been used to evaluate communicative abilities of persons with dementia, and some normative information has been published (Appel, 1982; Holland, 1980).

cative strategies, and carry them out, caregivers assume more of the responsibility for maintaining communication with the patient.

Patients in the early stages of dementia usually do not have major problems with verbal communication, and most have comprehension and speaking abilities sufficient for routine daily life situations. However, memory impairments may compromise the patient's retention of what is heard or read, comprehension may suffer in noisy and distracting contexts or if several people are talking, and intermittent word-retrieval failures may create annoying gaps in the patient's output even though they may not prevent communication.

The speech-language pathologist can help the patient determine which communicative functions have been compromised and which have been spared. The speech-language pathologist can then help the patient develop strategies for working around compromised functions and emphasizing intact ones. For example, a patient who cannot remember spoken instructions but who can read and write might compensate for the memory impairment by writing down the instructions and reading them when needed. The speech-language pathologist can help the patient differentiate communicative faults that actually interfere with communication from those that are primarily annoyances (e.g., word retrieval failures in which the patient comes up with synonyms are likely to be annoying but usually will not cause communication failure, whereas failing to provide the listener with referents for pronouns has more serious consequences). The patient can then focus his or her attention on the important aspects of communication and ignore the aberrations that are only annoyances. As the patient's communicative impairments worsen, the speech-language pathologist can provide emotional support and help the patient change his or her communicative strategies in accord with changes in the severity and nature of the communicative impairments. As the patient's competence diminishes, the responsibility for maintaining communication shifts to caregivers, and caregivers become the primary focus of intervention.

The speech-language pathologist works with caregivers to assist them in maintaining and enhancing the patient's communicative competence. The speech-language pathologist can inform caregivers about how the patient's impairments affect communication and how caregivers can modify communicative interactions to capitalize on the patient's strengths and circumvent his or her weaknesses. The speech-language pathologist may emphasize the importance of keeping messages short, simple, and concrete, of increasing message redundancy by repetition and paraphrase, of slowing speech rate to provide more time for the patient to process what he or she hears, and of confirming that the patient understands by having him or her repeat back what the caregiver says. As the patient's communicative abilities decline the speech-language pathologist helps caregivers adjust communicative interactions in response to the patient's diminished level of competence.

Helping the Patient Cope With Dementia

Memory Impairments.— Memory impairments usually are the most salient concern of patients in the initial stages of dementia, and helping the patient cope with

them can notably enhance both the patient's mental health and his or her competence in daily life. There are no known procedures for improving demented patients'
memory. Consequently, treatment is directed toward helping the patient find and
use compensatory techniques for remembering. Many of the compensatory techniques used with traumatically brain-injured patients' memory impairments are useful for patients with dementia. The following adjustments may help demented patients compensate for memory impairments.

1. Establish a routine schedule of activities that remains constant from day to
   day, in order to minimize demands on memory. Keep a written schedule of
   things to be done each day, and cross out or check off entries as they are
   completed.
2. Set an alarm clock to go off when specific things are to be done. Put a note
   by the clock to tell what is to be done when the alarm goes off.
3. Keep a list of important phone numbers near the telephone, with emer-
   gency numbers listed first, and the others listed in order of frequency of
   use.
4. Make up a checklist of things to be done when leaving the house (e.g., turn
   off lights, turn off the stove, get keys to house, etc.). Put the list by the exit
   used by the patient.
5. Keep personal possessions in a consistent location.
6. Keep things used at the same time or in the same activity together (e.g.,
   keep coffee pot, filters, coffee, and coffee measure on the same shelf).
7. Carry a card listing home address and the telephone numbers of at least
   two caregivers. Wear an identification bracelet containing the same information.

Disorientation and Confusion.—Occasional disorientation and confusion may
occur during the early stages of dementia, and may cause the patient emotional upset and anxiety disproportionate to their actual effects on the patient's life. Helping
the patient deal with disorientation and confusion in a constructive way, and reassur-
ing him or her that periodic disorientation and confusion are manageable are important aspects of support for the patient in the early stages of dementia. The following
adjustments may help the patient deal with disorientation and minimize confusion.

1. Keep a large calendar in a highly visible place. Cross off the current day
   before going to bed at night. (Caregivers may have to do this, if the patient
   can't remember to do so.)
2. Wear a digital calendar watch that shows time (preferably with a.m. and
   p.m. indicated) and date in a legible size. Some have built-in alarms that
   can be set to signal repetitive events, although most are too faint to be
   heard by patients with diminished hearing.
3. Have someone draw maps showing how to walk to nearby stores, shops,
   and businesses. The maps should be illustrated with pictorial representations
   of landmarks that can be used for orientation by the patient.

4. Put cards showing the contents of cabinets, dressers, and bureaus on doors and drawer fronts.

THE LONG HAUL: THE FAMILY AND THE DEMENTIA PATIENT

The speech-language pathologist, as a part of the professional team, is likely to work closely with the dementia patient's family, providing support and reassurance as well as information, guidance, and instruction. Understanding what the family is likely to experience as the patient's dementia progresses is crucial, if the speech-language pathologist's contribution to care and management are to be both appropriate and effective. The magnitude and the nature of the problems, stresses, and issues faced by the family inexorably increase as the patient's intellectual and behavioral dysfunction progress from annoying to enervating.

The Early Stages: Onset of Symptoms to Diagnosis

The first symptoms of dementia usually are subtle and may be overlooked by the family. The patient becomes forgetful, irritable, and inattentive, but remains oriented and socially appropriate. The first symptoms of dementia often are interpreted by family members as depression, stubbornness, or normal aging. The patient's gradual decline may continue, with family members unaware that something important is happening, until seizures or dyskinesia appear, or until a change in routine (e.g., going on vacation) leaves the patient disoriented, confused, and frightened.

During the very early stages of dementia, the patient's symptoms are primarily inconveniences, and families often spontaneously adapt to them. They no longer permit the patient to run errands unaccompanied, because they discover that he or she tends to get lost. They take away the patient's car keys because they sense that impaired judgment and slow reactions place the patient and other drivers in danger. They gradually assume responsibility for shopping, paying bills, housecleaning, and for legal and financial matters. They shape family routines around the patient's eccentricities. If the patient lives alone the family monitors the patient's condition with frequent telephone calls and visits, but gradually the family is forced to assume more and more responsibility for the patient, until the family decides that the patient must move in with a family member. This decision often is precipitated by a dramatic incident (e.g., the patient starts a fire by leaving a stove or iron unattended, gets lost and is picked up by the police, enters neighbors' houses uninvited and at inopportune times, or appears in public partially clothed or nude).

As the patient's dementia progresses it becomes apparent that something more ominous than normal aging is taking place. The patient's lapses of memory increase in frequency and duration, until they constitute a profound impairment in storing and retrieving new information. The patient begins to neglect self-care and has to be reminded, cajoled, or nagged to bathe, keep clothing clean, and maintain oral hygiene. Progressive impairments in judgment, attention, and memory put the patient and others at risk when the patient uses gas stoves, ovens, power tools, ladders, or other machinery. As the patient's confusion and disorientation progress, he or she may become progressively more anxious, depressed, or irritable. The patient may withdraw from interactions with family members and others. Periodic violent emotional outbursts may occur. The patient's usual sleep cycles may be disrupted, with frequent naps during the day and wakefulness and wandering during the night. Sometimes the patient's sleep cycle is reversed, and the patient sleeps all day and is awake all night. The patient may become indifferent to food and fail to maintain adequate caloric and fluid intake without supervision, or they may become gluttonous, eating continuously and indiscriminantly unless supervised.

As the family's concern deepens, they seek professional help in deducing what is wrong. When the diagnosis of dementia is made, it almost always precipitates a period of intense stress for the patient and family members, during which counseling and support for the patient and family is crucial. The patient needs help in dealing with feelings of grief and anger about what is happening, help with diffuse anxiety about the future, and a plan for coping with the future. The family needs information about what is happening to the patient and about what the course of the patient's illness is likely to be. The family, like the patient, needs help in dealing with the grief, anger, and anxiety that almost invariably follow the diagnosis.

The Middle Stages: Caring for the Demented Patient in the Home

Most demented patients are cared for by family members at home until the burden becomes intolerable and the patient is placed in a nursing home. The period of at-home care can range from 1 or 2 years to 10 or 15, depending on how rapidly the patient's dementia progresses and on the family's tolerance for the disruptions caused by the dementia. Clearly, caring for a dementia patient is "a long haul." During this time the patient and family members must cope with the patient's increasingly severe mental impairments and the disruptive effects of the impairments on family relationships and routines. The patient is frustrated and angry about the losses that have occurred, and worried and anxious about those yet to come. Patients at this stage often become depressed and apathetic and withdraw from family and friends, with intervals of self-imposed social isolation punctuated by angry outbursts over trivial incidents. Family members are distressed by the patient's increasing mental impairments and his or her unpredictable changes in mood. They may feel anger and resentment at the burden that has been imposed on them, although they often do not openly express or acknowledge these feelings and may feel guilty about them. Family relationships and routines are disrupted as caregivers become increasingly responsible for the patient and are forced to neglect other family activities and responsibilities.

As the patient's deterioration progresses and his or her appreciation of reality declines, depression and apathy often are replaced by hyperactivity, wandering, and stereotypic repetitive behaviors. The patient can no longer be left alone and requires continuous supervision. Family members have to take responsibility for bathing the patient and supervising his or her oral hygiene. When incontinence develops, the burden of caring for the patient escalates. Additional deterioration often brings verbal abusiveness, aggressiveness, and episodes of physical violence, further disrupting family relationships and increasing family members' anger, resentment, and guilt.

This phase of the patient's illness requires continuing education, support, and therapy for the family. Family members need education about why the patient behaves as he or she does, and about how disruptive behaviors can be controlled or eliminated by manipulating the patient's environment or by medications. Family members need help in setting up a safe, predictable, and stable environment for the patient. They may need help in dividing caregiving responsibilities among family members, and they may need encouragement and direction in taking advantage of respite-care and day-care services and support groups. As the burden of caring for the patient escalates, family members will need help in planning for and accomplishing nursing home placement for the patient. Throughout this phase of the patient's illness family members will need help in dealing with their feelings of resentment, anger, apprehension, and guilt, the latter becoming especially prominent as the family begins to contemplate the patient's nursing home placement.

The Late Stages: The Patient in a Nursing Home

Most demented patients spend their last years in a nursing home. Patients in the late stages of dementia typically are minimally oriented to their surroundings, do not communicate meaningfully with others, and sometimes do not recognize or remember friends or family members. Although the physical burden of caring for the patient has been removed by nursing home placement, the emotional burden carried by family members continues, often augmented by feelings of guilt over abandoning the patient to the care of strangers and by feelings of loss that accompany the patient's departure from home. As the patient's physical condition becomes more fragile, family members are faced with making decisions about whether heroic measures should be employed to sustain the patient's life. During this time family members need continuing help in resolving their often conflicting feelings about their own needs and their obligations to the patient, and in making decisions about when and how to terminate procedures for prolonging the patient's life.

The patient's death does not end the family's need for advice, support, and reassurance. The period of mourning following the death of the demented family member usually is brief, perhaps because the family has been mentally preparing for the patient's death for months or years. Although the mourning period may be short, the grief felt by family members may be intense, owing perhaps to the release of emotional tensions that have built up over the months and years of the patient's illness. Professional counseling and support during this period may help family members to acknowledge and understand their feelings and reactions to what they have been through, and may help them reconstruct and repair family relationships that have been damaged or distorted by the pressures of caring for the demented patient.

Helping Caregivers Cope With Dementia

Caregivers for demented patients face numerous problems related to the patient's declining intellect, mood swings, and changes in behavior. Although the decline in the patient's abilities cannot be arrested or reversed, the effects of the patient's intellectual impairments can be minimized, the patient's mood swings can be diminished, and distressing behaviors often can be controlled or eliminated by environmental manipulation and behavior modification techniques.

Rabins et al. (1982) surveyed the families of 55 patients with irreversible dementia to determine what they considered to be the major problems in caring for their demented family member. The results are summarized in Table 10–1. When the families were asked to identify the *most serious* problem caused by the patient's dementia, they ranked physical violence as the most serious, followed by memory disturbance, incontinence, catastrophic reactions, hitting, making accusations, and suspiciousness. Clearly, the perceived importance of a behavior problem is not determined only by its frequency of occurrence, but reflects the amount of emotional stress or inconvenience the behavior problem causes for family members.

Hostility, Verbal Abuse, and Physical Violence.— Combative, aggressive, and accusatory behaviors rank high on the list of problem behaviors in the report by Rabins et al. and in the general literature on management of patients with dementia. Caregivers need to understand that emotional outbursts, combativeness, and physical attacks often are predictable, based on previous incidents, are frequently preceded by warning signs, and often represent the patient's response to being pushed beyond his or her ability to deal with a situation or event. Many times such outbursts can be eliminated by removing their precipitating stimuli. For example, a man with dementia became violently angry when he saw his wife paying the monthly bills, perhaps because he thought that she was usurping his role as head of the household. The wife realized what precipitated her husband's outbursts and began paying the bills while her husband took his usual morning nap.

Many outbursts are preceded by warning signs, that if heeded can prevent the patient's emotional state from escalating out of control. Warning signs can be diverse and tend to be idiosyncratic. They range from subtle signs such as increased body rigidity, aversion of gaze, or increased respiration rate to more obvious behaviors such as crying and arguing. Teaching caregivers to recognize such warning signs and respond to them by slowing the pace of the activity, doing something else, or diverting the patient's attention can reduce the incidence of such outbursts.

If caregivers understand that the demented patient's outbursts may be an involuntary response to demanding or too-difficult situations, their responses to the outbursts are likely to change in constructive ways. They are less likely to regard the patient as stubborn and uncooperative and take the patient's emotional outbursts as a personal affront. They are more likely to look for what pushed the patient out of control and to eliminate or control the precipitating stimuli. Understanding that accusations and suspicion may be the patient's attempts to reconcile misplaced possessions, forgotten appointments, and unexpected changes in routine may lead caregivers to increase the predictability and orderliness of the patient's environment, rather than arguing with the patient about the accuracy of his or her suspicions.

Finally, caregivers should be aware that hostile and aggressive behavior can be caused by physical pain or illness. Consequently, medical evaluation of patients who exhibit sudden increases in aggressive behavior may be advisable. Some medications may cause increased aggressiveness. Consequently, changes in mood or toler-

TABLE 10–1.

Percentage of Families Reporting the
Occurrence of Behaviors and the Percentage
Considering the Behavior to Be a Problem*

Behavior	Occurrence (%)
BEHAVIORS MENTIONED	
Memory disturbance	100
Catastrophic reactions	87
Demanding and critical behavior	71
Night waking	69
Hiding things	69
Communication difficulties	68
Suspiciousness	63
Making accusations	60
Uncooperativeness at meals	60
Daytime wandering	59
Uncooperativeness at bathing	53
Hallucinations	49
Delusions	47
Physical violence	47
Incontinence	40
Unsafe cooking	33
Hitting	32
Unsafe driving	20
Unsafe or excessive smoking	11
Inappropriate sexual behavior	2
BEHAVIORS CONSIDERED A PROBLEM	
Physical violence	94
Memory disturbance	93
Catastrophic reactions	89
Incontinence	86
Delusions	83
Making accusations	82
Hitting	81
Suspiciousness	79
Uncooperativeness at bathing	74
Communication difficulties	74
Demanding and critical behavior	73
Unsafe driving	73
Hiding things	71
Daytime wandering	70
Unsafe or excessive smoking	67
Night waking	59
Uncooperativeness at meals	55
Unsafe cooking	44
Hallucinations	42
Inappropriate sexual behavior	0

*From Rabins PV, Mace NL, Lucas MJ: *JAMA* 1982;
248:333–336. Used by permission.

ance for frustration that occur when medications are begun or dosages are changed should be evaluated by a physician. In some cases medication may be needed to control a patient's physically violent behavior, but because of their depressive effects on the patient's alertness and general mental functioning, they should be prescribed only when behavioral methods fail to provide sufficient control.

Memory Impairments.—Caregivers can help the patient cope with his or her memory impairments by maximizing the orderliness and predictability of the patient's living environment. Keeping schedules and activities consistent from day to day lessens the amount that the patient has to remember in order to manage daily life activities. Keeping the patient's possessions in a consistent place and putting them away when they are not in use lessens the patient's need to remember where they are, and increases the likelihood that he or she will find them when they are needed. Providing a checklist of the day's activities and the patient's responsibilities for the day helps the patient keep track of what has been done and what yet needs to be done. Order, consistency, and predictability in the patient's daily life environment together with systematic use of schedules, lists, and check-offs can help the patient compensate for his or her memory impairments.

Sleep Disturbances.—Most people sleep less as they get older, and disrupted sleep patterns are particularly common in dementia. Helping the patient get a reasonable amount of sleep helps him or her begin each day well rested. It also makes it easier for the patient to deal with challenges and frustrations. Sleep medications are often prescribed, probably more often than necessary. Adjusting the patient's schedule and environment may normalize his or her sleep pattern and should be tried before medications are prescribed. Even when medications are prescribed, the changes in schedule and environment may enhance their effects and lower the dosage required. The following adjustments may help the patient sleep through the night.

1. Take fewer naps during the day. Do not nap after midafternoon.
2. Go to bed at the same time every night.
3. Get 20 to 30 minutes of mild exercise in the early evening. A brisk walk, if weather permits, is ideal.
4. Have a light snack (carbohydrates and milk are good) about an hour before going to bed.
5. Wear comfortable sleeping attire that does not constrict, twist, or bind.
6. Keep the bedroom door and windows closed to cut down on extraneous noise.
7. Keep the room dimly illuminated with a night light to avoid confusion and anxiety when awakening in the night.

Health Maintenance.—The mental impairments associated with dementing illness usually disrupt the patient's normal eating and drinking habits and his or her judgment regarding adequate nutrition and fluid intake. Consequently, maintaining adequate nutrition and fluid intake is an important part of the patient's general health care. Ensuring that the patient has properly fitting dentures and maintaining oral hygiene are important but sometimes overlooked aspects of patient care. Some patients in the later stages of a dementing illness develop swallowing problems, in which case compensatory swallowing techniques may be prescribed or alternatives to oral feeding may be recommended.

Other illnesses sometimes accompany dementia. Diabetes, heart disease, pulmonary disease, renal failure, or other diseases of internal organs may require medical care. Metabolic or chemical imbalances are common in normal and demented elderly patients. Demented patients are particularly susceptible to bacterial and viral infections; therefore, prevention and treatment of infections are important parts of the general program of health care. Providing hearing aids for the hard-of-hearing patient and properly fitting eyeglasses for those with impaired vision prevent sensory deprivation and contribute to the patient's constructive interaction with his or her environment. Providing canes, walkers, crutches, or wheelchairs provides physically impaired patients with the mobility needed to get around in their environment.

Financial and Legal Considerations.—Preservation of the patient's property and finances and safeguarding legal rights should be a major concern in the early stages of dementia. Because long-term care of demented patients is extremely costly, the patient's assets as well as those intended for the support of dependents and spouses may be exhausted unless they are protected by advance planning while the patient is still mentally competent to participate in making the plans. Some procedures for protecting the patient's assets can be accomplished without lawyers or the courts, while some (e.g., appointing guardians or conservators) cannot. However, the advice of a legal or financial professional should always be obtained when setting up any financial plan for a demented patient and his or her dependents.

Joint tenancy is established by entering the names of two (or more) people as joint owners of assets, usually bank accounts, securities, and real estate. In *joint tenancy with right of survivorship* the survivor becomes the owner of the property on the death of the other owner. Either tenant can deposit or withdraw funds from jointly held accounts, so that if one owner becomes incompetent or dies the other owner still has access to them. However, sale or transfer of jointly held securities or real property requires the signatures of all joint owners. Consequently, joint tenancy does not transfer control of these kinds of property when one of the joint tenants becomes incompetent or dies.

Power of attorney is an agreement in which the patient grants another person the legal right to carry out transactions in the patient's behalf. A power of attorney agreement does not require formal legal registration or court action, but it does require that the patient be mentally competent to enter into the agreement. A power of attorney can be revoked by the patient if he or she is mentally competent, or by a court if the patient is not competent. A traditional power of attorney terminates on the death or mental incompetence of the patient. Some states have provided for *durable powers of attorney* that remain in effect if the patient becomes mentally incompetent, making them useful for patients with progressive conditions such as dementia.

A *lifetime (intervivos) trust* is an agreement in which the patient transfers properties or assets to another person, who formally agrees to manage them for the patient and/or the patient's family. Like powers of attorney, lifetime trusts do not require legal registration or court action, but do require that the patient be mentally competent when the trust is set up. Trusts often are set up for defined periods of time, but for patients with progressive illness they usually extend for the patient's lifetime, and even beyond, in which case the trustee administers the property for the benefit of the survivors. Trusts are more sophisticated and flexible than powers of attorney, and in some cases may provide greater protection and preservation of assets than powers of attorney.

In *conservatorship* a court appoints a representative to manage the financial affairs of a person who is not competent to manage them. When the conservatorship is for a demented patient the conservator usually is the patient's spouse or another family member, although almost any adult or institution with an interest in the patient's welfare could serve. Conservatorships are established by a court following petition from a concerned person (usually the potential conservator) and require that the court find the patient not competent to manage his or her own financial affairs. The assets administered by the conservator must be used only for the benefit of the patient and his or her legal dependents. The conservatorship expires on the death of the patient.

In *guardianship* a court appoints a representative to make decisions about a legally incapacitated person's residence and physical and medical care. Guardianships resemble conservatorships in most aspects other than the nature of the guardian's responsibilities. In most cases the same person is appointed to be the patient's conservator and guardian, and makes decisions about both the patient's residence and care and manages his or her assets.

Chapter 11

Dysarthria

NEUROPATHOLOGY OF DYSARTHRIA

Weakness and Paralysis

Dysarthria is a generic label for a group of motor speech disorders caused by weakness, paralysis, slowness, incoordination, or sensory loss in the muscle groups responsible for speech. Speech depends on *respiration, phonation, articulation,* and *resonation.* Therefore, neurologic problems affecting muscle groups involved in these processes are likely to produce dysarthria, and the nature of the dysarthria will depend on which muscle groups are compromised and how they are compromised.

Weakness and paralysis of muscle groups involved in speech are the most frequent causes of dysarthria. The weakness or paralysis may arise from damage in the *central nervous system* (brain, brain stem, spinal cord), or the *peripheral nervous system* (peripheral motor or sensory nerves, nerve-muscle junctions, or the muscles themselves). The most common cause of muscle weakness or paralysis is destruction of nerves or neural fiber tracts, but they are sometimes caused by compression or inflammation of motor nerves. Because neural tissue does not regenerate, its destruction is irreversible and leads to persistent symptoms. However, compression and inflammation of nerves can be reversed, and symptoms often disappear with decompression or recovery from inflammation. However, prolonged compression or inflammation can lead to irreversible motor dysfunction.

Upper Motor Neuron Damage

Unilateral lesions in the primary motor cortex or the pyramidal tract (upper motor neuron) rarely produce persisting dysarthria (Darley et al., 1975). Immediately after the injury the patient may be mute, aphonic, or dysarthric, but these symptoms usually disappear within the first month. The muscles of the upper face, pharynx, and larynx are bilaterally innervated—muscles on both sides are innervated by both cerebral hemispheres. The muscles of the lower face, palate, and tongue are unilaterally innervated, receiving input only from the contralateral hemisphere (Fig 11–1).

From motor cortex

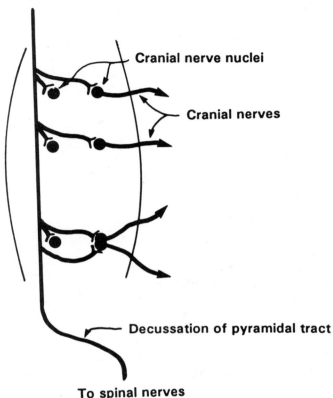

Cranial nerve nuclei

Cranial nerves

Decussation of pyramidal tract

To spinal nerves

FIG 11–1.
Diagram of cranial nerves and their nuclei. A lesion that destroys a cranial nerve nucleus usually also destroys descending pyramidal fibers. Cranial nerves with bilateral innervation will continue to function, and those with unilateral innervation (e.g., the lower face) will be paralyzed on the same side as the lesion. Because pyramidal fibers to spinal nerves are interrupted before they decussate, contralateral paralysis occurs in the spinal nerve distributions.

Consequently, unilateral pyramidal tract damage does not significantly affect muscles of the forehead and scalp, but may cause weakness or paralysis of the muscles of mastication, the lips, and the tongue. Bilateral lesions in the upper motor neuron can, and often do, produce dysarthria. The symptom-complex generated by bilateral upper motor neuron damage is called *pseudobulbar palsy.** Sometimes a patient develops pseudobulbar palsy after what seems to be unilateral upper motor neuron damage. In these cases, a previous "silent" (asymptomatic) injury usually has oc-

*"Palsy" is another, albeit old, name for paralysis. Another name for the brain stem is "the bulb." Paralysis caused by brain stem damage is sometimes called "bulbar palsy." The symptoms generated by bilateral upper motor neuron damage resemble in some respects those generated by brainstem damage; hence the term "pseudobulbar palsy."

curred. The second injury in combination with the first creates the pseudobulbar palsy. In pseudobulbar palsy, the facial muscles contralateral to the (second) lesion usually are paralyzed. The paralyzed muscles are spastic because the lesion is in the upper motor neuron. The affected muscles usually do not atrophy, and reflexes such as the jaw jerk and gag reflex are exaggerated. The arm and leg on the same side as the paralyzed facial muscles often are hemiplegic or hemiparetic.

Lower Motor Neuron Damage

Lesions of the brain stem (pons and medulla) almost always produce paralysis or paresis of facial, oropharyngeal, or laryngeal muscles, and involvement of the cranial nerves or cranial nerve nuclei almost always produces dysarthria. The general symptoms of lesions of cranial nerves or their nuclei are (1) flaccid paralysis of the muscles served by the nerve (on the same side as the lesion); (2) fasciculations (twitching) in the affected muscles; and (3) eventual atrophy of the muscles. The symptoms depend on whether the lesion affects only the cranial nerve or if the cranial nerve nucleus is involved. If only the cranial nerve is involved, the muscles served by the cranial nerve (on the same side as the lesion) are paralyzed and there is no hemiplegia or hemiparesis of either arm or leg. If the cranial nerve nucleus is damaged, spastic hemiparesis or hemiplegia of the contralateral arm and leg often follows, because the lesion that destroys the cranial nerve nucleus also destroys pyramidal tract fibers serving the arm and leg (see Fig 11–1). Because the pyramidal tract fibers serving the arm and leg decussate below the cranial nerve nuclei, lesions affecting cranial nerve nuclei in the left side of the brain stem create right-sided hemiplegia and vice versa.

Cranial Nerve Damage

If the *facial nerve (VII)* is damaged, weakness and flaccid paralysis of the ipsilateral face follow, involving the eyelid muscles and muscles of facial expression. Disruption of the sensory branch of the facial nerve leads to loss of taste in the anterior two thirds of the tongue. *Bell's palsy* is a relatively frequent (and in most cases reversible) facial nerve syndrome in which one-sided facial paralysis occurs. It is thought to be caused by inflammation of the facial nerve within the narrow passageway through which it exits the skull. Inflammation of the facial nerve causes swelling and compression within the passageway, suppressing its function. Paralysis and sensory loss in the ipsilateral face ensue. Bell's palsy usually resolves spontaneously within a few weeks. In some cases the palsy does not resolve, the facial muscles atrophy and droop, and the affected eye may have to be covered because of irritation caused by loss of the automatic eyeblink.

Damage to the *glossopharyngeal nerve (IX)* causes loss of the gag reflex. The muscles that elevate the palate and larynx and those that constrict the pharynx may be weakened or paralyzed (on the same side as the lesion). Tactile sensation to the posterior wall of the pharynx and back of the tongue may be diminished or abolished. Hypernasality and swallowing problems (dysphagia) are likely.

Damage to the *vagus nerve (X)* causes ipsilateral paralysis of the soft palate. If
the recurrent laryngeal branch of the vagus nerve is affected, unilateral vocal fold
paralysis follows. If the sensory branch of the vagus nerve is damaged, anesthesia of
the pharynx can occur, with consequent disruption of the mechanics of swallowing.

Damage to the *spinal accessory nerve (XI)* usually has no direct effects on
speech, because it innervates several muscle groups in the neck and shoulders,
rather than muscle groups directly involved in speech. Occasionally there may be
indirect effects of accessory nerve damage on speech, if muscle weakness causes
shoulder and head droop and compromises respiration and phonation. However,
dysarthria caused by isolated accessory nerve damage is rare (or nonexistent).

Damage to the *hypoglossal nerve (XII)* causes ipsilateral weakness of the tongue.
Patients with hypoglossal nerve damage have difficulty in protruding the tongue (it
deviates to the weak side)* and moving it laterally, and they misarticulate sounds
requiring tongue movement. Hypoglossal nerve damage sometimes contributes to
swallowing disabilities because the patient has difficulty controlling the movement of
food during chewing and has difficulty positioning the food before swallowing it.

Anterior Horn Cell Disease

Although cranial nerve dysfunction is the most common cause of dysarthria,
damage to spinal nerves may contribute to it. Diseases affecting the anterior horn
cells in the spinal cord and/or brain stem (e.g., poliomyelitis and amyotrophic lateral
sclerosis) cause symptoms typical of lower motor neuron disease—flaccid paralysis
and fasciculations. Diseases of the anterior horn cells usually cause progressive deterioration of the cells, generating increasing muscle weakness, diminution and loss of
reflexes, and increasing muscle flaccidity. Anterior horn cell disease affects speech
both directly and indirectly by interfering with articulatory movements, disabling
velopharyngeal valving, and compromising respiratory support. Anterior horn cell
diseases are almost always progressive (except for poliomyelitis). Consequently,
many patients require augmentative or alternative communication systems during
the final stages of their disease.

Spinal Nerve Disease

Spinal nerves may be the focus of inflammatory or destructive disease. Inflammatory nerve diseases (e.g., Guillain-Barré) usually are general rather than focal.
They often affect the longest nerve fibers first, and motor fibers before sensory ones.
Muscles in the limbs often are affected before the muscles in the torso, and distal
muscles of the limbs are affected before proximal limb muscles. Other spinal nerve
diseases produce symptoms typical of lower motor neuron disease—weakness, hypotonia, and diminished reflexes, with variable sensory impairment.

---

*It deviates to the weak side because the muscles on the strong side pull the tongue out, but the
paralyzed side lags behind.

Diseases of the Neuromuscular Junction

Diseases of the neuromuscular junction are characterized by abnormality in the neurotransmitters that are necessary for transmission of nerve impulses across synapses. The abnormality may be caused by deficiency or excess of neurotransmitters themselves, or by altered sensitivity of receptor cells to some neurotransmitters. *Myasthenia gravis* is the most common of these diseases. Myasthenia gravis is caused by autoimmune-mediated damage to the acetylcholine receptors on the muscle cells, resulting in a failure of neuromuscular transmission. Symptoms of myasthenia gravis include generalized fluctuating muscle weakness (with a predilection for the extraocular, bulbar, and proximal limb muscles), rapid fatigability of muscles, and quick recovery of strength when the muscles are rested.

Primary Diseases of Muscle (Myopathy)

Some diseases affect the muscle fibers themselves, and produce atrophy of muscle tissue. Myotonic dystrophy is a relatively common inherited myopathy that may affect speech. Myositis, an acquired inflammatory muscle disease, usually does not affect speech, but may affect respiratory muscles and produce swallowing problems in some cases.

SLOWNESS AND INCOORDINATION

The most likely sources for problems in coordination, rate, and timing of muscle movements are the *cerebellum* and the *extrapyramidal system*. When the cerebellum or the extrapyramidal system is damaged, the strength of muscle movements is largely unaffected, but their modulation and control are compromised.

Damage to the *cerebellum* causes disintegration of motor coordination and rhythm, usually with loss of muscle tone. Rapid alternating movements, such as alternately turning the hands palm up, then palm down, are slow and awkward. The range and force of movements are distorted (*dysmetria*). Although the average speed and velocity of movements may be normal, acceleration at the beginning of movements is slowed, and braking at the end of movements lags, causing overshoot of the target. Cerebellar damage causes movements to become jerky and segmented (*decomposition of movement*). In most cases, intentional movements are accompanied by tremor that disappears when the muscles are at rest. Cerebellar disease is also characterized by disorders of equilibrium and gait. The patient walks with feet apart, the rhythm of stepping is disturbed, step length is irregular, and the patient may lurch from side to side.

Damage to the *extrapyramidal system* abolishes voluntary muscle movements and creates abnormal movements. Extrapyramidal disease does not cause muscle weakness unless the pyramidal tract is also affected. However, control and integration of voluntary movements are disrupted. In some cases movements are abnormally slow (*hypokinetic*), and in others they may be abnormally quick and overactive (*hyperkinetic*).

The abnormal involuntary movements seen in extrapyramidal disease may take several forms. *Tremor* is a pattern of regular, cyclic, small-amplitude involuntary movements. Tremor is a physiologic phenomenon of normal muscles, but it is so slight that it cannot be seen. Normal tremor ranges in frequency from 8 to 13 Hz, and is present during waking and sleep. Pathologic tremor may appear in muscles at rest (*resting tremor*) or during volitional movement (*intention tremor*). Distal muscles are more likely to exhibit pathologic tremor than proximal muscles. Pathologic tremor is present in several extrapyramidal diseases—most notably Parkinson's disease. Pathologic tremor is visible to the eye, and is present only during waking. Rates of pathologic tremor vary from slow (less than 6 Hz in Parkinson's disease) to fast, as in familial tremor.

Chorea (from the Greek word for "dance") refers to involuntary movements that are quick, sometimes forceful, and abrupt (*choreiform movements*). Choreiform movements may resemble voluntary movements, and some patients may attempt to disguise them by incorporating them into voluntary movements. However, the strategy usually fails, for the combination of voluntary and involuntary movements usually appears grotesque and exaggerated. At rest, the muscles of patients with chorea tend to be hypotonic. *Ballism* (or *hemiballism* if it affects only one side of the body) is an extreme form of chorea. In ballism, the involuntary limb movements appear violent, and the limbs are flung wildly about.

In *athetosis* resting muscle groups are disturbed by slow, writhing, sinuous movements. Athetosis is especially prominent in the proximal limb muscles and neck. The movements are involuntary and purposeless, and often appear to flow from one muscle group to another. Athetoid movements usually are slower than choreiform movements, although in some cases it may be unclear which is which. In these cases, the disorder may be called *choreoathetosis*.

Dystonia is a condition in which muscle groups maintain abnormal involuntary contractions or postures over long durations. Because the contractions persist, and because they cause gross deformation, dystonia is sometimes called *torsion spasm*. Dystonia most frequently affects trunk, neck, and limb muscles, but any muscle group may be involved. In its less severe forms, dystonia may resemble athetosis.

In *myoclonus,* individual muscle groups contract sporadically and irregularly, in short bursts. The contractions may range from nearly imperceptible movements of a single muscle group to overt movements involving several muscle groups. Myoclonic movements typically are irregular in duration and rate, and they are most easily observed when the affected muscles are at rest. Myoclonus may be seen in epilepsy, dementia, and some cerebellar disorders. Sometimes it appears in isolation.

Rigidity is a prominent characteristic of many extrapyramidal diseases, including Parkinson's disease and Wilson's disease. In rigidity, the muscles are firm, tense, and resist both active and passive movement. Rigidity affects all muscle groups, but may be more prominent in flexors than in extensors. Tendon reflexes (e.g., the knee jerk) are not accentuated by rigidity. If rigidity affects the facial muscles, the patient exhibits an unchanging, expressionless, mask-like countenance, which is a prominent feature of advanced stages of Parkinson's disease. (Reduced automatic blinking may be a subtle early sign of Parkinson's disease.)

SENSORY LOSS

Damage to sensory branches of the cranial nerves or to the sensory cortex may impair sensation in the face, mouth, and neck. Such sensory disruptions sometimes cause transient speech disturbances, usually lasting less than 2 weeks. Persisting dysarthria from sensory disturbance alone is rare. However, if sensory disturbances are superimposed upon coexisting motor impairments, then the resulting dysarthria may be more severe than if the sensory problem were not present. A normal motor system usually has enough resilience to compensate for sensory disturbances, but an impaired one often does not.

EFFECTS OF NEUROLOGIC IMPAIRMENTS ON SPEECH PROCESSES

Neurologic impairments create dysarthria by affecting the physiologic processes involved in speech—*respiration, phonation, articulation, resonation,* and *prosody* in almost any combination. Most of the time several processes are affected, and there may be interactions among processes. Complex interactions among processes often make it difficult to determine which impairments are primary and which are secondary.

Upper Motor Neuron Disease

Significant problems with respiratory support for speech are not usually seen in dysarthrias caused by upper motor neuron disease (*spastic dysarthria*). However, disturbances of phonation, articulation, resonation, and prosody frequently occur. Spasticity of laryngeal muscles contributes to what Darley et al. (1975) called "strained-strangled-harsh" voice quality. Spasticity of articulatory muscles leads to imprecise consonant articulation, especially for complex movements requiring rapid sequences of movements. Spasticity of velopharyngeal muscles may prevent the velum from occluding the velopharyngeal port, contributing to hypernasality. These patients' vocal pitch tends to be low and variations in pitch and loudness diminish, contributing to monotonous vocal quality.

Lower Motor Neuron Disease

Problems in respiratory support for speech are common in disease of the lower motor neuron, the neuromuscular junction, or the muscle fibers themselves. The patient's weak and flaccid respiratory muscles fail to fully inflate the lungs, and when the patient speaks they fail to provide normal amounts of breath pressure at the vocal folds. The patient's respiratory insufficiency may be further complicated by weak and flaccid laryngeal muscles, which fail to bring the vocal folds into close approximation for phonation, wasting the already insufficient air supply. Consequently, patients with lower motor neuron disease usually speak in short utterances, with frequent pauses for breath. Their voice intensity usually is weak and breathy, particularly at the end of utterances. Their vocal pitch tends to be low and monotonous.

Extrapyramidal Disease

In *Parkinson's disease,* muscle rigidity causes respiration to be shallow, and the patient speaks in short utterances with noticeable pauses between utterances. The patient's voice quality is likely to be strained and breathy, because rigid laryngeal muscles fail to move the vocal folds into proper adduction. The loudness of the patient's voice usually is reduced, sometimes to inaudibility. Articulation is markedly imprecise and indistinct, as rigid articulatory muscles fail to reach full excursion, with frequent rushes of rapid and indistinct speech in which most consonant articulation disappears. Speech rate usually is highly variable, with periods of normal rate interspersed with rushes of rapid and indistinct speech, punctuated by inappropriately placed pauses.

In *dyskinesia,* respiration may be periodically disrupted by involuntary movements, causing involuntary changes in breath pressure at the glottis, with consequent abrupt changes in vocal intensity. Articulatory accuracy often falls victim to the dyskinesic movements, causing periods of essentially normal articulation to alternate with intervals of articulatory inaccuracy. Speech prosody also is affected. Speech rate is slowed, loudness and pitch variations are exaggerated by dyskinesic movements of respiratory muscles, and inappropriately placed pauses and explosive articulation interrupt the flow of speech.

Cerebellar Disease

Patients with cerebellar disorders often fall victim to anomalies of force, timing, and amplitude of movements in the muscle groups involved in speech. Uncontrollable changes in breath pressure at the glottis may produce irregular, sometimes explosive changes in pitch and loudness. Ataxic articulatory muscles create similar irregular disruptions of articulation. The patient's speech may be alternately normal and hypernasal.

EVALUATION OF DYSARTHRIA

Dysarthric patients are referred to speech-language pathologists because their speech sounds abnormal to physicians, nurses, family members, or to the patients themselves. The speech-language pathologist's assessment of a dysarthric patient usually has five purposes:

1. To determine whether the patient's speech is abnormal.
2. To evaluate the nature and severity of the abnormalities.
3. To determine the cause(s) of the abnormalities.
4. To determine if treatment is appropriate.
5. To identify potential directions for treatment, if treatment is appropriate.

Because dysarthria is a problem with talking, it seems logical that one should look to the mouth for its source. The mouth is the appropriate place to start, but the search must also extend down to the throat, chest, and abdomen, and up into the pharynx and nasal cavities. In order to talk we must breathe, so assessment of dysarthria includes assessment of respiration. In order to talk we must produce voice, so assessment of dysarthria includes assessment of vocal fold function. In order to talk normally, we must be able to direct the voice either through the mouth or through the nose, so assessment of dysarthria includes assessment of the muscles of the posterior pharynx and the soft palate. In order to speak intelligibly, we must shape the breath stream into consonants and vowels, so assessment of dysarthria includes assessment of how well the tongue, lips, and jaw move, and how accurately they reach their targets. Assessment of dysarthria requires assessment of *respiration, phonation, resonation,* and *articulation.* However, one cannot consider these four processes piece-by-piece, because they interact. Respiratory anomalies may disrupt phonation and articulation, and anomalies in resonation often affect articulation. For these reasons, assessment of dysarthria is as much a search for interactions among processes underlying speech as it is a diagnosis of anomalies within each process.

Evaluation of Breath Support for Speech

Characteristics of Normal Respiration.— In neurologically normal adults, respiration for biologic purposes and respiration for speech differ in subtle but important ways. In normal passive breathing, the diaphragm provides most of the respiratory drive by contracting during inhalation. This contraction compresses the abdominal contents downward, increases the volume of the chest cavity, and generates negative pressure in the lungs. Muscles in the chest wall and shoulder girdle contribute by elevating the shoulders and rib cage, thus further increasing the volume of the chest cavity and adding to the negative pressure in the lungs. Outside atmospheric pressure then forces air into the lungs. Expiratory force for exhalation is generated by a combination of torque generated by the expanded rib cage as it seeks to return to its resting position, and upward pressure on the bottom of the diaphragm by compressed abdominal contents as they seek to regain their normal volume. During normal passive breathing most expiratory force is provided by the elasticity of the rib cage and pressure generated by compressed abdominal organs. During speech, active contraction of abdominal muscles to increase upward pressure on the diaphragm is necessary, because the elasticity of the rib cage and the pressure exerted by compressed abdominal contents by themselves do not generate enough breath pressure for speech (Hixon, 1987).

During passive breathing, normal adults inflate their lungs to about 20% of total capacity, but when they speak they increase the amount of air in their lungs to 35% to 60% of total capacity (Hixon, 1987). The usual respiratory pattern during speech consists of quick inhalation to about 60% of lung capacity, followed by slow exhalation until the lungs reach about 30% of total capacity, when the speaker takes another breath. The normal ratio of inhalation to exhalation is about 1:6. That is, the expiratory phase lasts about six times as long as the inspiratory phase (Yorkston et al., 1988).

Preliminary Observation of Respiration.—Visual evaluation of the patient's posture and general appearance often provide important information about potential sources of respiratory insufficiency. If the patient is slouched and bent over, and his or her head droops forward, the chest cavity will be compressed and respiration for speech may be compromised.

Observation of the patient's resting respiration rate and depth of respiration can also provide information about potential respiratory problems. Normal resting respiration rates range from 12 to 20 cycles per minute, but the variability in the normal adult population is substantial. Normal respiration is not accompanied by overt movement of the shoulders or head. Fast, shallow breathing in the absence of exertion or elevated emotions may be a sign of weakness in the muscles of respiration, and suggests that the patient may have difficulty speaking with normal loudness and phrase length. Irregularities in breathing rate (cyclical changes in resting breathing rate) may be caused by cerebellar or extrapyramidal system pathology. Irregular breathing patterns may produce comparable aberrations in phonation and articulation.

Assessment of Respiration for Speech.—The clinician's first objective should be to determine whether comprehensive evaluation of respiratory function is necessary. This usually is accomplished by asking the patient to produce sustained phonation and to repeat syllables. If the patient can sustain phonation of an open vowel ("ah") with normal loudness for 4 to 5 seconds without undue effort, and can say at least three consonant-vowel syllables on a single breath with normal loudness, respiration probably is adequate for intelligible speech, and direct work on respiration is not likely to be needed.

If the patient fails these tests, one cannot immediately conclude that the problem is with respiratory support, because sustained phonation requires not only that the patient impound an adequate reservoir of air, but that he or she has enough strength in the respiratory muscles to generate subglottic air pressure and enough laryngeal muscle movement and strength to maintain the vocal folds in adduction against the pressure of the breath stream. Problems with vocal fold adduction usually are obvious during phonation. If the vocal folds are not closing, the patient's voice sounds weak and breathy. If the vocal folds are hypertonic, the patient's voice sounds harsh and strangled.

Measuring Respiratory Pressure and Flow.—Sophisticated (and expensive) instruments are available for measuring respiratory pressure and flow. They are not commonly available clinically. However, two inexpensive and relatively simple instruments for measuring intraoral breath pressure and flow can be constructed.

Netsell and Hixon (1978) described a U-tube manometer that is suitable for measuring intraoral breath pressure (Fig 11–2). The manometer is a U-shaped glass tube fastened to a board. The U-tube is approximately half-filled with colored water and calibrated in centimeters (see Netsell and Hixon, 1978, for specifications). A flexible tube is attached to one end of the U-tube. A rigid T-shaped tube serves as a mouthpiece and leak tube. The patient blows into the mouthpiece, and breath pres-

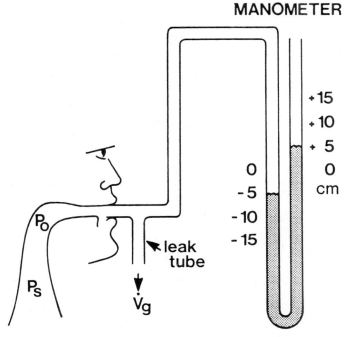

MANOMETER

FIG 11–2.
A U-tube manometer. The patient blows into the mouthpiece. A leak tube permits a constant amount of air to escape. The height of the liquid in the U-tube is related to the amount of breath pressure the patient can sustain. (From Netsell R, Hixon TJ: A noninvasive method for clinically estimating subglottal air pressure. *Journal of Speech and Hearing Disorders.* 1978; 43:326–330. Used by permission.)

sure displaces the column of water. The leak tube provides a constant escape for the airstream so that the person being tested must maintain continuous air flow in order to sustain displacement of the water. According to Netsell and Hixon, an individual who can maintain a 5 cm displacement of the water column for 5 seconds has sufficient breath pressure for most speech requirements (the "5 for 5 rule").

Hixon et al. (1982) suggest a similar but simpler device. A tall drinking glass (12 cm or more) is filled with water. The glass is calibrated in centimeters (Fig 11–3). A drinking straw is affixed to the glass so that it reaches a given depth (for example, 5 cm). An individual blowing into the straw must maintain breath pressure equal to the depth to which the straw is inserted in the water to generate a stream of bubbles at the end of the straw. By inserting the straw to 5 cm, one can evaluate whether a patient meets the "5 for 5" rule.

Assessment of Phonation

Phonation Time and Voice Quality.— The typical first step in evaluating phonation is to ask the patient to sustain an open vowel ("ah") for as long as he or she

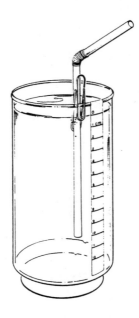

FIG 11–3.
A water glass manometer. The deeper the straw is in the water, the more breath pressure is needed to sustain a string of bubbles at the deep end of the straw. (From Hixon TJ, Hawley JT, Wilson KJ: An around-the-house device for the clinical determination of respiratory driving pressure. *Journal of Speech and Hearing Disorders.* 1982; 47:413–415. Used by permission.)

can. The clinician times the duration of the patient's phonation. Phonation times below 12 to 15 seconds in duration are considered abnormally low, and suggest problems either with glottal valving or with breath support for speech (see above). During this phase of the examination, the clinician also evaluates the loudness, pitch, and quality of the patient's voice.

Damage to cranial nerves, especially the pharyngeal branch of the vagus nerve, causes weakness or paralysis of laryngeal muscles. As a consequence, problems in adduction of the vocal folds may be seen, and the patient's voice may be breathy and weak, with abnormally low pitch. Inability to strongly adduct the vocal folds may contribute to inefficient use of the airstream. However, if the problems are limited to laryngeal muscles, respiratory support for speech ordinarily is sufficient to maintain at least 4 to 5 seconds of phonation.

Bilateral damage to the upper motor neuron often causes strained, strangled, harsh voice quality (Darley et al., 1975). Spastic laryngeal muscles constrict the glottal valve, increasing its resistance to airflow and reducing maximum phonation duration. However, most patients with upper motor neuron pathology have sufficient respiratory drive to produce 5 to 10 seconds of sustained phonation.

Cerebellar damage often generates sudden perturbations in vocal pitch and loudness caused by ataxic laryngeal muscles. However, most patients with cerebellar pathology can produce 5 to 10 seconds of sustained phonation, although voice quality is likely to be abnormal, and both loudness and quality may fluctuate. Anomalies in coordination of respiration and vocal fold adduction may cause aspiration of voice sounds or strained, strangled voice quality at the onset of phonation.

Extrapyramidal diseases often affect vocal fold adduction, shortening phonation time and affecting voice quality. Patients with *Parkinson's disease* typically have breathy, hoarse voices and their maximum phonation time is reduced by rigidity of laryngeal muscles. Patients with Parkinson's disease often begin phonation normally, but as phonation continues their voice often deteriorates, either into a voiceless whisper or a strained squeak. Patients with *dyskinesias* often produce alterations in vocal pitch, loudness, and quality as they sustain phonation. The alterations may be slow or rapid, continuous or intermittent, depending on the nature of the patient's movement disorder. Patients with *tremor* usually produce regular, cyclic perturbations of pitch and loudness. Patients with *chorea* produce irregular prolonged distortions of vocal pitch and loudness. Maximum phonation times for patients with extrapyramidal disease range from substantially reduced (3 to 4 seconds) to normal, depending on the efficiency of glottal valving and the degree to which respiratory muscles are affected.

Vocal Flexibility and Coordination.—Assessing phonation time and voice quality provide important information about the efficiency of laryngeal valving and respiratory support for speech. However, since continuous phonation requires only that the vocal folds be adducted and maintained in a constant state of tension, the results of such tests do not provide much information about how well the laryngeal muscles can accomplish the more intricate movements of connected speech. The latter information is obtained by asking the patient to change vocal pitch and loudness in response to the examiner's requests. Typical tasks for this purpose include:

1. Asking the patient to count aloud from 1 to 10, progressively changing loudness from a whisper to a shout and vice versa.
2. Asking the patient to sing a musical scale (do-re-mi . . .) going from low pitch to high and from high to low.
3. Asking the patient to count aloud, starting with the lowest pitch that he or she can produce and continuing with increasingly higher pitch until the patient can go no higher.
4. Asking the patient to utter short sequences of numbers aloud, alternating loud and soft voice or high and low pitch.
5. Asking the patient to repeat sentences at (a) a whisper, (b) normal loudness, and (c) a shout.
6. Asking the patient to read a paragraph or story aloud, with exaggerated stress patterns.

The changes in pitch and loudness achieved by the patient in these tasks may be compared with what the patient does in connected speech (e.g., reading aloud and conversational speech). Many patients whose pitch and loudness in connected speech is abnormally restricted can produce greater variety in pitch and loudness in structured tasks when the focus is on pitch and loudness changes. When this is true, the clinician's task may emphasize transfer of vocal variety from structured tasks to less structured environments.

The clinician may also assess the patient's ability to coordinate respiration with the onset of phonation. This can be done by:

1. Asking the patient to utter a series of short vowels ("uh- uh-uh," "ee-ee-ee").
2. Asking the patient to alternate aspirate-vowel and voiced continuant-consonant pairs ("huh-muh—huh-muh").
3. Asking the patient to alternate voiced and voiceless consonant-vowel pairs ("puh-buh—puh-buh").

Vocal flexibility is almost always reduced by nervous system pathology sufficient to produce significant dysarthria. The causes for the loss of flexibility vary, depending on the location of the pathology. Constricted range of pitch and loudness can be caused by upper motor neuron, lower motor neuron, extrapyramidal, or cerebellar pathology. Problems with coordination of respiration and voice onset are most often caused by extrapyramidal or cerebellar pathology.

Evaluation of Velopharyngeal Function.—Velopharyngeal structures serve to isolate the pharyngeal and oral cavities from the nasal cavity during swallowing and during production of nonnasalized speech sounds. Although the exact means by which velopharyngeal closure is achieved differs somewhat across individuals (Yorkston et al., 1988), closure usually involves (1) movement of the velum (soft palate) up and back to meet the posterior pharyngeal wall, and (2) movement of the lateral pharyngeal walls toward the midline to meet the sides of the velum. Occasionally the posterior pharyngeal wall may move forward toward the velum (Croft et al., 1981). When normal speakers produce nonnasal sounds, velopharyngeal muscles contract, closing the nasopharyngeal opening and preventing the escape of air from the oral cavity through the nasal cavity. When the speaker produces nasal sounds, the velopharyngeal muscles relax, opening the nasopharyngeal opening and allowing part of the airstream to pass through the nasal cavity, adding nasal resonance to these sounds.

The clinician first estimates the adequacy of velopharyngeal function as the patient sustains phonation and repeats syllables, listening for *hypernasality, nasal escape of air,* and *imprecise consonants* during production of denasal sounds, especially those requiring interruption or constriction of the airstream (stop consonants such as /p/ and /b/ and continuants such as /s/ and /sh/).

Judgment of *hypernasality* is one of the clinician's most difficult tasks. Such judgments often are unreliable, in part because they are affected by other speech characteristics (Moll, 1968). The more severe a patient's articulatory deviations are, the more likely it is that the patient will be judged hypernasal. Furthermore, patients who speak loudly tend to be judged more hypernasal than those who speak softly (Yorkston et al., 1988). However, no satisfactory substitute for subjective judgments of hypernasality exists.

One of the easiest tests for hypernasality is to alternately pinch and release the nostrils as the patient produces a sustained vowel. If the patient is hypernasal, the sound of the vowel changes as the nostrils are occluded and opened. However, this test does not always predict hypernasality in connected speech. Some patients can successfully occlude the velopharyngeal opening during sustained phonation, but cannot do so during the more complicated movement patterns of connected speech. One can, of course, pinch and release the patient's nostrils as he or she produces connected speech. If the hypernasality is dramatic, changes in vocal resonance will be apparent. Moderate hypernasality may not be apparent, and mild hypernasality will not be. Fortunately, moderate hypernasality, either by itself or in combination with mild articulatory imprecision, usually does not cause speech to be grossly unintelligible. Direct treatment of hypernasality usually is reserved for those patients in whom velopharyngeal incompetence is so severe that it precludes intelligible production of consonants requiring oral impoundment or constriction of the airstream.

The primary means of assessing *nasal escape of air* is also perceptual—the clinician listens for sounds of air escaping through the nose as the patient sustains phonation or repeats syllables, phrases, or sentences. Other techniques have been used (feathers or small pieces of tissue on a card held under the nose, a cold mirror held under the nose), but they usually yield positive results only when nasal emission is very great. Instrumentation that measures nasal emission is available, but it is expensive and not available in most clinics. Consequently, the clinician's ears and eyes remain the most frequently used instrument for measuring nasality.

Certain patterns of *consonant imprecision* may suggest velopharyngeal incompetence. Consonants in which the airstream is restricted (continuants such as /s/, /sh/) or momentarily occluded (stops such as /b/, /p/) may be produced weakly, with nasal emission of air. Voiced consonants such as /b/ or /d/ may sound weak and hypernasal. When articulation of consonants depending on increased oral breath pressure (stops and continuants) seems markedly poorer than articulation of more "open" consonants (such as /h/, /l/, /r/), velopharyngeal incompetence may be present.

Evaluation of Articulation.— Syllable and phrase repetition are the primary vehicles for assessing dysarthric patients' articulatory accuracy. The syllables and phrases are chosen to highlight the contribution of the various articulatory structures to the overall speech product. Lip closure is evaluated by asking the patient to repeat bilabial consonant-vowel combinations ("pa-pa-pa," "ba-ba-ba"). Tongue tip elevation is evaluated by asking the patient to repeat tongue-tip alveolar-ridge combinations ("ta-ta-ta-," "da-da-da-"). Elevation of the back of the tongue is evaluated by asking the patient to repeat high-back-consonant combinations ("ka-ka-ka-," "ga-ga-ga-"). Articulatory flexibility and coordination is evaluated by asking the patient to repeat strings of syllables in which articulation points change ("pa-ta-ka, da-ba-ga"). Articulatory accuracy in connected speech is estimated by asking the patient to repeat multisyllabic words ("gingerbread-gingerbread-gingerbread," "artillery-artillery-artillery"), phrases ("the Republican convention"), and sentences ("Nelson Rockefeller drives a Lincoln Continental").

Comprehensive inventories of articulation rarely are administered to dysarthric patients. There appear to be two reasons for this. First, articulatory problems in dysarthria frequently are only part of a constellation of respiratory, phonatory, and resonance disturbances. Consequently, clinicians are not interested so much in what sounds are in error, but in what impaired speech processes account for the *pattern* of articulatory impairment. Second, the goal of most treatment for dysarthric patients is intelligibility rather than articulatory accuracy. Because articulatory accuracy exhibits only a general relationship to intelligibility, measuring intelligibility usually provides more therapeutically valuable information than measuring articulatory accuracy. Yorkston et al. (1988) offer several objections to the use of traditional articulation inventories with dysarthric speakers. They assert that (1) a judge's perceptions of articulatory accuracy may not accurately reflect the adequacy of the patient's articulatory movements; (2) articulation inventories fail to discriminate between sounds that are accurate and sounds that are distorted but still within phoneme boundaries; and (3) when judges know the target words, as in traditional articulation inventories, they are likely to overestimate the patient's articulatory accuracy. Yorkston et al. (1986) advocate use of the *Phoneme Identification Task* to eliminate some of these problems. In the *Phoneme Identification Task,* the speaker is tape recorded as he or she produces a list of single words and sentences. The list is designed to elicit 57 target phonemes. A judge (not the examiner) then listens to the tape recording and identifies the target phonemes with the following procedure. A word or sentence is played. The judge is given a card showing a word with the target phoneme missing (e.g., "ma_"), and is asked to identify the missing phoneme. Then the judge rates the patient's production of the perceived phoneme using a four-point scale, ranging from "no basis for a guess," to "correct, undistorted."

Evaluation of Intelligibility.—Yorkston and Beukelman (1981) published an assessment tool called *Assessment of Intelligibility of Dysarthric Speech* (AIDS). The test has two sections. One measures single-word intelligibility; the other assesses sentence intelligibility and speaking rate. In the *single word task* (part 1), a speaker's production of 50 single words is tape recorded. Each word is selected by the examiner (before the test) from a pool of 12 similar-sounding words. One or more judges (not the examiner) then listen to the tape and either (1) write down each word that they hear, or (2) choose each word that they hear from a set of 12 words that are similar in sound to the target word. In the *sentence task* (part 2) the speaker says aloud 22 sentences, ranging in length from 5 to 15 words (2 sentences at each length). The examiner chooses the sentences (before the test) from a large pool of sentences. One or more judges (not the examiner) then listen to the recording and write down the sentences that they hear. Judges' transcriptions are then scored by the examiner to yield several measures: (1) a percent intelligibility score; (2) speech rate for sentences (words per minute); (3) intelligible words per minute; (4) unintelligible words per minute; and (5) communicative efficiency ratio (intelligible words per minute divided by "normal" speech rate—190 words per minute).

Assessment of Intelligibility of Dysarthric Speech appears to be a sensitive and reliable estimator of speech intelligibility, if administered and scored according to instructions. The measures obtained are useful for predicting a speaker's intelligibility in daily life, for measuring changes in intelligibility over time, and in planning treatment to improve a speaker's intelligibility. Patients who are both aphasic and dysarthric may have difficulty with the sentence production part of AIDS because of reading problems or problems in auditory comprehension and retention. Consequently, the test may not be appropriate for patients who are both dysarthric and moderately or severely aphasic.

TREATMENT OF DYSARTHRIA

Dysarthria is caused by various neurologic or physical disturbances that cause weakness, slowness, clumsiness, incoordination, diminished range of movement, or sensory loss in speech structures. Some patients do not have the muscle strength or range of movement needed for normal speech. Others may have the muscle strength but not the coordination. Still others may lack the respiratory support necessary for normal speech. Consequently, there is no single treatment for dysarthria.

Treatment of dysarthria must take into account both the causes of a patient's dysarthria and the nature of the speech disturbances. Some treatment procedures may be concerned with causative mechanisms, while others may focus on the speech disturbances themselves. The goal of dysarthria treatment is to maximize the dysarthric patient's communicative effectiveness and efficiency. This goal might be achieved in various ways: by improving the physiologic support for speech; by direct work on speech; by environmental control, education, and counseling; by providing compensatory techniques or alternatives to speech for communication; by providing prosthetic facilitation of speech; or by medical or surgical intervention.

Treatment of dysarthric patients often approaches speech indirectly, by improving sensory and motor functions within physiologic processes that serve speech, rather than directly, by working on speech itself. Indirect treatment procedures include sensory stimulation, muscle strengthening, modifying muscle tone, and modifying respiration. Direct procedures include modifying phonation, resonation, articulation, and prosody. For most dysarthric patients, treatment is a combination of direct and indirect procedures. If a patient is severely dysarthric and can produce little or no volitional speech or speech sounds, treatment is likely to be directed toward enhancing physiologic support for speech. If a patient can produce some voice, approximate a few vowel sounds, and produce a few articulatory movements, the physiologic processes underlying speech can be enhanced by working on production of speech sounds. Nonspeech exercises to strengthen muscles and increase their agility and range of movement may also be appropriate, but primarily as an adjunct to direct work on speech. The more severe the patient's dysarthria, the more likely it is that the clinician will work to strengthen muscles and improve sensory function outside the context of speech. Patients with mild or moderate dysarthria may get their muscles strengthened and their sensory functions improved, but almost always this will be accomplished by controlled experiences with speaking, rather than by stimulation of oral structures or movement exercises in isolation.

T2. **Indirect Treatment Procedures**

Sensory Stimulation.—The intent of sensory stimulation is to increase the dysarthric patient's motor control by increasing the amount and fidelity of sensory feedback from oral structures. Stimulation may include brushing, stroking, vibrating, or applying ice to the patient's lips, tongue, pharyngeal walls, or soft palate. There is little empirical evidence that sensory stimulation improves motor performance in dysarthria, and its use remains controversial, except, perhaps, for stimulation of the soft palate. Rosenbek and LaPointe (1985) suggest that massage and lifting of the soft palate concurrent with the patient's attempts to raise it may improve velopharyngeal competence. Johns (1985) reports that movement of the lateral pharyngeal walls toward the midline sometimes increases after installation of palatal prostheses. He attributes this to increased sensory feedback generated by contact of the pharyngeal walls with the prosthesis. However, Dworkin and Johns (1980), after reviewing various approaches to managing velopharyngeal insufficiency, assert that neither stimulation or muscle strengthening are likely to be effective if the insufficiency is caused by neurologic impairment. It may be that a clinician's willingness to use stimulation when velopharyngeal closure is deficient results as much from the paucity of other methods for remediation as from the clinician's belief that stimulation actually works. Nevertheless, stimulation of the soft palates and pharyngeal walls of dysarthric patients with gross velopharyngeal incompetence is likely to continue, at least until something better comes along.

Muscle Strengthening.—Muscle strengthening exercises are intended to improve the dysarthric patient's respiration, phonation, articulation, and resonance by enhancing movement of weakened muscles. There is no conclusive evidence confirming the efficacy of muscle strengthening in treating dysarthria, but it appears to have positive effects for at least some patients (Powers and Starr, 1974; Yules and Chase, 1969; Massengill et al., 1968). Rosenbek and LaPointe (1978) suggest that muscle strengthening is most appropriate for patients whose dysarthria is severe and whose physiologic support for speech is substantially compromised. They recommend muscle strengthening when (1) changes in posture, muscle tone, and respiration, phonation, articulation, and prosody will leave the patient unintelligible; (2) the patient will remain in treatment for several weeks; and (3) the patient is able and willing to carry out assignments outside the clinic. In practice, muscle strengthening usually is reserved for severely dysarthric patients who can produce little intelligible speech, or can produce it only in fragments and under ideal conditions.

It is important that clinicians not exaggerate the importance of muscle strength for producing adequate speech movements. Most speech movements do not require forceful muscle activity to produce intelligible speech. In fact, forceful articulatory movements, such as those seen in ataxia, dystonia, and chorea, may actually diminish intelligibility. Agility and range of movement almost always are more important for intelligible speech than strength. Consequently, muscle strengthening exercises that include movement (*isotonic* exercise) are likely to be more effective than those requiring exertion against stationary resistance (*isometric* exercise). (However, isotonic exercises that require a patient to increase the range and accuracy of articulatory movements also strengthen muscles.) Rosenbek and LaPointe (1985) suggest that isometric exercises are more likely to be appropriate early in treatment with severely dysarthric patients, and that isotonic exercises are more likely to be appropriate later with less severely dysarthric patients. As a general rule, the clinician should move from isometric to isotonic movements as soon as the patient can accomplish short sequences of simple movements. Muscle strengthening activities should lead into agility and range of motion exercises as soon as the muscle groups have sufficient strength to carry out the exercises at low levels of speed and efficiency.

Muscle strengthening by itself is most appropriate for severely dysarthric patients. If a patient can produce a vowel or two and approximate a few consonants, muscle strengthening usually is supplemented by direct work on speech production. Patients whose muscles do not have the strength, agility, or range of movement to talk but who can produce a few speech sounds will usually develop increased strength, agility, and range of movement in the muscle groups needed for speech more quickly (and more efficiently) if they are talking than if they are moving speech structures in nonspeech movement drills.

Modification of Muscle Tone.—Some dysarthric patients exhibit abnormalities in muscle tone that interfere with speech intelligibility. Some are *hypertonic*. Hypertonicity appears as *spasticity* when patients have upper motor neuron pathology, and as *rigidity* in Parkinson's disease. Both kinds of hypertonicity are constant over time and uniform across affected muscle groups. Hypertonicity also appears as a consequence of extrapyramidal diseases such as dystonia and chorea. In these disorders muscle tone tends to wax and wane within a given muscle group and may move from muscle group to muscle group. Abnormally diminished muscle tone (hypotonicity) is usually seen following lower motor neuron or peripheral nervous system pathology. Hypotonicity is almost always constant over time and does not move from one muscle group to another.

A variety of procedures for relaxing hypertonic muscles have been reported in the literature. *Progressive relaxation* often is used to reduce the hypertonic patient's overall level of muscle tension. *Shaking* (Froeschels, 1943) and *chewing* exercises (Froeschels, 1952) continue to be used to accomplish local relaxation of muscle groups involved in speaking. In some cases supine posture may be helpful for hypertonic patients because it helps to lower overall muscle tension. *Biofeedback,* in which the electrical activity within certain muscle groups is amplified and converted to auditory or visual signals that are monitored by the patient, is a promising new approach to selective relaxation of certain muscle groups. Netsell and Cleeland (1973), Hand et al. (1979), and Rubow et al. (1984) have reported positive results for such procedures. When hypertonicity is caused by extrapyramidal pathology (such as Parkinson's disease) medications to reduce muscle tone may be more effective than behavioral treatment. In fact, hypertonicity related to extrapyramidal disease usually is not very responsive to behavioral treatment.

Hypotonicity (as in flaccid dysarthria) typically is treated by raising the patient's overall level of muscle tension. Simply asking the patient to increase his or her overall level of effort sometimes improves the intelligibility of patients with flaccid dysarthria (Rosenbek and LaPointe, 1985). If this approach is not effective, the patient's general level of muscle tension may be increased by asking him or her to push or pull against a stationary resistance while speaking. Pushing down on a table or on the arms of a chair or wheelchair or clasping the hands together and pulling may increase overall muscle tone and improve the speech intelligibility of hypotonic patients.

Posture and Speaking Position.—Modifying the dysarthric patient's posture and speaking position may sometimes improve his or her speech, especially when general muscle weakness is present, as in generalized neuropathies. Straightening the slouching patient's spine and neck and bringing his or her head to an upright position by means of braces or supports may improve the mechanical relationships among the structures involved in speech, with beneficial consequences for the quality of the patient's speech. Postural adjustments may help the patient compensate for weak muscles and stabilize the "platform" from which speech movements are carried out. Cervical collars, body braces, slings, and restraints, singly or in combination, may be used to get a weak patient into a more efficient position for speech and to help the patient maintain that position. Posture and positioning are most often useful with weak or flaccid patients who have difficulty sitting up and keeping their head erect.

When the patient has been positioned in a better speaking posture, stabilization and support of certain muscle groups may further enhance the intelligibility of the patient's speech. If a patient's neck muscles are weak, a cervical collar or neck brace may stabilize the patient's head. Girdles, stomach bands, or stomach boards (Rosenbek and LaPointe, 1985) may be used to stabilize and support weak abdominal muscles. Stomach boards are boards, usually fastened to a wheelchair, against which the patient can press his or her abdomen to compress it and generate greater expiratory pressure for speech. Girdles and stomach bands compress the abdomen, compensating for weak abdominal muscles and providing a firm base for exhalation during speech. Patients with movement disorders may wear cervical collars, neck braces, or body braces to limit involuntary movements.

Posturing, positioning, stabilization, and support should be carried out *only* in collaboration with a physician, because changes in posture or bracing, banding, and belting may predispose the patient to medical complications. For example, abdominal banding or girdling may restrict respiration and predispose patients to pneumonia. Cervical collars and neck braces may compress muscles and nerves in the patient's neck and shoulders, compromising their function.

Respiratory Capacity and Efficiency.— Respiratory capacity is most likely to be a problem for patients with generalized weakness, as in demyelinating diseases, diseases of the spinal cord, and diseases involving the neuromuscular junction. Increasing respiratory capacity may improve these patients' speech, but only if they can use the breath stream efficiently. In most cases, outright respiratory capacity is far less important to speech than efficient use of the airstream. If a patient's glottal valving, nasopharyngeal porting, and articulation are poor, increasing respiratory capacity will do little for the intelligibility of their speech.

Treatment procedures for enhancing respiratory support take several forms. Postural adjustments, positioning, and stabilization may improve the mechanical background for respiration. Muscle strengthening activities may be directed toward the muscles of respiration. Sometimes techniques for increasing muscle tone (such as pushing and bearing down) are employed to increase respiratory drive. Training in more efficient glottal valving and increasing articulatory precision may have indirect positive effects on respiratory support.

Exercises that deal directly with respiration also may be appropriate. Controlled exhalation, in which the patient slowly exhales a uniform stream of air over a period of time, may improve respiratory capacity and enhance control of exhalation. In most cases, direct treatment of respiration is an early phase of treatment, and the focus of treatment usually moves to speech production as soon as the patient achieves basic respiratory support for speech.

Direct Treatment Procedures

In direct treatment procedures, dysarthric patients produce speech under controlled conditions. (Technically, one cannot treat "speech"—one treats speech by changing the amplitude, speed, or accuracy of movements that generate speech. Consequently, even "direct" treatment procedures are indirect, in this sense.) Treatment of dysarthric patients usually includes both indirect and direct procedures, and indirect procedures tend to fade into direct procedures, as, for example, when controlled exhalation gives way to controlled phonation. Direct treatment procedures, too, tend to overlap and merge one into another, as when controlled phonation progresses into simple articulation drills. Direct treatment procedures may address phonation and respiratory support, resonation, articulation, and prosody, either singly or in combination.

Speech activities to enhance phonation and respiratory support emphasize efficient laryngeal valving of the airstream and adjusting utterance length to the patient's respiratory capacity. Controlled phonation is the primary vehicle for increasing dysarthric patients' laryngeal efficiency. In the early stages of treatment, the patient may be asked to produce prolonged vowels, and to gradually increase their duration. Production of vowels may lead to controlled production of strings of vowels or consonant-vowel syllables, with the length of the strings gradually increasing. Gradual changes in intensity may then be superimposed on the strings to further enhance respiratory control. When the patient can say short phrases, treatment may focus on the concept of "optimal breath group" (Linebaugh, 1983). The optimal breath group for a given patient is the number of syllables that he or she can produce comfortably on one breath. This approach entails (1) determining the patient's optimal breath group; (2) teaching the patient to keep the number of syllables per breath within his or her optimal breath group; and (3) gradually increasing the length of the patient's optimal breath group by means of drills.

When laryngeal valving is compromised by spastic laryngeal muscles, procedures for reducing laryngeal tension, including relaxation, massage or vibration of the larynx, or providing postural support may be combined with work on voice production. When laryngeal muscles are flaccid, pushing and bearing down during phonation may be incorporated into voice drills, and in some cases visual feedback, such as that provided by a VU meter or an oscilloscope tracing may be used to help the patient control (and increase) the loudness of his or her phonation.

The resonance of speech is affected by the size and configuration of the oral and nasal cavities, and the amount of communication between the two. Although aberrations in the shape of the oral cavity may change the resonance characteristics of speech, such changes are primarily cosmetic, affecting the quality of speech rather than its intelligibility. (However, aberrations in the shape of the oral cavity are produced by abnormal positions of the articulators, so that articulatory errors usually are superimposed upon the resonance abnormalities. The combination of the two can sometimes destroy intelligibility.) By far the most important resonance aberration in dysarthria is hypernasality, caused by failure to close the velopharyngeal opening between the oral and nasal cavities. This failure has two effects. It produces excessive nasal resonance. More importantly, it distorts or destroys sounds that require oral breath pressure (stops, such as /p/, /b/, /t/, and /d/, and affricates, such as /f/, /v/, /s/, and /z/), because the air required to produce them escapes through the nose.

 Velopharyngeal insufficiency is most common in flaccid dysarthria.* Increasing velopharyngeal competence can create dramatic improvements in intelligibility for many hypernasal patients. Several behavioral techniques for ameliorating hypernasality exist. These usually involve ear training to teach the patient to recognize hypernasality, and some combination of movement facilitation (pushing, bearing down, biofeedback), to help the patient do something about the hypernasality when he or she hears it. Behavioral remediation of hypernasality usually is successful only when hypernasality is mild. If it is moderate or severe, prosthetic or surgical management usually is necessary.

Improving the dysarthric patient's *articulation* was for many years the core of treatment for dysarthria. Dysarthria was considered to be little more than defective articulation. However, as Rosenbek and LaPointe (1985) assert, "Articulation is being forced to share its popularity with other speech processes . . . and dysarthria is coming to mean speech—not articulation—deficit." Most dysarthric patients receive articulation treatment. However, few receive *only* articulation treatment.

Treatment procedures for improving articulation include *imitation, phonetic derivation* (deriving sounds that the patient cannot say from those that he or she can say), *phonetic placement* (physically adjusting or positioning the articulators), and *sequential repetition* of sounds, syllables, and words. In most cases, articulation exercises focus on speech movements (production of syllables or words), rather than on fixed positions (individual sounds). Only when a patient's dysarthria is severe is he or she likely to be drilled in producing fixed articulatory positions. When a patient's articulatory movements are imprecise, he or she may be taught to exaggerate them,

*In ataxic dysarthria, velopharyngeal closure may be poorly coordinated with other speech movements, but therapeutic attention usually is focused on control of respiration, articulation, pitch, and intensity, rather than on velopharyngeal valving itself.

making them more precise. Sometimes when a patient cannot produce an articulatory movement or position, a compensatory movement or substitute position may be taught. Work on articulatory precision often is combined with slowing the patient's speech rate. Slowing speech rate allows the patient more time to make articulatory movements, and it allows the patient's listeners more time to decode what the patient is saying.

Activities for changing the *prosodic* characteristics of dysarthric patients' speech may focus on rate, loudness, or pitch (intonation). Changes in patients' *speech rate* can be produced by changes in articulation rate (the rate at which individual speech sounds are produced) or by increasing the number or duration of pauses in the patient's speech. Most dysarthric speakers have great difficulty changing articulation rate. Consequently, most rate manipulations are performed with pauses. If a patient is trained to produce "optimal breath groups," pauses may occur automatically. However, in many cases, the pauses will not be at syntactic or semantic boundaries. In these cases it may be helpful to teach the patient to mark the boundaries with pauses. Teaching a patient to put pauses at syntactic or semantic boundaries makes it easier for listeners to segment the patient's utterances into meaningful units. If the patient is perceptive and alert, he or she may be taught to monitor listeners and to pause (and repeat or paraphrase) when the patient perceives that the listener does not understand.

There are several techniques for controlling dysarthric patients' speech rate. In most of them the patient speaks in unison with an external timing stimulus. The clinician may tap, gesture, or speak along with the patient. The patient may speak to the beat of a metronome or a flashing light. The patient may tap, drop beads in a cup, gesture, or produce other nonoral movements in unison with speaking. Teaching the patient to speak with exaggerated articulation and to exaggerate emphatic stress (contrastive stress drill—see below) also may slow the patient's speech rate.

When loudness is a problem in dysarthria, it usually is a case of too little, rather than too much. A few dysarthric patients talk too loudly, but most talk too softly. The loudness of dysarthric patients' speech may be enhanced by improving respiratory support, increasing the efficiency of phonation, or increasing articulatory precision. Sometimes a patient still speaks too softly after these activities have produced all the gains in loudness that they are likely to, and exercises specific to increasing vocal intensity may be needed. These exercises may include (1) teaching the patient an appropriate "breath group"; (2) positioning, bracing, or banding; (3) counting, saying the alphabet, or other sequences with increasing or decreasing loudness across the sequences; and (4) contrastive stress drill. In contrastive stress drill (Rosenbek and LaPointe, 1985), the clinician gives a sentence such as "Bob hit Bill" and then asks questions such as "who hit Bill?," "what did Bill do?," and so on. The patient answers each question, putting emphatic stress on elements that answer the questions (e.g., "Bob *hit* Bill"). If adequate vocal intensity cannot be obtained by means of behavioral treatment, amplification may be provided. However, as Rosenbek and LaPointe (1985) caution, amplification is appropriate only when the patient's articulation is good. Amplifying unintelligible speech only produces louder unintelligible speech.

Increasing *vocal pitch range* may be appropriate for some patients, particularly those with flaccid dysarthria. Control of *pitch changes* may be important for patients with ataxic dysarthria. Techniques for increasing pitch range include (1) phonation with gradually rising and falling pitch; (2) counting, saying the alphabet, numbers, days of the week, or other sequences with gradually rising or falling pitch across the sequences; (3) contrastive drill, using questions (for rising pitch) and assertions (for falling pitch). Techniques for controlling pitch changes include (1) continuous phonation while keeping pitch constant; and (2) continuous phonation with slowly rising or falling pitch.

ENVIRONMENTAL CONTROL AND EDUCATION

Most dysarthric speakers eventually discover that intelligibility in the speech clinic, where the rooms are quiet and well-lighted and they are face-to-face with the clinician, is no guarantee of intelligibility in daily life, where rooms may be poorly lit and noisy, and where listeners may not always be nearby and/or looking. Skilled clinicians know that this is likely to occur, and they teach patients how to compensate for less-than-ideal speaking conditions. They also teach them how they can control their speaking environment to be maximally intelligible. When a dysarthric speaker reaches reasonable levels of intelligibility in the controlled environment of the clinic, the treatment program is broadened to include education and training in maximizing communication in less-than-ideal speaking situations. This requires *control* and *compensation*.

The patient can be taught ways to *control* the speaking environment to minimize adverse effects on speech intelligibility. The most effective controls involve ambient noise, lighting, and the spatial relationships between the dysarthric speaker and his or her listener(s). Keeping ambient noise levels low should be a primary requirement for the dysarthric speaker and those around him or her. Turning the television set down or off and closing windows or doors to shut out outside noise are simple but effective ways to diminish ambient noise. Berry (1983) suggests that families obtain remote controls for television sets, and that draperies or other acoustic treatments be employed to control ambient noise levels in dysarthric speakers' homes.

Controlling lighting and the position of the dysarthric speaker relative to his or her listeners may also enhance the dysarthric speaker's communicative effectiveness. Whenever it is practical the dysarthric speaker should arrange room lighting so that his or her face is well-lighted, and he or she should sit or stand so that listeners can see the dysarthric speaker's face. Arranging conditions so that listeners can "lip-read" will almost always enhance the dysarthric speaker's intelligibility.

Dysarthric speakers should be taught to monitor their listeners' comprehension by maintaining eye contact and periodically asking listeners whether they understand. They also can be taught to repeat, simplify, paraphrase, and exaggerate articulatory movements in ongoing speech (especially when the patient perceives comprehension failure). Those around the dysarthric speaker may be taught to control the situational variables discussed above, to indicate (either gesturally or verbally) to the speaker when they do not understand what he or she is saying, and to ask the dysarthric speaker to slow down, exaggerate articulatory movements, repeat, paraphrase, or simplify when they fail to communicate.

Prosthetic Intervention.—Hypernasality caused by palatal insufficiency may sometimes be reduced by installation of a palatal lift prosthesis. A palatal lift prosthesis is constructed by a prosthodontist, usually in collaboration with a speech pathologist. It consists of a plate that covers the hard palate that is attached to the teeth by means of wires. Attached to the rear of the plate is the palatal lift itself, usually made of acrylic and shaped to fit the patient's oropharynx. The lift portion of the appliance mechanically pushes the palate up and back, providing improved closure of the nasopharyngeal opening. After the lift is constructed and fitted to the patient's mouth, its position is adjusted by the prosthodontist in collaboration with the speech pathologist to produce the optimum reduction of hypernasality without creating excessive hyponasality.

The literature (Netsell and Rosenbek, 1985; Rosenbek and LaPointe, 1985; Yorkston and Beukelman; 1988) suggests that patients with the following characteristics are the best candidates for palatal lift prostheses.

1. Patients who are extremely hypernasal, who cannot achieve velopharyngeal closure, and for whom behavioral intervention has been unsuccessful.
2. Patients whose soft palates and pharyngeal muscles are not spastic. Spastic muscles resist displacement and may dislodge the prosthesis.
3. Patients who have teeth to which the prosthesis can be anchored. Occasionally prostheses have been fitted to dentures, but the results generally are unsatisfactory.
4. Patients who have reasonably good articulation and phonation. Hypernasal patients with severe articulatory or phonatory deficits will generally remain as unintelligible after the prosthesis is fitted as they were before.
5. Patients who are likely to cooperate by wearing the lift and caring for it. Some severely involved patients may not tolerate the discomfort associated with wearing the prosthesis, and some unmotivated patients may not put up with the inconvenience of wearing the prosthesis and caring for it.
6. Patients who do not have swallowing difficulties. Palatal prostheses sometimes may interfere with swallowing.
7. Patients without degenerative disease. Although fitting a prosthesis to such patients may provide temporarily increased intelligibility, the effects are in most cases likely to be transitory and eventually overcome by the progression of the disease.

Amplification.—Patients who cannot generate enough vocal intensity to be intelligible may be helped by portable amplifiers. The patient wears either a throat-mounted or headset-mounted microphone that is connected to a small amplifier and speaker that can be worn in a pocket or on a strap or belt. Such devices are useful with patients with weak voices but reasonably good articulation.

MEDICAL AND SURGICAL TREATMENT

Medical Treatment.—Some conditions causing dysarthria are treatable with medications. When they are, medical treatment precedes behavioral intervention, and when medical treatment is successful, behavioral intervention may not be needed. Medically treatable conditions causing dysarthria include extrapyramidal diseases such as parkinsonism, irritative and inflammatory processes causing peripheral nerve dysfunction, and some metabolic and nutritional disturbances.

Parkinson's disease is caused by deficiencies in certain neurotransmitters (dopamines) and often responds well to medications such as levodopa (L-dopa) that replenish the missing neurotransmitters. These medications often diminish or eliminate the motor symptoms of the disease, including dysarthria. Movement disorders (such as chorea and dystonia) sometimes respond favorably to tranquilizers and related medications, although complete remission of symptoms with such medications is unusual. Some facial paralyses and neuralgias are treatable with steroids. (However, such conditions rarely cause significant dysarthria.) Neurologic diseases caused by abnormalities in central nervous system metabolism, such as Wilson's disease, may be medically treatable. When medical treatment of a dysarthric patient's neurologic disease is effective, his or her dysarthria often improves enough to make direct treatment of dysarthria unnecessary. However, in many cases medical treatment decreases but does not eliminate a patient's dysarthria, so that behavioral treatment of the patient's dysarthria is necessary in conjunction with medical treatment.

Teflon Injections and Surgical Treatment.—Sometimes when structural anomalies or insufficiencies produce dysarthria, surgical management is appropriate. When dysphonia is caused by inability to adduct the vocal folds, injection of Teflon into the vocal folds may improve voice quality. In most cases, surgical intervention does not completely resolve the speech abnormalities and behavioral intervention is necessary after surgery. Teflon injections into the posterior pharyngeal walls have been employed to remediate velopharyngeal insufficiency (Lewy et al., 1965; Bluestone et al., 1968). Such injections probably are most useful in cases of mild to moderate hypernasality when behavioral modification of hypernasality has not been successful.

Surgical remediation of velopharyngeal insufficiency appears efficacious in some cases of severe velopharyngeal incompetence, although the general opinion seems to be that surgery is a last resort, to be tried only after less dramatic approaches have failed. The most frequent surgical procedure for remediating velopharyngeal insufficiency is the posterior pharyngeal flap. In this procedure, bands of muscle tissue are lifted from the posterior pharyngeal walls and one end of each band is attached to the soft palate. When the pharyngeal wall muscles contract, the bands shorten, pulling the soft palate toward the pharyngeal walls. Pharyngeal flap procedures are most common in management of palatal insufficiency for children with cleft palates. Their use to treat hypernasality in dysarthria is controversial. Gonzalez and Aronson (1970) assert that prosthetic management of velopharyngeal insufficiency usually produces better results than surgery. Hardy et al. (1961) make a similar assertion regarding management of velopharyngeal insufficiency in children. Miniami et al. (1975) did pharyngeal flaps on five dysarthric patients with "palatal paresis," and reported that the results were disappointing in terms of resolution of hypernasality. However, Johns (1985), after reviewing the literature and summarizing his own experience with surgical remediation of velopharyngeal insufficiency, concluded that surgical management "holds great promise for a large number of dysarthric patients."

AUGMENTATIVE AND ALTERNATIVE COMMUNICATION

Many severely dysarthric patients never regain enough speech to communicate even simple messages by talking. Nonspeech communication systems may enable many of these patients to communicate with those around them. Nonspeech communication systems can be either *augmentative* or *alternative*. *Augmentative systems* supplement what the patient can say and permit the patient to communicate more elaborate messages, or simple messages with greater intelligibility. *Alternative systems* replace speech as a means of communication. There are four major categories of nonspeech communication systems: (1) communication boards and communication books; (2) mechanical and electronic devices; (3) gesture and pantomime; and (4) sign language.

Selection of an alternative communication system for a given patient requires consideration of the patient's perceptual, motor, and linguistic abilities, because different systems require different abilities and different levels of skill within those abilities. Some systems require that the user point to symbols or operate a keyboard. Patients with poor manual dexterity may not be able to use such systems. Some systems require that the user spell, read, or arrange words into phrases or sentences. Patients with linguistic impairments may not be able to use them.

Communication Boards and Communication Books.—Communication boards and communication books are similar in content but dissimilar in form. A communication board is an array of symbols on a durable surface. A communication book is a collection of symbols arranged in book form. The symbols in both can be pictures, letters, words, phrases, or some combination of the four. To communicate, the patient points to the symbols, either singly or in sequence. Figure 11–4 shows examples of two kinds of communication boards. At the top is a simple board containing pictorial symbols and printed words. At the bottom is a more complex board containing letters, numerals, and words.

In general, communication boards and books containing letters, words, and phrases are best suited for patients without substantial linguistic impairments. The board shown at the **top** of Figure 11–4 would be usable by many linguistically impaired patients because its symbols are nonverbal. The board shown at the bottom of Figure 11–4 would be inappropriate for linguistically impaired patients, but would be appropriate for dysarthric patients without major linguistic impairment, as long as they have the motor ability to point to the symbols on the board.

NO   YES

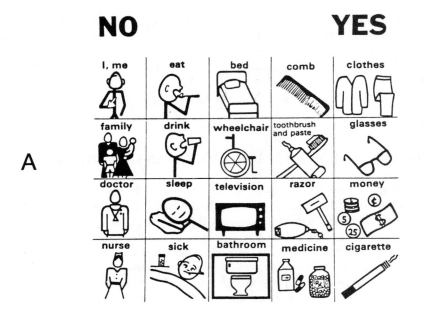

A

B

I CAN HEAR PERFECTLY			PLEASE REPEAT AS I TALK (THIS IS HOW I TALK BY SPELLING OUT THE WORDS)							WOULD YOU PLEASE CALL	
A	AN	HE	AM	ARE	ASK	BE	BEEN	BRING	CAN	ABOUT	ALL
HER	I	IT	ME	COME	COULD	DID	DO	DOES	DON'T	AND	ALWAYS
MY	HIM	SHE	DRINK	GET	GIVE	GO	HAD	HAS	HAVE	ALMOST	AS
THAT	THE	THESE	IS	KEEP	KNOW	LET	LIKE	MAKE	MAY	AT	BECAUSE
THEY	THIS	WHOSE	PUT	SAY	SAID	SEE	SEEN	SEND	SHOULD	BUT	FOR FROM
WHAT	WHEN	WHERE	TAKE	TELL	THINK	THOUGHT		WANT		HOW	IF IN
WHICH	WHO	WHY	WAS	WERE	WILL	WISH	WON'T	WOULD	-ED	OF	ON OR
YOU	WE	YOUR	-ER	-EST	-ING	-LY	-N'T	-'S	-TION	TO	UP WITH

A		B	C		D		E		F		G	AFTER AGAIN
	H			I		J		K	L		M	ANY EVEN
N		O		P		Qu		R		S	T	EVERY HERE
	U		V		W		X		Y		Z	JUST MORE
1		2		3		4		5		6	7	ONLY SO
	8		9		10		11		12		30	SOME SOON
												THERE VERY

SUN. MON. TUES. WED. THUR. FRI. SAT. BATHROOM	PLEASE THANK YOU GOING OUT		$¢½(SHHH!!)?
	MR.	MRS.	MISS	START OVER
	MOTHER	DAD	DOCTOR	END OF WORD

IS MY NAME

FIG 11–4.
A picture communication board **(A)** suitable for a patient with moderate to severe language impairment. **B** is a more complex board containing words and phrases that would be appropriate for a patient with good language abilities and sufficient finger and arm dexterity to point to letters and words at a reasonably rapid rate.

Versions of communication boards that do not require the user to directly select symbols have been developed. The simplest of these is the *eye gaze board*. Eye gaze boards can be used when speechless patients have good language abilities but cannot move their limbs to directly select symbols from a board (e.g., patients who are quadriplegic after cervical spinal cord injuries). Eye gaze boards allow such patients to "point" to symbols by looking at them. Message recipients watch the patient's eye movements and read aloud what they believe the patient is looking at. The patient signals correct choices, usually by blinking. Because it is difficult for message recipients to tell exactly where a patient is looking, eye gaze boards have to be relatively large, with large spaces between symbols. For this reason the number of symbols that can be put on an eye gaze board is limited. Most eye gaze boards contain an alphabet, numbers, and perhaps a few key words or phrases. Many are printed on transparent plastic sheets, or have cutouts through which message recipients can monitor the patient's eye movements.

Mechanical and Electronic Devices.—Mechanical and electronic devices for augmenting or replacing speech differ in cost, complexity, portability, and output. They range in cost from less than $100.00 to several thousand dollars. They range in portability from small hand-held devices to large units that cannot be carried. The most common units are portable electronic devices that translate keyboard inputs into messages that are either displayed on electronic readouts, printed on paper tape, or translated into speech-like output. Some generate literal representations of what is entered on the keyboard, and what the auditor sees is what the user has entered. Other units translate codes entered by the user into programmed output messages; for example, a three-digit code entered by the user might generate a five- or six-word phrase. Many (especially the hand-held devices) require finger dexterity and coordination to operate keyboards, and most require that the user read, spell, or remember codes, making them unsuitable for use with most aphasic patients or patients with poor motor control.

Gesture and Pantomime.—Some dysarthric patients may be taught gesture or pantomime to augment speech, but usually other systems (communication boards, electronic devices) provide better communication.

Sign Languages.—Sign languages sometimes can be taught to patients who are not too aphasic to learn them. Sign languages that require spelling and syntactic abilities usually are less practical for brain-damaged persons than languages requiring less linguistic ability. *Amer-Ind* (American Indian sign) Skelly, 1979) contains signs that do not depend heavily on verbal skills. Consequently, they can be learned by some patients with linguistic impairments. Most Amer-Ind signs are comprehensible to message recipients without extensive training. A major problem with many sign languages is that the signs are not comprehensible to message recipients without training, so patients who use them cannot communicate with untrained persons.

Silverman (1983) has discussed other considerations when one is choosing an alternative or augmentative system for a patient.

1. The *cost* of the system may be important when resources for purchasing it are limited.

2. The amount of *training* needed for the patient to learn to use the system may be important. If the system is to be a permanent replacement or augmentation for speech, then extensive training might be justified. If the system is for temporary use, or if an alternative means of communication is needed immediately, then systems requiring extensive training will not be appropriate.

3. *Interference,* or the extent to which using the system interferes with other activities, may be important. A system that requires the patient to sit at a terminal and use both hands to operate it would be more disruptive to other activities than a portable system that can be operated with one hand.

4. The *intelligibility* of the output of the system will affect both the time required to make it functional and the generality with which it can be used by the patient. Systems that generate output that is intelligible to untrained message recipients require less time to become operational and will be useful in more different places than systems producing symbols whose meanings message recipients must be taught. Systems that print messages on paper tape or in liquid crystal displays cannot be used in the dark, over the telephone, or when patient and auditor are more than a few feet apart. Systems that generate messages on illuminated displays can be used in the dark, but not over the telephone or at a distance. Systems that generate speech-like output may be unintelligible in noisy environments, and may not be intelligible over the telephone, depending on the fidelity of the system's output.

5. The *acceptability* of the system to user and message recipients is likely to affect the extent to which it will be used in daily life. If the device or system is too cumbersome, complicated, or unnatural, it may be discarded in favor of less cumbersome (and less effective) ways to communicate.

Providing a patient with a system to augment or replace speech requires (1) careful assessment of the patient's communicative needs and physical and mental capabilities; (2) selection of the best system for the patient, based on the relationships between the patient's communicative needs, the patient's abilities, and the characteristics of the system; (3) training the patient to use the system; (4) training those around the patient to help the patient use the system efficiently; (5) periodic reassessment, to ensure that the system is still appropriate for the patient and that the patient is still using the system.

Apraxia of Speech

NEUROPHYSIOLOGY OF THE APRAXIAS

Liepmann (1900) described two major categories of apraxia—*ideational apraxia* and *ideomotor apraxia*. Liepmann characterized *ideational apraxia* as a disruption of the *ideas* needed to *understand* the use of objects. Persons exhibiting ideational apraxia are unable to carry out movement sequences that lead to a given result (e.g., *2.* filling a pipe and lighting it). According to Liepmann, ideational apraxia is caused by damage in the left parietal lobe, and always affects both sides of the body. Patients with ideational apraxia are unable to carry out the movement sequences even if they are given real objects to use in the movements.

Ideomotor apraxia represents disruption of the *plans* needed to *demonstrate* actions. According to Liepmann, ideomotor apraxia is caused by frontal lobe damage, and the apraxia may be either unilateral or bilateral. Patients with ideomotor apraxia *2.* usually can carry out movement sequences if they are given real objects to use in the movements. Several varieties of ideomotor apraxia have been identified, including *buccofacial apraxia, limb apraxia,* and *apraxia of speech.* (A fourth, so-called *dressing apraxia* sometimes seen in right hemisphere pathology, is not a true apraxia.)

In *buccofacial apraxia* (oral nonverbal apraxia) the patient is unable to execute *1.* volitional sequences of movements with the tongue, jaw, lips, and other oral structures. Buccofacial apraxia is tested by asking the patient to demonstrate movements such as whistling, blowing dust off a shelf, sucking up through a straw, and sniffing a flower. In *limb apraxia* the patient is unable to carry out sequences of preplanned *1.* volitional movements involving the arm, wrist, and hand. Limb apraxia usually is bilateral, but the presence of hemiplegia usually masks the limb apraxia on one side. Limb apraxia is more severe *distally* (away from the torso) than *proximally* (near the torso), so that patients with limb apraxia perform shoulder and elbow movements better than they perform wrist and finger movements. Limb apraxias are tested by asking the patient to demonstrate movement sequences such as flipping a coin, winding a watch, thumbing a ride, using a hammer, and waving good-bye.

For many years, the presence of apraxia was taken as evidence for damage in the premotor cortex, regarded as the center for motor planning. In recent years this view of the etiology of apraxia has been questioned. Buckingham (1979), for example, has postulated two different models for apraxia: the "center" model and the "disconnection" model. According to the "center" model (which Buckingham has called the "Mayo" model, because it was developed by Darley and associates at Mayo Clinic), apraxia is caused by damage to the cortical "center" for praxis. According to the "disconnection" model, apraxia is caused by disconnection of those parts of the left hemisphere that can comprehend spoken commands from those parts that can plan and carry out responses to the commands. Although patients with either kind of apraxia exhibit articulatory disturbances in speech, the key difference, according to Buckingham, is in their responses to nonverbal requests for movements of the "apraxic" body parts. Patients with "center" apraxia are unable to execute requested movements whether the movements are requested verbally or nonverbally (for example, by showing a picture depicting the requested movement) because the "center" for planning the movements is damaged. Patients with "disconnection" apraxia, on the other hand, are unable to perform movements in response to verbal requests, but will be able to do them if the requests are made nonverbally, because making the request nonverbally bypasses the pathways involved in transmission of the request from the language comprehension area.

Both sides of the body are routinely tested for limb apraxias, unless one side is paralyzed. The nondominant limb is tested first, because limb apraxia sometimes is unilateral, and if so the nondominant limb will be the unilaterally apractic one. If a patient were unilaterally apractic, and one tested the (unaffected) dominant limb first, the patient might then perform the movement sequence with the apractic nondominant limb by watching the performance of the dominant limb and mimicking it with the nondominant limb.

The relationship between dominance and unilateral apraxia is explainable by a connectionistic model. According to this model, the left hemisphere pathways from the primary auditory cortex to Wernicke's area and via the arcuate fasciculus to the premotor and motor cortex are crucial for performing motor movements in response to spoken commands. (In order to keep things simple, the patient is assumed to be right-handed.)

According to the model, the spoken request for a movement is perceived at the primary auditory cortex (Fig 12–1, *1*). The message then goes to Wernicke's area (*2*) where its meaning is deduced. A response to the message then goes, via the arcuate fasciculus to the premotor cortex (*3*), where the plan for the requested movement sequence is drawn up. If the patient is to carry out the movement sequence with the right hand and arm, the plan is sent from the premotor cortex to the primary motor cortex in the left hemisphere (*4*). If the patient is to carry out the movement sequence with his or her left hand, then the plan is sent from the left hemisphere premotor cortex across the corpus callosum to the motor cortex in the right hemisphere (*5*). (The left premotor area for the hand and arm apparently plans movement sequences for both sides of the body, just as Broca's area seems to plan all speech movements.)

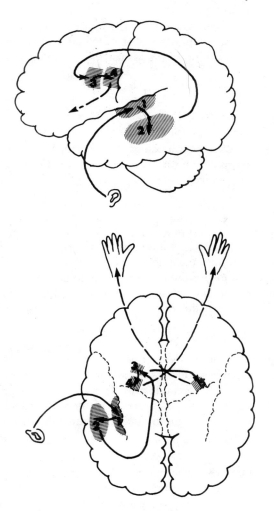

FIG 12–1.
A connectionistic explanation for apraxia. The spoken command is perceived by the primary auditory cortex *(1)*, comprehended by Wernicke's area *(2)*, sent via the arcuate fasciculus to Broca's area *(3)*, where the plan for the movements is formulated and sent to the primary motor cortex. If the movement is to be carried out by the opposite limb, the plan is sent to the motor cortex in the same hemisphere *(5)*. If the movement is to be carried out by the limb on the same side, the plan is sent across the corpus callosum to the motor cortex in the other hemisphere.

Destruction of Wernicke's area, interruption of the pathway that carries information from Wernicke's area to the premotor area, or destruction of the left premotor area causes bilateral limb apraxia, because the motor cortex in both hemispheres is cut off from the message. If the pathways from the left primary auditory cortex through the left premotor cortex are spared, but the crossing fibers that connect the premotor cortex in the left hemisphere with the motor cortex in the right hemisphere are interrupted, then unilateral apraxia of the left hand occurs, because the left hand is isolated from both the meaning of the instructions and the motor plans for the response.

DIAGNOSIS OF APRAXIA

In arriving at a diagnosis of apraxia, the examiner must be careful to exclude other possible explanations for the movement disabilities observed. Alternative explanations include the following.

Paralysis or Weakness.—Apractic individuals usually can perform movements when they are unplanned, when they are a spontaneous response to natural occurrences in the environment, or when they occur as parts of automatic movement sequences. The presence of automatic and unplanned movements rules out weakness and paralysis as explanations for the disorder. The apractic patient may be unable to show the examiner how one would use a hammer when asked to pretend that he is using it, but usually performs the movements when given a hammer, some nails, and a board.

Sensory Loss.—Absent or decreased sensation in the body parts involved should make the examiner cautious about diagnosing apraxia, especially if the movements do not appear in their unplanned, automatic form. Sensory loss, by itself, is probably not a likely explanation for movement disorders, including apraxia. However, its presence demands that the examiner exclude it as a potential cause for what seems to be an apraxia.

Comprehension Deficit.—The examiner must be certain that inability to comprehend the instructions used in testing for apraxia is not misinterpreted as apraxia. One can estimate a patient's comprehension and at the same time test his or her "knowledge" of the movement pattern by demonstrating a series of different movement sequences, asking the patient with each sequence, "Am I [for example] using a hammer?" If the patient responds appropriately to such questions, one can assume that auditory comprehension and knowledge of the movements requested are good enough to eliminate them as explanations for any movement disabilities observed.

Incoordination.—Patients with incoordination generally will perform requested movement sequences, but with clumsiness and distortion. These patients can be distinguished from those exhibiting apraxia by the consistent presence of clumsiness and incoordination in unplanned, automatic movements, and by clumsiness and distortion of movements in activities such as walking or movements that involve proximal muscles.

EVALUATING PATIENTS WITH APRAXIA OF SPEECH

Error Patterns in Apraxia of Speech

Articulation.—Darley et al. (1975) and Wertz et al. (1984b), among others, have described error patterns that are characteristic of apraxia of speech. These error patterns define relationships between articulatory or linguistic characteristics and error probabilities. Knowledge of these relationships is important when treatment activities for apractic speakers are formulated.

Wertz et al. (1984b) describe the following error patterns: (1) Substitution errors are more frequent than distortion, omission, or addition errors. Many substitution errors involve substituting a more difficult sound for an easier one. However, recent physiologic and acoustic studies of voice onset, phoneme duration, and movement patterns suggest that what listeners perceive as substitutions may actually be extreme phonetic distortion errors (Kearns and Simmons, 1988). (2) Errors are more likely to be errors in placement of the articulators than errors of voicing, manner, or resonance. (3) Most errors resemble the target sound. (4) Consonant clusters are more likely to be in error than single consonants. (5) Front-of-the-mouth sounds (labial and alveolar sounds) are more likely to be correct than sounds produced at other locations.

Wertz et al. (1984b) suggest that the following characteristics are true for apractic speakers as a group but may not always be true for a given apractic speaker: (1) Voiceless sounds are more frequently substituted for voiced sounds than vice versa. (2) *Anticipatory errors* (producing a sound before it occurs in a word or phrase, as in "thoothbrush" for "toothbrush") usually are more frequent than either *perseverative errors* (saying a sound again, later in a word or phrase, when it is not appropriate, as in "manina" for "manila") or *metathetic errors* (transposition of adjacent sounds, as in "tevelision" for "television"). (3) Consonant errors are more frequent than vowel errors.

Consistency.—Darley et al. (1975), Wertz et al. (1984b), Kearns and Simmons (1988) and others have identified articulatory inconsistency as one of the hallmarks of apraxia of speech. This inconsistency is seen (heard) as correct articulation of given phonemes at one time and incorrect articulation of the same phonemes at another. Inconsistency in articulation often is related to variations in the context in which the phonemes are produced. A given phoneme may be articulated correctly in one phonemic context (e.g., when the same phoneme is repeated in words or phrases, as in "*D*on did the *d*ishes"), and misarticulated in another (e.g., when contrasting phonemes occur in words or phrases, as in "*D*on bought the *d*ishes"). Apractic patients' articulation characteristically is better in naturalistic situations than in artificial ones. An apractic patient's articulation of "good-bye" is likely to be better when he is actually leaving than when he is asked by a clinician to say it in the middle of a treatment session. This phenomenon is related to what Darley et al. (1975) referred to as "islands of fluent, error-free speech," in which the patient produces occasional fluent words, phrases, or sentences in the midst of effortful, struggling speech. Such periods of fluent speech in an overall context of nonfluency help to differentiate apraxia of speech from the dysarthrias, in which such intermittent periods of correct articulation do not occur.*

Apraxia of Speech Versus Aphasia.—Apraxia of speech in its pure form, unaccompanied by aphasia, is very rare. It most often occurs in association with nonfluent (Broca's) aphasia, and, in fact, descriptions of the speech output of patients with Broca's aphasia usually resemble those for apraxia of speech (Goodglass and Kaplan, 1983a; Wertz et al., 1984b). When apraxia of speech accompanies Broca's aphasia, the patient's speech often is *agrammatic* as well as apractic; that is, "function" words (articles, conjunctions, prepositions, verb auxiliaries, and grammatical morphemes) are left out, and the patient's speech consists primarily of "content" words (nouns, verbs, adjectives, adverbs), giving their speech a "telegraphic" character. A patient with Broca's aphasia produced the following speech sample when talking about the attempted assassination of President Reagan.

> Um. . .Reagan. . . .um. . . .President. . . .Reagan. . . .shod. . . .was. . .
> shod. . .um. . .yestuhday. . .um. .um. . . .New Yoak Cidy. . .uh. . . .
> hospidal. . .be oh-kay. . . .nod bad. . .

TREATMENT OF APRAXIA OF SPEECH

General Concepts

Patients with apraxia of speech have difficulty organizing and carrying out sequential speech movements. Most patients with significant apraxia of speech are also aphasic, with problems comprehending and formulating language. Consequently, a test battery for apractic patients should include language tests, and treatment of language impairments often is carried out concurrently with treatment for apraxia of speech. Treatment of apractic patients' speech production impairments will be discussed in this section. Treatment of their language impairments resembles treatment of language impairments for patients who are aphasic but not apractic, discussed elsewhere in this book.

According to Rosenbek and Wertz (1972), treatment for patients with apraxia of speech should:

> Concentrate on the disordered articulation and, therefore, be different from the language stimulation and auditory and visual processing therapies appropriate to the aphasias† . . . . Emphasize the relearning of adequate points of articulation and the sequencing of articulatory gestures. . . . Provide conditions such that the apraxic patient can advance from limited, automatic-reactive speech to appropriate, volitional purposive communication.

---

*The primary exceptions are dysarthrias accompanying cerebellar ataxia and some dysarthrias caused by extrapyramidal disease.

†Rosenbek and Wertz were addressing treatment of apraxia per se. This does not imply that "therapies appropriate to the aphasias" are not appropriate for patients who are both apractic and aphasic.

It is important that many (probably most) apractic speakers can produce individual sounds and one-syllable words correctly, but that their problems arise when they *8.* must create sequential articulatory movements. As the number of syllables in an utterance increases and as the articulatory complexity of utterances increases, so does the effortfulness and struggle of the patient's speech behavior.

Apraxic speakers' problems are not caused by inability to hear or discriminate the sounds of speech. Consequently, it is unnecessary and unproductive to provide "ear training" or "auditory discrimination training" for patients with apraxia of speech. Early studies of apractic speakers suggested that they often were deficient in oral sensation and oral form identification (Guilford and Hawk, 1968; Larimore, *10.* 1970; Rosenbek et al., 1973b), but subsequent studies have failed to support these conclusions (Deutsch, 1981; Square and Weidner, 1976). The evidence suggests that sensory anomalies may coexist with apraxia of speech, but are not strongly related to its severity. Consequently, work on oral sensation is unlikely to be of much help to these patients.

Candidacy for Treatment

Apraxia of speech can occur in isolation (a rare occurrence) but usually it occurs in combination with aphasia that ranges anywhere from mild to severe. Whether an apractic patient will benefit from treatment depends both on the severity of his or her *11.* apraxia and the severity of any accompanying aphasia. The more severe the impairments are (beyond the first 3 or 4 weeks postonset), the poorer the prognosis for recovery. Patients who, a month or more postonset, have no volitional speech, emit stereotypic speech responses ("mi-mi-mi," "fa-la-fa-la," etc.), and are severely aphasic are unlikely to recover functional speaking abilities, even with extensive treatment.

Patients With Severe Apraxia of Speech

Characteristics at Intake.—Patients with severe apraxia of speech usually have no volitional speech. Many emit stererotypic speech responses during the first month or two postonset. These stereotypic responses usually disappear by 2 months postonset, unless the patient is severely aphasic. Most patients with severe apraxia of speech also exhibit moderate to severe buccofacial and limb apraxia. They are almost always hemiparetic or hemiplegic, and most are at least moderately aphasic.

Progression of Treatment.—Treatment of severely apractic patients begins at elemental levels. Many cannot phonate voluntarily. Most of those who can phonate *12* cannot modify their phonation to produce vowels, and few can produce consonant-vowel syllables. Consequently, early stages of treatment usually are concerned with developing volitional vocalization and a small repertoire of vowels and consonant-vowel syllables. Treatment procedures make use of phonetic placement (mechanical *13.* positioning of the patient's articulators), and phonetic derivation (deriving a new *13.* sound from one that the patient can make). Severely apractic speakers usually are

13. poor imitators. Consequently, imitation drills may not be appropriate, although integral stimulation ("Watch me and do what I do") may be useful in some cases. Some severely apractic speakers occasionally utter single words, but the words are likely to have little or no communicative value and are likely not to be under the speaker's volitional control. Helm and Barresi (1980) have suggested that such words can be *12.* incorporated into treatment activities and brought under the patient's control, and have described a program for incorporating such involuntary utterances into treatment.

Alternative communication devices (communication boards, communication books) frequently are necessary to provide a means of communication for patients *12'* with severe apraxia of speech, at least on a temporary basis. Severely apractic patients' use of gestural communication may also be emphasized and trained. Education and counseling of those who care for the patient are crucial aspects of treatment for severely apractic patients.

Outcome.— Only a small proportion of patients who remain severely apractic at 3 or more months postonset develop even rudimentary functional speech. In many of these cases, alternative communication systems may be appropriate. Patients with *13.* severe apraxia of speech who are also severely aphasic frequently are placed in nursing homes. For these patients, it may be particularly important to develop some form of rudimentary communication between the patient and those who care for him or her.

Patients With Moderate Apraxia of Speech

Characteristics at Intake.— Patients with moderate apraxia of speech usually have some volitional speech at 1 to 2 months postonset. These patients may emit *14b.* stereotypic utterances for a short time immediately after onset, but they disappear as the patient recovers. Many exhibit mild to moderate buccofacial and limb apraxia. Almost all are hemiparetic or hemiplegic. Mild to moderate aphasia often is present.

Progression of Treatment.— Because patients with moderate apraxia of speech usually have some volitional speech, treatment can begin at the syllable, word, or phrase level. These patients can be active participants in treatment — they are motivated to recover, they can work independently, and they can learn and generalize learning to new situations. They can collaborate with the clinician in setting goals and *Ha'* designing and carrying out treatment procedures, and they may take responsibility for independent practice. Patients with moderate apraxia of speech usually move quickly from single-syllable to multiple-syllable speech production. Consequently, treatment activities can emphasize volitional control of sequenced articulatory movements, along with manipulations of rate, pauses, and intonation.

Wertz et al. (1984b) recommend contrastive stress drills for the early phases of *Ha* treatment for patients with moderate apraxia of speech, and suggest that oral reading may be suitable in later phases of treatment. Relaxation training in conjunction with speech retraining may help many of these patients to speak better and with less effort. Many patients with moderate apraxia of speech can learn a problem-solving approach to communication, in which they (1) learn to anticipate difficult words and difficult speaking situations; (2) recognize communication failure when it occurs; and (3) respond to communication failure in a planned and systematic way.

Outcome.—Most patients with moderate apraxia of speech regain some functional speech. Many continue slow improvement in speech ability over many years, even after formal treatment has ended. Most return to their homes after discharge from the hospital, and most function independently in common daily life activities. A few, whose work does not depend heavily on speech, may return to work, but most will not.

Patients With Mild Apraxia of Speech

Many patients who exhibit only mild apraxia of speech by the end of the first month or so postonset spontaneously recover enough speech to be functional talkers in daily life. Most patients with mild apraxia of speech are only mildly aphasic, if they are aphasic at all. Patients with mild apraxia of speech usually profit from instruction in strategic approaches to communication and how best to deal with the inconveniences created by their communication disabilities.

Treatment usually involves repetition drills and formulation and production of phrases, sentences, and extended speech. The emphasis is on improving articulatory agility and accuracy and on developing appropriate prosody and rate. Patients with mild apraxia of speech almost always return home. Some may return to work. Almost all communicate independently in most daily life situations.

Stimulus Manipulations Affecting Response Accuracy in Apraxia of Speech

Visibility, Length, and Articulatory Complexity.—The visibility and articulatory complexity of speech movements strongly affect their difficulty for apractic speakers. More visible and less complex movements are easier for apractic speakers. Visibility and complexity interact to some extent, because more visible movements tend to be less motorically complex than less visible movements. As word length increases, the probablility of apractic speech errors also increases (Shankweiler and Harris, 1966; Johns and Darley, 1970), although short words with complex articulatory sequences may be more difficult than long words without complex sequences. Apractic errors seem to increase as the distance between successive points of articulation increases (Wertz et al., 1984b), although this last clinical observation has not been experimentally verified.

Rate and Delay.—In general, the faster the rate at which articulatory sequences must be produced, the more difficulty an apractic speaker will have in producing the sequences. If delay intervals are imposed between the clinician's model and the apractic speaker's opportunity to imitate the model, imitation usually is more difficult than if no delay is imposed.

Context.—The characteristics of the word or phrase in which a particular sound is located may affect the likelihood that it will be produced correctly by an apractic speaker. There is some evidence suggesting that the first sound in a word is more likely to be produced correctly than subsequent sounds (Shankweiler and Harris, 1966; Trost and Canter, 1974). However, others have failed to confirm this effect (Johns and Darley, 1970; LaPointe and Johns, 1975; Dunlop and Marquardt, 1977).

Prompting.—The nature of prompts (or "cues") provided to apractic patients is likely to affect their success in producing speech. In general, the probability of successful responses increases as more information about target responses is provided by the prompts or cues. Love and Webb (1977) studied the effects of four different prompts on picture naming by patients with Broca's aphasia (and apraxia of speech). The prompts were (1) the complete target word; (2) a sentence with the target word missing; (3) the first sound of the target word; and (4) the printed target word. They found that, on the average, providing the complete word was most successful in eliciting the target word. Providing the initial syllable was next most effective, followed by sentence completion and printed words, in that order. Each of these differences was statistically significant except the one between sentence completion and printed words. Love and Webb do not report whether individual subjects all generated the same hierarchy as the group (it is doubtful that they did). Furthermore, Love and Webb's subjects' may have been both apractic and aphasic, with word retrieval impairments complicating their attempts to produce spoken words (a probability to which Love and Webb allude). However, Love and Webb's results do show that prompts can have strong effects on the accuracy of apractic speakers' word retrieval and production of single words.

Rosenbek et al. (1973a) proposed an eight-step continuum of prompts for treatment of patients with apraxia of speech. The continuum gradually reduces the salience of prompts while gradually increasing reponse requirements.

1. The clinician and patient produce the target utterance in unison.
2. The clinician produces the target utterance. The patient then produces the utterance while the clinician silently mouths the utterance with the patient.
3. The clinician produces the utterance. The patient says the utterance.
4. The clinician produces the utterance. The patient says the utterance several times in succession.
5. The patient is given the target utterance printed on a card and reads it aloud.
6. The printed utterance is given to the patient to study and then is taken away. The patient then says the utterance.
7. The clinician asks a question that is answerable with the target utterance. The patient says the target utterance.
8. The clinician and patient interact in a role-playing situation in which given target utterances are appropriate. The patient says the target utterances at appropriate times.

Stimulus Modality.— Most treatment programs for apractic patients manipulate the modalities in which stimuli are delivered, although not all do so systematically. In spite of the frequently encountered claim that multimodality stimulation is better than unimodality stimulation, no experimental evidence exists to support it, and it almost certainly does not apply to *every* apractic patient seen for treatment.

Visual stimulation in apraxia treatment consists primarily of two techniques— the ubiquitous "watch me and do what I do" technique, and the use of mirrors (or sometimes videotapes) in which the patient watches himself or herself speak, with or without the clinician alongside. The former is almost always helpful. The latter may be helpful with some patients, but may be counterproductive with others.

Emphasizing the patient's attention to *tactile and kinesthetic stimuli* during speech may in many cases improve the accuracy of apractic patients' speech. (This does not imply that tactile stimulation by itself, outside of speech activity, is likely to be beneficial.)

Although the *auditory modality* is not usually written about in treatment of apraxia of speech (Wertz et al., 1984, is an exception), most treatment programs depend heavily on the patient's ability to listen to his or her own speech. Most clinicians spend little or no time training auditory discrimination as a separate skill. However, most encourage apractic patients to listen to themselves to tell when a given utterance is adequate (not necessarily "correct").

Meaningfulness.— In general, the more meaningful a given speech response is, the easier it will be for an apractic speaker. Consequently, most clinicians structure treatment around meaningful words, phrases, and sentences. However, Dabul and Bollier (1976) recommend that treatment for patients with apraxia of speech should begin by concentrating on production of *nonmeaningful* articulatory sequences in order to teach the patient volitional control of speech production before he or she attempts meaningful words. There is no conclusive evidence for either position. Majority opinion at this time seems to favor using real words as soon as possible.

Automacity.— Overlearned sequences (counting, reciting the alphabet, reciting the days of the week) may be surprisingly easy for some patients who are severely apractic. In such cases, repeated production of such sequences may help to increase oral agility and oral motor control in preparation for work on more volitional speech production.

Context.— The context in which a word is produced usually affects how difficult it is for an apractic patient to say. Placing a word in a frequently occurring phrase usually makes it easier. For example, the word "coffee" usually is easier if it is elicited by a phrase such as "I want a cup of _____." than if it is elicited by a picture. Situational context may also affect apractic speakers' success. Most speak better to friends and relatives (and speech clinicians) than they do to strangers. Most speak better face-to-face than on the telephone. Most speak better when they express their own knowledge, opinions, and wishes than they do when they must speak about things prescribed by others (by speech clinicians, for example).

Reorganization

Rosenbek et al. (1976) and Rosenbek (1978) have discussed the uses of two kinds of reorganization in treatment programs for patients with apraxia of speech—*intersystemic reorganization* and *intrasystemic reorganization*. In *intersystemic reorganization,* behaviors that are not ordinarily part of a given motor performance are introduced into the performance in order to improve it. For a patient with apraxia of speech, intersystemic reorganization may include activities such as tapping or pantomiming along with speech movements.

Rosenbek et al. (1976) proposed the following sequence of activities for intersystemic reorganization. First, a set of simple, meaningful, and easily recognizable gestures is compiled for the patient. The patient is taught to recognize each gesture and its verbal equivalent when they are produced by the clinician. Then the patient is taught to imitate the gesture. (Rosenbek et al. stress the importance of feedback from the clinician at this stage, because they have observed that many apractic patients have difficulty judging the adequacy of their own gestures.) During this stage the clinician may manipulate the patient's hand and arm to bring about the gesture, or the patient may be given real objects to use in the movement. When the patient can produce each gesture without effort, he or she is taught to combine each gesture with a word or phrase. When the patient can reliably and appropriately produce speech and gesture combinations both in and out of the clinic, the gestures may be gradually deemphasized. However, Rosenbek et al. recommend that even at this stage patients should be encouraged to continue using gestures for self-prompting and self-correction of errors. According to Rosenbek et al., patients who cannot learn gestures, those who cannot learn to pair gestural and speech responses, and those who are severely aphasic are not candidates for intersystemic reorganization. According to Rosenbek et al., patients who are severely aphasic usually do no better when treated with intersystemic reorganization than when they are treated with other procedures.

Intrasystemic reorganization is accomplished by using different components of the same system to produce or enhance movements, usually by shifting the locus of control from one level of the system to another. The shift in control usually is from automatic to volitional. The typist who slows down and types words syllable by syllable when typing unfamiliar or complicated words is employing intrasystemic reorganization to decrease errors. (The typist who subvocally spells the word is using intersystemic reorganization.) Many treatment activities for apractic patients qualify as intrasystemic reorganization, even though they are not labeled as such. Teaching patients to speak slowly and with consciously controlled articulatory movements is one example of intrasystemic reorganization. Teaching them to speak with exaggerated prosody and teaching them to concentrate on kinesthetic feedback during speech are two other examples.

There are no reliable data to support the efficacy of reorganization in eliciting speech from apractic patients, or in generating speech that apractic patients are likely to use in daily life communication, and there are no data comparing reorganization with other treatments. Anecdotal reports suggest that reorganization is effective in eliciting speech from many apractic patients, and that it makes meaningful changes in the daily life communicative ability of some of them.

Melodic Intonation Therapy

Melodic intonation therapy (MIT) (Sparks et al., 1974; Sparks and Holland, 1976) was designed to elicit speech from severely aphasic (and apractic) patients who have little or no volitional speech by increasing the participation of the nondominant hemisphere in speech activities. Melodic intonation therapy places the patient in structured drills in which phrases are produced with exaggerated stress, rhythm, and pitch, and the patient taps out the rhythm of each phrase as he or she produces it.

In MIT the patient is trained to utter propositional phrases and sentences, using sung intonation patterns that are similar to the natural intonation patterns of the spoken phrases or sentences. First, the clinician intones sentences and helps the patient tap the stress patterns of the sentences in unison with the clinician's utterances. Then, the patient and clinician intone the sentences and tap their stress patterns together. Finally, the clinician gradually fades his or her participation in production and tapping, until the patient is intoning and tapping them without assistance in response to the clinician's intoned model.

When the patient's simultaneous intonation and tapping have stabilized, speech production moves away from melody toward more natural prosody. First, there is a transition from melodic intonation to *sprechgesang* (speech song), in which words are no longer sung, but are spoken with exaggerated inflection. The next transition is from sprechgesang to spoken prosody.

According to Sparks et al. (1974), MIT is appropriate for patients with the following characteristics:

1. Auditory comprehension is better than verbal expression. (Spontaneous recognition and self-correction of errors by the patient is considered a favorable sign.)
2. The patient is emotionally stable and has good attention span.
3. The patient has severely impaired verbal output. He or she has little or no ability to name, repeat, or complete sentences.
4. The patient makes vigorous attempts at self-correction.
5. The patient emits clearly articulated, stereotyped utterances.

There are no controlled evaluations of the efficacy of MIT, either by itself or relative to other treatment approaches. Anecdotal reports suggest that MIT is effective in eliciting speech from patients who otherwise cannot produce volitional speech. The most significant problem with MIT appears to be extension of speech learned in the clinic to daily life. Little generalization of what patients learn in MIT to other activities usually occurs until the patient is in the final stages of MIT, and many patients do not make it to the final stages. (A particularly difficult transition seems to be the transition from sung phrases to sprechgesang.)

Many severely apractic patients never regain enough volitional speech to permit them to communicate even simple messages by talking. Nonspeech communication systems may help some of them to communicate with those around them. However, most severely apractic patients also have signficant aphasia, which may compromise their ability to use alternative communication systems that depend on verbal skills.

Some patients with apraxia of speech may learn gesture and pantomime as part of re-organization (Rosenbek, 1978). The gestures and pantomime may function both as a substitute for speech and as a facilitator for the patient's production of speech. Some patients with apraxia of speech may learn to use sign languages such as Amer-Ind, either temporarily as they are reacquiring speech or as a permanent substitute. Producing such signs may also facilitate speech through intersystemic reorganization. (See pages 269–272 for a discussion of alternative and augmentative communication systems.)

Bibliography

Adamovich BB, Brooks RA: A diagnostic protocol to assess the communication deficits of patients with right hemisphere damage, in Brookshire R (ed): *Clinical Aphasiology Conference Proceedings.* Minneapolis, BRK Publishers, 1981, pp 244–253.

Adams RD, Victor M: *Principles of Neurology.* New York, McGraw-Hill, 1981.

Albert ML, Feldman RG, Willis AL: The "subcortical dementia" of progressive supranuclear palsy. *J Neurol Neurosurg Psychiatry* 1974; 37:121–130.

Albert ML: A simple test of visual neglect. *Neurology* 1973; 23:658–664.

Albert ML, Goodglass H, Helm NA, et al: *Clinical Aspects of Dysphasia.* New York, Springer-Verlag, 1981.

Appell J, Kertesz A, Fishman M: A study of language functioning in Alzheimer patients. *Brain Lang* 1982; 17:73–81.

Barton M, Maruszewski M, Urrea D: Variation of stimulus context and its effect on word finding ability in aphasics. *Cortex* 1969; 5:351–365.

Basso A, Capitani E, Vignolo LA: Influence of rehabilitation on language skills in aphasic patients: A controlled study. *Arch Neurol* 1979; 36:190–196.

Bayles KA: Management of neurogenic communication disorders associated with dementia, in Chapey R (ed): *Language Intervention Strategies in Adult Aphasia,* ed 2. Baltimore, Williams and Wilkins, 1986.

Bayles KA, Kaszniak AW, Tomoeda C: *Communication and Cognition in Normal Aging and Dementia.* Boston, College-Hill, 1987.

Bayles KA, Tomoeda C: *Arizona Battery for Communication Disorders of Dementia (Research Edition).* Tuscon, Canyonlands Publishing, 1991.

Benson DF: Aphasia rehabilitation. *Arch Neurol* 1979; 36:187–189.

Benton AL: *The Revised Visual Retention Test,* ed 4. New York, Psychological Corporation, 1974.

Benton AL, Smith KC, Lang M: Stimulus characteristics and object naming in aphasic patients. *J Commun Disord* 1972; 5:19–24.

Bernstein-Ellis E, Wertz RT, Dronkers NF: PICA performance by traumatically brain injured and left hemisphere CVA patients, in Brookshire RH (ed): *Clinical Aphasiology Conference Proceedings.* Minneapolis, BRK Publishers, 1985.

Berry W: Treatment of hypokinetic dysarthria, in Perkins WH (ed): *Dysarthria and Apraxia.* New York, Thieme-Stratton, 1983, pp 91–99.

Bisiach E: Perceptual factors in the pathogenesis of anomia. *Cortex* 1966; 2:90–95.

Bluestone CD, Musgrave RH, McWilliams BJ, et al: Teflon injection pharyngoplasty. *Cleft Palate J* 1968; 5:19–26.

Boning RA: *Specific Skills Series.* Baldwin, NY, Barnell-Loft, 1976.

Borkowski JG, Benton AL, Spreen O: Word fluency and brain damage. *Neuropsychologia* 1967; 5:135–140.

Brenneise-Sarshad R, Nicholas LE, Brookshire RH: Effects of apparent listener knowledge on aphasic and non-brain-damaged speakers' narrative discourse. *J Speech Hear Disord* 1991; 56:168–176.

Brooks N: Closed head trauma: Assessing the common cognitive processes, in Lezak M (ed): *Assessment of the Behavioral Consequences of Head Trauma.* New York, AR Liss, 1989.

Brookshire RH: Effects of trial time and inter-trial interval on naming by aphasic subjects. *J Commun Disord* 1971; 3:289–301.

Brookshire RH: Effects of task difficulty on naming performance of aphasic subjects. *J Speech Hear Res* 1972; 15:551–558.

Brookshire RH: Consequences in speech pathology: Incentive and feedback functions. *J Commun Disord* 1973; 6:1–5.

Brookshire RH: Differences in responding to auditory verbal materials among aphasic patients. *Acta Symbolica* 1974; 3:1–17.

Brookshire RH: Effects of prompting on spontaneous naming of pictures by aphasic subjects. *J Can Speech Hear Assoc* 1975, autumn, pp 63–71.

Brookshire RH: Effects of task difficulty on sentence comprehension performance of aphasic subjects. *J Commun Disord* 1976; 9:167–173.

Brookshire RH: Auditory comprehension and aphasia. In Johns DF (ed): *Clinical Management of Neurogenic Communicative Disorders.* Boston, Little, Brown, 1978, pp 103–128.

Brookshire RH: *An Introduction to Aphasia,* ed 2. Minneapolis, BRK Publishers, 1979.

Brookshire RH, Krueger K, Nicholas L, et al: Analysis of clinician-patient interactions in aphasia treatment, in Brookshire RH (ed): *Clinical Aphasiology Conference Proceedings.* Minneapolis, BRK Publishers, 1977, pp 181–187.

Brookshire RH, Nicholas LE: Effects of clinician request and feedback behavior on responses of aphasic individuals in speech and language treatment sessions, in Brookshire RH (ed): *Clinical Aphasiology Conference Proceedings.* Minneapolis, BRK Publishers, 1978, pp 40–48.

Brookshire RH, Nicholas LE: Comprehension of directly and indirectly pictured verbs by aphasic and nonaphasic listeners, in Brookshire RH (ed): *Clinical Aphasiology Conference Proceedings.* Minneapolis, BRK Publishers, 1982, pp 200–206.

Brookshire RH, Nicholas LE: Comprehension of directly and indirectly stated main ideas and details in discourse by brain–damaged and non-brain-damaged listeners. *Brain Lang* 1984a; 21:21–36.

Brookshire RH, Nicholas LE: Consistency of the effects of slow rate and pauses on aphasic listeners' comprehension of spoken sentences. *J Speech Hear Res,* 1984b, 27:323–328.

Brookshire RH, Nicholas LE: Consistency of the effects of rate of speech on brain-damaged subjects' comprehension of information in narrative discourse, in Brookshire RH (ed): *Clinical Aphasiology.* Minneapolis, BRK Publishers, 1985, vol 15, pp 262–271.

Brookshire RH, Nicholas LE, Krueger KM: Sampling of speech pathology treatment activities: An evaluation of momentary and interval sampling procedures. *J Speech Hear Res* 1978; 21:652–667.

Brownell H, Potter HH, Bihrle AM, et al: Influence of deficits in right-brain-damaged patients. *Brain Lang* 1986; 27:310–321.

Bryan KL: *The Right Hemisphere Language Battery.* Leicester, England, Far Communications, 1989.

Bryden MP, Ley RG: Right hemispheric involvement in imagery and affect, in Penecman E (ed): *Cognitive Processing in the Right Hemisphere.* New York, Academic Press, 1983.

Buckingham HW: Explanation in apraxia with consequences for the concept of apraxia of speech. *Brain Lang* 1979; 8:202–226.

Burns MS, Halper AS, Mogil SI: *Clinical Management of Right Hemisphere Dysfunction.* Rockville, Md, Aspen, 1985.

Busch C, Brookshire RH: Aphasic adults' auditory comprehension of yes-no questions. 1982, unpublished manuscript.

Butfield E, Zangwill OL: Re-education in aphasia: A review of 70 cases. *J Neurol Neurosurg Psychiatry* 1946; 9:75–79.

Canter GJ: Dysarthria, apraxia of speech, and literal paraphasia: Three distinct varieties of articulatory behaviors in the adult with brain damage. Presented at the annual convention of the American Speech and Hearing Association, Detroit, 1973.

Caplan LR: *Stroke.* CIBA Clinical Symposia, Summit, NJ, CIBA Pharmaceutical Company, 1988.

Cappa SF, Cavalotti G, Guidotti M, et al: Subcortical aphasia: Two clinical CT-scan correlation studies. *Cortex* 1983; 19:227–242.

Cappa SF, Cavalotti G, Vignolo L: Phonemic and lexical errors in fluent aphasia: Correlation with lesion site. *Neuropsychologia* 1981; 19:171–177.

Cappa SF, Vignolo LA: "Transcortical" features of aphasia following left thalamic hemorrhage. *Cortex* 1979; 15:121–130

Caramazza A: The logic of neuropsychological research and the problem of patient classification in aphasia. *Brain Lang* 1984; 21:9–20.

Caramazza A, Zurif EB: Dissociation of algorithmic and heuristic processes in language comprehension: Evidence from aphasia. *Brain Lang* 1976; 3:572–582.

Carrow E: *Test for Auditory Comprehension of Language.* Boston, Teaching Resources Corporation, 1973.

Carrow E: *Test for Auditory Comprehension of Language.* Boston, Teaching Resources Corporation, 1984.

Carrow-Woodfolk E: *Test for Auditory Comprehension of Language.* Allen, Tex, DLM Teaching Resources, 1985.

Chall JS: *Stages of Reading Development.* New York, McGraw-Hill, 1983.

Chapey R: The assessment of language disorders in adults, in Chapey R (ed): *Language Intervention Strategies in Adult Aphasia,* ed 2. Baltimore, Williams & Wilkins, 1986.

Chapey R, Rigrodsky S, Morrison EB: Aphasia: A divergent semantic interpretation. *J Speech Hear Disord* 1977; 42:287–295.

Cicone M, Wapner W, Gardner H: Sensitivity to emotional expressions and situations in organic patients. *Brain Lang* 1980; 16:145–158.

Clark HH, Haviland SE: Comprehension and the given-new contract, in Freedle RO (ed): *Discourse Comprehension and Production.* Norwood, NJ, Ablex, 1977.

Cohn R, Neumann MS, Wood NH: Prosopagnosia: A clinicopathological study. *Ann Neurol* 1977; 1:177–182.

Collins M: *Diagnosis and Treatment of Global Aphasia.* San Diego, College-Hill, 1986.

Collins M: *Global Aphasia.* San Diego, College-Hill Press, 1990.

Corlew MM, Nation JE: Characteristics of visual stimuli and naming performance in aphasic adults. *Cortex* 1975; 11:186–191.

Correia L, Brookshire RH, Nicholas LE: Aphasic and non-brain-damaged adults' descriptions of aphasia test pictures and gender-biased pictures. *J Speech Hear Disord* 1990; 55:713–720.

Craik FI, Lockhart RS: Levels of processing: A framework for memory research. *J Verbal Learn Verbal Behav* 1972; 11:671–684.

Croft CB, Shprintzen RJ, Rakoff SJ: Patterns of velopharyngeal valving in normal and cleft palate subjects: A multi-view videofluoroscopic and nasendoscopic study. *Laryngoscope* 1981; 91:265–271.

Culton GL: Spontaneous recovery from aphasia. *J Speech Hear Res* 1969; 12:825–832.

Cummings JL: Cortical dementias, in Benson DF, Blumer D (eds): *Psychiatric Aspects of Neurologic Disease.* New York, Grune and Stratton, 1983.

Cummings JL, Benson DF: *Dementia: A Clinical Approach.* Boston, Butterworths, 1983.

Dabul B, Bollier B: Therapeutic approaches to apraxia. *J Speech Hear Disord* 1976; 41:268–276.

Darley FL: *Evaluation of Appraisal Techniques in Speech and Language Pathology.* Reading, Mass, Addison-Wesley, 1979.

Darley FL, Aronson AE, Brown JR: *Motor Speech Disorders.* Philadelphia, WB Saunders, 1975.

Davis GA, Wilcox MJ: *Adult Aphasia Rehabilitation: Language Pragmatics.* San Diego, College-Hill, 1985.

Deal JL, Deal LA: Efficacy of aphasia rehabilitation:Preliminary results, in Brookshire RH (ed): *Clinical Aphasiology Conference Proceedings.* Minneapolis, BRK Publishers, 1978, pp 66–77.

Delis DC, Wapner W, Gardner H, et al: The contribution of the right hemisphere to the organization of paragraphs. *Cortex* 1983; 19:43–50.

DeRenzi E, Faglioni P, Previdi P: Increased susceptibility of aphasics to a distractor task in the recall of verbal commands. *Brain Lang* 1978; 6:14–21.

DeRenzi E, Ferrari C: The Reporter's Test: A sensitive test to detect expressive disturbances in aphasics. *Cortex* 1978; 14:279–283.

DeRenzi E, Vignolo LA: The Token Test: A sensitive test to detect receptive disturbances in aphasics. *Brain* 1962; 85:665–678.

Deutsch SE: Oral form identification as a measure of cortical sensory dysfunction in apraxia of speech and aphasia. *J Commun Dis* 1981; 14:65–71.

Dewitt LD, Grek AJ Buonanno FS, et al: MRI and the study of aphasia. *Neurology* 1985; 35:861–865.

Diggs CC, Basili AG: Verbal expression of right CVA patients. *Brain Lang* 1987; 30:130–147.

Diller L, Weinberg J: Differential aspects of attention in brain-damaged persons. *Percept Mot Skills* 1977; 35:71–81.

Doyle P, Goldstein H, Bourgeois M: Experimental analysis of syntax training in Broca's aphasia: A generalization and social validation study. *J Speech Hear Disord* 1987; 52:143–155.

Dunlop JM, Marquardt TP: Linguistic and articulatory aspects of single word production in apraxia of speech. *Cortex* 1977; 13:17–29.

Dunn LM: *Peabody Picture Vocabulary Test*. Circle Pines, Minn, American Guidance Service, 1965.

Dunn LM, Markwardt FC: *Peabody Individual Achievement Test*. Circle Pines, Minn, American Guidance Service, 1970.

Dworkin JP, Johns DF: Management of velopharyngeal incompetence in dysarthria: A review. *Clin Otolaryngol* 1980; 5:61–74.

Efron R: Temporal perception, aphasia, and déjà vu. *Brain* 1963; 86:403–423.

Eisenberg HM, Weiner RL: Input variables: How information from the acute injury can be used to characterize groups of patients for studies of outcome, in Levin HS, Grafman J, Eisenberg HM (eds): *Neurobehavioral Recovery From Head Injury*. New York, Oxford University Press, 1987.

Eisenson J: *Examining for Aphasia*. New York, The Psychological Corporation, 1954.

Eisenson J: *Adult Aphasia: Assessment and Treatment*. New York, Appleton-Century-Crofts, 1973.

Eisenson J: Personal communication, 1990.

Faber MM, Aten FL: Verbal performance in aphasic patients in response to intact and altered pictorial stimuli, in Brookshire RH (ed): *Clinical Aphasiology Conference Proceedings*. Minneapolis, BRK Publishers, 1979, pp 177–186.

Friedman WA: *Head Injuries*. CIBA Clinical Symposia, Summit, NJ, CIBA Pharmaceutical Company, 1983.

Froeschels E: A contribution to pathology and therapy of dysarthria due to certain cortical lesions. *J Speech Hear Disord* 1943; 8:301–321.

Froeschels E: Chewing method as therapy. *Arch Otolaryngol* 1952; 61:427–435.

Gainotti G, Tiacci C: Patterns of drawing disability in left and right hemisphere patients. *Neuropsychologia* 1970; 8:379–384.

Gardner H, Albert ML, Weintraub S: Comprehending a word: The influence of speed and redundancy on auditory comprehension in aphasia. *Cortex* 1975; 11:155–162.

Gardner H, Brownell HH, Wapner W, et al: Missing the point: The role of right hemisphere in the processing of complex linguistic materials, in Perecman E (ed): *Cognitive Processing in the Right Hemisphere.* New York, Academic Press, 1983.

Gleason JB, Goodglass H, Green E, et al: The retrieval of syntax in Broca's aphasia. *Brain Lang* 1975; 2:451–471.

Gloning I, Gloning K, Haub C, et al: Comparison of verbal behavior in right-handed and non-right-handed patients with anatomically verified lesion of one hemisphere. *Cortex* 1969; 5:43–52.

Goldman R, Fristoe M, Woodcock RW: *Goldman-Fristoe-Woodcock Test of Auditory Discrimination.* Circle Pines, Minn, American Guidance Service, 1970.

Gonzalez J, Aronson A: Palatal lift prosthesis for treatment of anatomic and neurologic palatopharyngeal insufficiency. *Cleft Palate J* 1970; 7:91–104.

Goodglass H, Blumstein SE, Gleason JB, et al: The effect of syntactic encoding on sentence comprehension in aphasia. *Brain Lang* 1979; 7:201–209.

Goodglass H, Kaplan E: *The Boston Naming Test.* Philadelphia, Lea and Febiger, 1983a.

Goodglass H, Kaplan E: *The Boston Diagnostic Aphasia Examination.* Philadelphia, Lea and Febiger, 1972.

Goodglass H, Kaplan E: *The Boston Diagnostic Aphasia Examination.* Philadelphia, Lea and Febiger, 1983b.

Goodglass H, Kaplan E, Weintraub S, et al: The tip of the tongue phenomenon in aphasia. *Cortex* 1976; 12:145–153.

Goodglass H, Stuss DT: Naming to picture versus description in three aphasia subgroups. *Cortex* 1979; 15:199–211.

Gordon MC: Some effects of stimulus presentation rate and complexity on perception and retention in brain-damaged patients. *Cortex* 1970; 6:273–286.

Gordon WA, Ruckdeschel-Hibard M, Egelko S, et al: *Evaluation of the Deficits Associated With Right Brain Damage: Normative Data on the Institute of Rehabilitation Medicine Test Battery.* New York, Department of Behavioral Sciences, NYU Medical Center, 1984.

Graham DI, Adams JH, Doyle D: Ischemic brain damage in fatal non-missile head injuries. *J Neurol Sci* 1978; 39:213.

Graham RK, Kendall BS: The memory for designs test: Revised general manual. *Percept Mot Skills (Suppl)* 1960; 11:147–188.

Grant DA, Berg EA: A behavioral analysis of degree of reinforcement and ease of shifting to new responses in a Weigl-type card sorting problem. *J Exp Psychol* 1948; 38:404–411.

Gray L, Hoyt P, Mogil S, et al: A comparison of clinical tests of yes/no questions in aphasia, in Brookshire RH (ed): *Clinical Aphasiology Conference Proceedings.* Minneapolis, BRK Publishers, 1977, pp 265–268.

Guilford AM, Hawk AM: A comparative study of form identification in neurologically impaired and normal subjects. *Speech and Hearing Science Research Reports.* Ann Arbor, Mich, University of Michigan, 1968.

Hagen C, Malkamus D: Interaction strategies for language disorders secondary to head trauma. Presented at the American Speech-Language-Hearing Association, Atlanta, 1979.

Halpern H, Darley FL, Brown JR: Differential language and neurologic characteristics in cerebral involvement. *J Speech Hear Disord* 1973; 38:162–173.

Hammill DD: *Detroit Test of Learning Aptitudes.* Austin, Tex, Pro-Ed, 1966.

Hand CR, Burns MO, Ireland E: Treatment of hypertonicity in muscles of lip retraction. *Biofeedback Self Regul* 1979; 4:171–176.

Hanna G, Schell LM, Schreiner R: *The Nelson Reading Skills Test.* Chicago, Riverside Publishing Company, 1977.

Hardy JC, Rembolt RR, Spreisterbach DC, et al: Surgical management of palatal paresis and speech problems in cerebral palsy. *J Speech Hearing Disord* 1961; 26:320–327.

Haskins S: A treatment procedure for writing disorders, in Brookshire RH (ed): *Clinical Aphasiology Conference Proceedings.* Minneapolis, BRK Publishers, 1976; pp 192–199.

Heath PD, Kennedy P, Kapur N: Slowly progressive aphasia without generalized dementia. *Ann Neurol* 1983; 13:687–688.

Hecaen H, Angelergues R: Agnosia for faces. *Arch Neurol* 1962; 7:92–100.

Hecaen H, Assal G: A comparison of constructive deficits following left and right hemisphere lesions. *Neuropsychologia* 1970; 8:289–303.

Heilman KM, Watson RT, Valenstein E: Neglect and related disorders, in Heilman K, Valenstein E (eds): *Clinical Neuropsychology,* ed 2. New York, Oxford University Press, 1985.

Helm NA, Barresi B: Voluntary control of involuntary utterances: A treatment approach for severe aphasia, in Brookshire RH (ed): *Clinical Aphasiology Conference Proceedings.* Minneapolis, BRK Publishers, 1980, pp 308–315.

Helm-Estabrooks NA: "Show me the . . . whatever": Some variables affecting auditory comprehension scores of aphasic patients, in Brookshire RH (ed): *Clinical Aphasiology Conference Proceedings.* Minneapolis, BRK Publishers, 1981, pp 105–107.

Helm-Estabrooks N, Ramsberger G, Morgan AR et al: *Boston Assessment of Severe Aphasia.* Tuscon: Communication Skill Builders, 1989.

Hixon TJ: *Respiratory Function in Speech and Song.* San Diego, College-Hill, 1987.

Hixon TJ, Hawley JL, Wilson JL: An around-the-house device for the clinical determination of respiratory driving pressure. *J Speech Hear Disord* 1982; 47:413–415.

Holland AL: Some practical considerations in aphasia rehabilitation, in Sullivan M, Kommers MS (eds): *Rationale for Adult Aphasia Therapy.* Lincoln, Nebraska, University of Nebraska Medical Center, 1977.

Holland AL: *Communicative Abilities in Daily Living.* Baltimore, University Park Press, 1980.

Holland AL, McBurney DH, Moossy J, et al: The dissolution of language in Pick's disease with neurofibrillary tangles: A case study. *Brain Lang* 1985; 24:36–58.

Hooper HE: *The Hooper Visual Organization Test Manual.* Los Angeles, Western Psychological Services, 1958.

Hooper HE: *The Hooper Visual Organization Test.* Los Angeles, Western Psychological Services, 1983.

Horner J, LaPointe LL: Evaluation of learning potential of a severe aphasic adult through analysis of five performance variables, in Brookshire RH (ed): *Clinical Aphasiology Conference Proceedings.* Minneapolis, BRK Publishers, 1979, pp 101–114.

Jastak S, Wilkinson GS: *Wide Range Achievement Test—R.* Wilmington, Del, Jastak Associates, 1984.

Jennett B: Assessment of the severity of head injury. *J Neurol Neurosurg Psychiatry* 1976; 39:647–655.

Jerger J, Weikers N, Sharbrough F, et al: Bilateral lesions of the temporal lobe: A case study. *Acta Otolaryngol (Stockh)* 1969; 258:1–51.

Johns D (ed): *Clinical Management of Neurogenic Communication Disorders.* Boston, Little, Brown, 1985.

Johns DF, Darley FL: Phonemic variability in apraxia of speech. *J Speech Hear Res* 1970; 13:556–583.

Johns DF, LaPointe LL: Neurogenic disorders of output processing: Apraxia of speech, in Whitaker H, Whitaker HA (eds): *Studies in Neurolinguistics*. New York, Academic Press, 1976, vol 1, pp 161–200.

Kaplan E, Goodglass H, Weintraub S: *The Boston Naming Test*. Philadelphia, Lea and Febiger, 1983.

Kay T, Silver SM: Closed head trauma: Assessment for rehabilitation, in Lezak M (ed): *Assessment of the Behavioral Consequences of Head Trauma*. New York, AR Liss, 1989.

Kazdin AE: *Single-Case Research Designs: Methods for Clinical and Applied Settings*. New York, Oxford University Press, 1982.

Kearns K, Hubbard DJ: A comparison of auditory comprehension tasks in aphasia, in Brookshire RH (ed): *Clinical Aphasiology Conference Proceedings*. Minneapolis, BRK Publishers, 1977, pp 32–45.

Kearns KP, Salmon SJ: An experimental analysis of auxiliary and copula verb generalization in aphasia. *J Speech Hear Disord* 1984, 49:152–163.

Kearns KP, Simmons NN: Group therapy for aphasia: A survey of VA Medical Centers, in Brookshire RH (ed): *Clinical Aphasiology Conference Proceedings*. Minneapolis, BRK Publishers, 1985, pp 176–183.

Kearns KP, Simmons NN: Motor speech disorders: The dysarthrias and apraxia of speech, in Lass NJ, McReynolds LV, Northern JL, et al (eds): *Handbook of Speech-Language Pathology and Audiology*. Philadelphia, BC Decker, 1988.

Keenan JS, Brassel EG: *Aphasia Language Performance Scales*. Murfreesboro, Tenn, Pinnacle Press, 1975.

Kertesz A: *Aphasia and Associated Disorders: Taxonomy, Localization, and Recovery*. New York, Grune and Stratton, 1979.

Kertesz A: *Western Aphasia Battery*. New York, Grune and Stratton, 1982.

Kertesz A: Personal communication, 1990.

Kimelman MDZ, McNeil MR: An investigation of emphatic stress comprehension in aphasia: A replication. *J Speech Hear Res* 1987; 30:295–300.

Kintsch W: *The Representation of Meaning in Memory*. Hillsdale, NJ, Lawrence Erlbaum, 1974.

Knopman DS, Selnes OA, Niccum N, et al: Recovery of naming in aphasia: Relationship to fluency, comprehension, and CT findings. *Neurology* 1984; 34:1461–1470.

Knopman D, Selnes OA, Niccum N, et al: A longitudinal study of speech fluency in aphasia: CT correlates of recovery and persistent nonfluency. *Neurology* 1983; 33:1170–1178.

Kreindler A, Gheorghita N, Voinescu I: Analysis of verbal reception of a complex order with three elements in aphasics. *Brain* 1971; 94:375–386.

LaPointe LL: Base-10 programmed stimulation: Task specification, scoring, and plotting performance in aphasia therapy. *J Speech Hear Disord* 1977; 42:90–105.

LaPointe LL, Johns DF: Some phonemic characteristics in apraxia of speech. *J Commun Disord* 1975; 8:259–269.

LaPointe LL, Holtzapple P, Graham LF: The relationship among two measures of auditory comprehension and daily living communication skills, in Brookshire RH (ed): *Clinical Aphasiology Conference Proceedings*. Minneapolis, BRK Publishers, 1985, pp 38–46.

LaPointe LL, Horner J: *Reading Comprehension Battery for Aphasia*. Tigard, Ore, CC Publications, 1979.

Larimore HW: Some verbal and nonverbal factors associated with apraxia of speech. Doctoral dissertation, University of Denver, 1970.

Lasky EZ, Weidner WE, Johnson JP: Influence of linguistic complexity, rate of presentation, and interphrase pause time on auditory-verbal comprehension of adult aphasic patients. *Brain Lang* 1976; 3:386–395.

Lee L: *Northwestern Syntax Screening Test*. Evanston, Ill, The Northwestern University Press, 1971.

Lenneberg E: *Biological Foundations of Language*. New York, Wiley, 1967.

Levin HS, Benton AL, Grossman RG: *Neurobehavioral Consequences of Closed Head Injury*. New York, Oxford University Press, 1982.

Levin HS, O'Donnell VM, Grossman RG: The Galveston Orientation and Amnesia Test: A practical scale to assess cognition after head injury. *J Nerv Ment Dis* 1979;167:675–684.

Lewy R, Cole R, Wepman J: Teflon injection in the correction of velopharyngeal insufficiency. *Ann Otol Rhinol Laryngol* 1965; 78:874.

Ley RG, Bryden MP: Hemispheric differences in processing emotions and faces. *Brain Lang* 1979: 7:127–138.

Lezak MD: *Neuropsychological Assessment,* ed 2. New York, Oxford University Press, 1983.

Liepmann H: Das krankheitsbild der apraxia. *Monatsschr Psychiatrie Neuroligie* 1900; 7.

Liles BZ, Brookshire RH: The effects of pause time on auditory comprehension of aphasic subjects. *J Commun Disord* 1975; 8:221–236.

Lincoln NB, Mulley GP, Jones AC, et al: Effectiveness of speech therapy for aphasic stroke patients: A randomized controlled trial. *Lancet* 1984; 1:1197–1200.

Linebaugh CW: Treatment of anomic aphasia, in Perkins WH (ed): *Language Handicaps in Adults.* New York, Thieme-Stratton, 1983, pp 35–43.

Love RJ, Webb WJ: The efficacy of cueing techniques in Broca's aphasia. *J Speech Hear Disord* 1977; 42:170–178.

Luria AR: Neuropsychological analysis of focal brain lesions, in Wolman BB (ed): *Handbook of Clinical Psychology.* New York, McGraw-Hill, 1965.

Luria AR: *Traumatic Aphasia.* The Hague, Netherlands, Mouton, 1970.

MacGinitie WH: *Gates-MacGinitie Reading Test.* Chicago, Riverside Publishing Co, 1978.

Marshall RC: Word retrieval behavior of aphasic adults. *J Speech Hear Disord* 1976; 41:444–451.

Marshall JC, Newcombe F: Patterns of paralexia: A psycholinguistic approach. *J Psycholinguist Res* 1973; 2:175–199.

Martino AA, Pizzamiglio L, Razzano C: A new version of the Token Test for aphasics: A concrete objects form. *J Commun Disord* 1976; 9:1–5.

Massengill R, Quinn GW, Pickrell KL, et al: Therapeutic exercise and pharyngeal flap. *Cleft Palate J* 1968; 5:44–52.

McKeever WF, Dixon MF: Right-hemisphere superiority for discriminating memorized from unmemorized faces: Affective imagery, sex, and perceived emotionality effects. *Brain Lang* 1981; 12:246–260.

McNeil MR, Prescott TE: *Revised Token Test.* Baltimore, University Park Press, 1978.

Meadows JC: The anatomical basis of prosopagnosia. *J Neurol Neurosurg Psychiatry* 1974; 37:489–501.

Mesulam MM: A cortical network for directed attention and unilateral neglect. *Ann Neurol* 1981; 10:309–325.

Mesulam MM: Slowly progressive aphasia without generalized dementia. *Ann Neurol* 1982; 11:592–598.

Metter EJ, Riege WH, Hanson WR, et al: Correlations of glucose metabolism and structural damage to language function in aphasia. *Brain Lang* 1984; 21:187–207.

Metter, EJ, Riege WH, Hanson WR, et al: Comparisons of metabolic rates, language and memory in subcortical aphasias. *Brain Lang* 1983; 19:33–47.

Meyer BJF: *The Organization of Prose and Its Effects on Memory.* Amsterdam, North-Holland, 1975.

Mills RH, Knox AW, Juola JF, et al: Cognitive loci of impairments of picture naming by aphasic subjects. *J Speech Hear Res* 1979; 22:73–87.

Miniami RT, Kaplan EN, Wu G, et al: Velopharyngeal incompetency without overt cleft palate. *Plast Reconstr Surg* 1975; 55:573–587.

Mohr JP, Pessin MS, Finkelstein S, et al: Broca aphasia: Pathologic and clinical aspects. *Neurology* 1978; 28:311–324.

Mohr JP, Walters WC, Duncan GW: Thalamic hemorrhage and aphasia. *Brain Lang* 1975; 2:3–17.

Moll KL: Speech characteristics of individuals with cleft lip and palate, in Spriesterbach DC, Sherman D (eds): *Cleft Palate and Communication* New York, Academic Press, 1968.

Murdoch BE: *Acquired Speech and Language Disorders.* New York, Chapman and Hall, 1990.

Myers PS: Profiles of communication deficits in patients with right cerebral hemisphere damage: Implications for diagnosis and treatment, in Brookshire RH (ed): *Clinical Aphasiology Conference Proceedings.* Minneapolis, BRK Publishers, 1979.

Myers PS: Visual imagery in aphasia treatment: A new look, in Brookshire RH (ed): *Clinical Aphasiology Conference Proceedings.* Minneapolis, BRK Publishers, 1980, pp 68–77.

Myers PS: Treatment of right hemisphere communication disorders, in Perkins WH (ed): *Language Handicaps in Adults.* New York, Thieme-Stratton, Inc, 1983.

Myers PS: Right hemisphere impairment, in Holland AL (ed): *Language Disorders in Adults.* San Diego, College-Hill Press, 1984.

Myers PA: Influence failure: The underlying impairment in right hemisphere communication disorders. Presented at the Clinical Aphasiology Conference, Santa Fe, NM, June 1990.

Naeser MA, Alexander MP, Helm-Estabrooks N., et al: Aphasia with predominantly subcortical lesion sites: Description of three capsular putamenal aphasia syndromes. *Arch Neurol* 1982; 39:2–14.

Naeser MA, Hayward RW, Laughlin SA, et al: Quantitative CT scan studies in aphasia: I. Infarct size and CT numbers. *Brain Lang* 1981a; 12:140–164.

Naeser MA, Hayward RW, Laughlin SA, et al: Quantitative CT scan studies in aphasia: II. Comparison of right and left hemispheres. *Brain Lang* 1981b; 12:165–189.

Nelson MJ: *The Nelson Reading Test.* Boston, Houghton-Mifflin, 1962.

Netsell R, Cleeland C: Modification of lip hypotonia in dysarthria using EMG feedback. *J Speech Hear Disord* 1973; 38:131–140.

Netsell R, Hixon TJ: A noninvasive method for clinically estimating subglottal air pressure. *J Speech Hear Disord* 1978; 43:326–330.

Netsell R, Rosenbek JC: Treating the dysarthrias, in Darby J (ed): *Speech and Language Evaluation in Neurology: Adult Disorders.* New York, Grune and Stratton, 1985.

Nicholas LE, Brookshire RH: Syntactic simplification and context: Effects on sentence comprehension by aphasic adults, in Brookshire RH (ed): *Clinical Aphasiology Conference Proceedings.* Minneapolis, BRK Publishers, 1983, pp 166–172.

Nicholas LE, Brookshire RH: Consistency of the effects of rate of speech on brain-damaged adults' comprehension of narrative discourse. *J Speech Hear Res* 1986; 29:462–470.

Nicholas LE, MacLennan DL, Brookshire RH: Validity of multiple-sentence reading comprehension tests for aphasic adults. *J Speech Hear Disord* 1986; 51:82–87.

Ojemann GA: Language and the thalamus: Object naming and recall during and after thalamic stimulation. *Brain Lang* 1976; 2:101–120.

Osgood C, Miron M: *Approaches to the Study of Aphasia.* Chicago, University Park Press, 1963.

Pang D: Physics and pathophysiology of closed head injury, in Lezak M (ed): *Assessment of the Behavioral Consequences of Head Trauma.* New York, AR Liss, 1989.

Parkhurst BG: The effects of time altered speech stimuli on the performance of right hemiplegic adult aphasics. Presented at the annual convention of the American Speech and Hearing Association, New York, 1970.

Pashek GV, Brookshire RH: Effects of rate of speech and linguistic stress on auditory paragraph comprehension by aphasic individuals. *J Speech Hear Res* 1982; 25:377–382.

Pasternak KF, LaPointe LL: Aphasic-nonaphasic performance on the Reading Comprehension Battery for Aphasia (RCBA). Presented to the annual convention of the American Speech Language and Hearing Association, Toronto, 1982.

Pimental PA, Kingsbury NA: *Neuropyschological Aspects of Right Brain Injury.* Austin, Pro-Ed, 1989.

Pirozzolo FJ, Kerr KL: Neuropsychological assessment of dementia, in Pirozzolo FJ, Maletta GJ (eds): *The Aging Nervous System.* New York, Praeger Publishers, 1980, pp 175–186.

Podraza BL, Darley FL: Effect of auditory prestimulation on naming in aphasia. *J Speech Hear Res* 1977; 20:669–683.

Poeck K: What do we mean by "aphasic syndromes?" A neurologist's view. *Brain Lang* 1983; 20:79–89.

Poeck K, Huber W, Willmes K: Outcome of intensive language rehabilitation in aphasia. *J Speech Hear Disord* 1989; 54:471–479.

Poeck K, Pietron H: The influence of stretched speech presentation on Token Test performance of aphasic and right brain damaged subjects. *Neuropsychologia* 1981; 19:133–136.

Polinko PR: Working with the family: The acute phase, in Ylvisaker M (ed): *Head Injury Rehabilitation: Children and Adolescents*. San Diego, College-Hill, 1985.

Poppelreuter W: *Die psychischen schodigringendurch kopfschuss im kriege:* 1914/1916. Leipzig, Verlag von Leopold Voss, 1917.

Porch BE: *Porch Index of Communicative Ability*. Palo Alto, Calif, Consulting Psychologists Press, 1967.

Porch BE: Multidimensional scoring in aphasia testing. *J Speech Hear Res* 1971; 14:776–792a.

Porch BE: *Porch Index of Communicative Ability*. Palo Alto, Calif, Consulting Psychologists Press, 1981a.

Porch BE: Therapy subsequent to the PICA, in Chapey R (ed): *Language Intervention Strategies in Adult Aphasia*. Baltimore, Williams and Wilkins, 1981b, pp 283–296.

Porec JP, Porch BE: The behavioral characteristics of "simulated" aphasia, in Brookshire RH (ed): *Clinical Aphasiology Conference Proceedings*. Minneapolis, BRK Publishers, 1977, pp 297–301.

Porteus SD: *The Maze Test and Clinical Psychology*. Palo Alto, Calif, Pacific Books, 1959.

Powers GL, Starr CD: The effects of muscle exercise on velopharyngeal gap and nasality. *Cleft Palate J* 1974; 11:28–40.

Rabins PV, Mace NL, Lucas MJ: The impact of dementia on the family. *JAMA* 1982; 248:333–336.

Raven JC: *The Standard Progressive Matrices*. New York, The Psychological Corporation, 1960.

Raven JC: *The Coloured Progressive Matrices*. New York, The Psychological Corporation, 1965.

Reitan RM, Tarshes EL: Differential effects of lateralized brain lesions on the Trail Making Test. *J Nerv Ment Dis* 1959; 129:257–262.

Rivers DL, Love RJ: Language performance on visual processing tasks in right hemisphere lesion cases. *Brain Lang* 1980; 10:348–366.

Rochford G, Williams M: Studies in the development and breakdown in the use of names: IV. The effects of word frequency. *J Neurol Neurosurg Psychiatry* 1965; 28:407–413.

Robin D, Schienberg S: Subcortical lesions and aphasia. *J Speech Hear Disord* 1990; 55:90–100.

Rosenbek JC: Treating apraxia of speech, in Johns DF (ed): *Clinical Management of Neurogenic Communication Disorders.* Boston, Little, Brown, 1978, pp 191–241.

Rosenbek JC, Collins MJ, Wertz RT: Intersystemic reorganization for apraxia of speech, in Brookshire RH (ed): *Clinical Aphasiology Conference Proceedings.* Minneapolis, BRK Publishers, 1976, pp 255–260.

Rosenbek JC, LaPointe LL: The dysarthrias: Description, diagnosis, and treatment, in Johns DF (ed): *Clinical Management of Neurogenic Communication Disorders.* Boston, Little, Brown, 1978, pp 251–310.

Rosenbek JC, LaPointe LL: The dysarthrias: Description, diagnosis, and treatment, in Johns DF (ed): *Clinical Management of Neurogenic Communication Disorders,* ed 2. Boston, Little, Brown, 1985, pp 97–152.

Rosenbek JC, LaPointe LL, Wertz RT: *Aphasia: A Clinical Approach.* Boston, Little, Brown, 1989.

Rosenbek JC, Lemme ML, Ahern MB, et al: A treatment for apraxia of speech in adults. *J Speech Hear Disord* 1973a; 38:462–472.

Rosenbek JC, Merson RM: Measurement and prediction of severity of apraxia of speech. Presented to the annual convention of the American Speech and Hearing Convention, Chicago, 1971.

Rosenbek JC, Wertz RT: Treatment of apraxia of speech in adults, in Wertz RT, Collins M (eds): *Clinical Aphasiology Conference Proceedings.* Minneapolis, Minnesota, BRK Publishers, 1972, pp 191–198.

Rosenbek JC, Wertz RT, Darley FL: Oral sensation and perception in apraxia of speech and aphasia. *J Speech Hear Res* 1973b; 16:22–36.

Rubens AB: The role of changes within the central nervous system during recovery from aphasia, in Sullivan M, Kommers MS (eds): *Rationale for Adult Aphasia Therapy.* Lincoln, Neb, University of Nebraska Medical Center, 1977, pp 28–43.

Rubow RT, Rosenbek JC, Collins MJ, et al: Reduction of hemifacial spasm in dysarthria following EMG feedback. *J Speech Hear Disord* 1984; 49:26–33.

Russell EW: A multiple scoring method for the assessment of complex memory functions. *J Consult Clin Psychol* 1975; 43:800–809.

Russell WR: *The Traumatic Amnesias.* New York, Oxford University Press, 1971.

Russell WR, Nathan PW: Traumatic amnesia. *Brain* 1946; 69:183–187.

Salvatore AP, Thompson C: Treatment of global aphasia, in Chapey, R (ed): *Language Intervention Strategies in Adult Aphasia,* ed 2. Baltimore, Williams and Wilkins, 1986.

Sands E, Sarno MT, Shankweiler D: Long term assessment of language function in aphasia due to stroke. *Arch Phys Med Rehabil* 1969; 50:202–207.

Sarno MT: *The Functional Communication Profile.* New York, New York University Medical Center Monograph Department, 1969.

Sarno MT, Levita E: Natural course of recovery in severe aphasia. *Arch Phys Med Rehabil* 1971; 52:175–178.

Sarno MT, Silverman M, Sands E: Speech therapy and language recovery in severe aphasia. *J Speech Hear Res* 1970; 13:607–623.

Schuell HM: A short examination for aphasia. *Neurology* 1957; 7:625–634.

Schuell HM: *The Minnesota Test for Differential Diagnosis of Aphasia.* Minneapolis, University of Minnesota Press, 1965.

Schuell HM: *The Minnesota Test of Differential Diagnosis of Aphasia.* Minneapolis, University of Minnesota Press, 1972.

Schuell HM, Jenkins JJ: Reduction of vocabulary in aphasia. *Brain* 1961; 84:243–261.

Schuell HM, Jenkins JJ, Jimenez-Pabon E: *Aphasia in Adults.* New York, Harper and Row, 1965.

Schuell HM, Jenkins JJ, Landis L: Relationship between auditory comprehension and word frequency in aphasia. *J Speech Hear Res* 1961; 4:30–36.

Selnes OA, Knopman DS, Niccum N, et al: Computed tomographic scan correlates of auditory comprehension deficits in aphasia: A prospective recovery study. *Ann Neurol* 1983; 13:558–566.

Selnes OA, Knopman DS, Niccum N, et al: The critical role of Wernicke's area in sentence repetition. *Ann Neurol* 1985; 17:549–557.

Shankweiler D, Harris KS: An experimental approach to the problem of articulation in aphasia. *Cortex* 1966; 2:277–292.

Shewan CM: *The Auditory Comprehension Test for Sentences.* Chicago, Biolinguistics Clinical Institutes, 1979.

Shewan CM, Canter GJ: Effects of vocabulary, syntax, and sentence length on auditory comprehension in aphasic patients. *Cortex* 1971; 7:209–226.

Shewan CM, Kertesz A: Reliability and validity characteristics of the Western Aphasia Battery (WAB). *J Speech Hear Disord* 1980; 45:308–324.

Shewan CM, Kertesz A: Effects of speech and language treatment on recovery from aphasia. *Brain Lang* 1984; 23:272–299.

Silverman FH: Dysarthria: Communication augmentation systems for adults without speech, in Perkins WH (ed): *Dysarthria and Apraxia.* New York, Thieme-Stratton, 1983, pp 115–121.

Skelly M: *Amer-Ind Gestural Code.* New York, Elsevier, 1979.

Sparks R, Helm NA, Albert ML: Aphasia rehabilitation resulting from melodic intonation therapy. *Cortex* 1974; 10:303–316.

Sparks R, Holland AL: Method: Melodic intonation therapy for aphasia. *J Speech Hear Disord* 1976; 41:287–297.

Spreen O, Benton AL: *Neurosensory Center Comprehensive Examination for Aphasia.* Victoria BC, Neuropsychology Laboratory, University of Victoria, 1977.

Square PA, Weidner WE: Oral sensory perception in adults demonstrating apraxia of speech. Presented to the American Speech and Hearing Association, Houston, 1976.

Stachowiak FJ, Huber W, Poeck K, et al: Text comprehension in aphasia. *Brain Lang* 1977; 4:177–195.

Stanton K, Yorkston KM, Talley-Kenyon V, et al: Language utilization in teaching reading to left neglect patients, in Brookshire RH (ed): *Clinical Aphasiology Conference Proceedings.* Minneapolis, BRK Publishers, 1981.

Stedman's Medical Dictionary. Baltimore, Williams and Wilkins, 1990.

Stokes TF, Baer DM: An implied technology of generalization. *J Appl Behav Anal* 1977; 10:349–367.

Stone CP, Girdner J, Albrecht R: An alternate form of the Wechsler Memory Scale. *J Psychol* 1946; 22:199–206.

Teasdale G, Jennett B: Assessment and prognosis of coma after head injury. *Acta Neurochir (Wien)* 1976; 34:45–55.

Teasdale G, Mendelow D: Pathophysiology of head injuries, in Brooks N (ed): *Closed Head Injury: Psychological, Social, and Family Consequences.* Oxford, Oxford University Press, 1984.

Thompson C, Byrne M: Across setting generalization of social conventions in aphasia, in Brookshire RH (ed): *Clinical Aphasiology Conference Proceedings.* Minneapolis, BRK Publishers, 1984, pp 132–144.

Thurstone LL: *A Factorial Study of Perception.* Chicago, University of Chicago Press, 1944.

Tomlinson BE, Henderson G: Some quantitative cerebral findings in normal and demented old people, in Terry R, Gerskor S (eds): *Neurobiology of Aging*. New York, Raven, 1976.

Toppin CJ, Brookshire RH: Effects of response delay and token relocation on Token Test performance of aphasic subjects. *J Commun Disord* 1978; 11:65–78.

Trost JE, Canter GJ: Apraxia of speech in patients with Broca's aphasia: A study of phoneme production accuracy and error patterns. *Brain Lang* 1974; 1:63–79.

Trupe EH: Reliability of rating spontaneous speech in the Western Aphasia Battery: Implications for classification, in Brookshire RH (ed): *Clinical Aphasiology Conference Proceedings*. Minneapolis, BRK Publishers, 1984, pp 55–69.

Tweedy JR, Shulman PD: Toward a functional classification of naming impairments. *Brain Lang* 1982; 15:193–206.

Ulatowska HK, Doyel AW, Freedman-Stern RF: Production of procedural discourse in aphasia. *Brain Lang* 1983; 18:315–341.

VanDemark AA, Lemmer EC, Drake ML: Measurement of reading comprehension in aphasia with the RCBA. *J Speech Hear Res* 1982; 47:288–291.

Van Zomeren AH, Brouwer WH, Deelman BG: Attentional deficits: The riddles of selectivity, speed, and alertness, in Brooks N (ed): *Closed Head Injury: Psychological, Social, and Family Consequences*. Oxford, Oxford University Press, 1984.

Vignolo LA: Evolution of aphasia and language rehabilitation: A retrospective study. *Cortex* 1964; 1:344–367.

Wagenaar E, Snow CE, Prins RS: Spontaneous speech of aphasic patients: A psycholinguistic analysis. *Brain Lang* 1975; 2:281–303.

Walker-Batson D, Devous MD, Bonte FJ, et al: Single-photon emission tomography (SPECT) in the study of aphasia: A preliminary report, in Brookshire RH (ed): *Clinical Aphasiology Conference Proceedings*. Minneapolis, BRK Publishers, 1987.

Waller MR, Darley FL: The influence of context on the auditory comprehension of paragraphs in aphasic subjects. *J Speech Hear Res* 1978; 21:732–745.

War Department: *The Trail-Making Test*. 1944.

Warrington EK, James M: Disorders of visual perception in patients with localized cerebral lesions. *Neuropsychologia* 1967; 5:253–266.

Wechsler D: A standardized memory scale for clinical use. *J Psychol* 1945; 19:87–95.

Wechsler D: *Wechsler Adult Intelligence Scale*, ed 4. Baltimore, Williams and Wilkins, 1955.

Wechsler D: *Wechsler Adult Intelligence Scale—Revised*. New York, Psychological Corporation, 1981.

Wegner ML, Brookshire RH, Nicholas LE: Comprehension of main ideas and details in coherent and noncoherent discourse by aphasic and nonaphasic listeners. *Brain Lang* 1984; 21:37–51.

Weidner WE, & Lasky EZ: The interaction of rate and complexity of stimulus on the performance of adult aphasic subjects. *Brain Lang* 1976; 3:34–40.

Weisenburg TH, McBride KE: *Aphasia*. New York, Commonwealth Fund, 1935.

Wener DL, Duffy JR: An investigation of the sensitivity of the Reporter's Test to expressive language disturbances (abstract), in Brookshire RH: (ed) *Clinical Aphasiology Conference Proceedings*. Minneapolis, BRK Publishers, 1983, pp 15–17.

Wepman JM: *Recovery From Aphasia*. New York, Ronald Press, 1951.

Wepman JM: Aphasia therapy: A new look. *J Speech Hear Disord* 1972; 37:203–214.

Wepman JM: *Auditory Discrimination Test*. Chicago, Language Research Associates, 1978.

Wertz RT: Neuropathologies of speech and language: An introduction to patient management, in Johns DF (ed): *Clinical Management of Neurogenic Communication Disorders*. Boston, Little, Brown, 1978, pp 1–101.

Wertz RT, Aten JL, LaPointe LL, et al: Comparison of clinic, home, and deferred treatment for aphasia. Presented at the annual convention of the American Speech Language and Hearing Association, San Francisco, 1984a.

Wertz RT, et al: Veterans Administration Cooperative Study on Aphasia: A comparison of individual and group treatment. *J Speech Hear Res* 1981; 24:580–594.

Wertz RT, et al: A comparison of clinic, home, and deferred language treatment for aphasia: A VA cooperative study. *Arch Neurol* 1986; 43:653–658.

Wertz RT, Keith RL, Custer DD: Normal and aphasic behavior on a measure of auditory input and a measure of verbal output. Presented at the annual convention of the American Speech and Hearing Association, Chicago, 1971.

Wertz RT, LaPointe LL, Rosenbek JC: *Apraxia of Speech in Adults: The Disorder and Its Management*. Orlando, Grune and Stratton, 1984b.

West JF: Auditory comprehension in aphasic adults: Improvement through training. *Arch Phys Med Rehabil* 1973; 54:78–86.

West JF, Kaufman GA: Some effects of redundancy on the auditory comprehension of adult aphasics. Presented at the annual convention of the American Speech and Hearing Association, San Francisco, 1972.

Whitely AM, Warrington EK: Prosopagnosia: A clinical, psychological, and anatomical study of three patients. *J Neurol Neurosurg Psychiatry* 1977; 40:395–403.

Wiegel-Crump C, Koenigsknecht RA: Tapping the lexical store of the adult aphasic: Analysis of the improvement made in word retrieval skills. *Cortex* 1973; 9:411–418.

Willanger R, Danielson UT, Ankerhaus J: Visual neglect in right-sided apoplectic lesions. *Acta Neurol Scand* 1981; 64:310–326.

Williams SE: Factors influencing naming performance in aphasia: A review of the literature. *J Commun Disord* 1983; 16:357–372.

Williams SE, Canter GJ: The influence of situational context on naming performance in aphasic syndromes. *Brain Lang* 1982; 17:92–106.

Wilson B, Cockburn J, Baddeley A: *The Rivermead Behavioral Memory Test.* Reading, Thames Valley Test Co, 1985.

Wyke M, Holgate D: Colour naming defects in dysphasic patients: A qualitative analysis. *Neuropsychologia* 1973; 11:451–461.

Yorkston KM: Treatment of right hemisphere damaged patients: A panel presentation, in Brookshire RH (ed): *Clinical Aphasiology Conference Proceedings.* Minneapolis, BRK Publishers, 1981.

Yorkston KM, Beukelman DR: *Assessment of Intelligibility of Dysarthric Speech.* Tigard, Ore, CC Publications, 1981.

Yorkston KM, Beulkelman DR, Bell KR: *Clinical Management of Dysarthric Speakers.* San Diego, College-Hill, 1988.

Yorkston KM, Dowden PA, Beukelman DR, et al: A Phoneme Identification Task as a measure of perceived articulatory adequacy. Presented at the third biennial Clinical Dysarthria Conference, Tucson, 1986.

Yorkston KM, Marshall RC, Butler M: Imposed delay of response: Effects on aphasics' auditory comprehension of visually and nonvisually cued material. *Percept Mot Skills* 1977; 44:647–655.

Yules RB, Chase RA: A training method for reduction of hypernasality in speech. *Plast Reconstr Surg* 1969; 43:180–185.

Index